Mayo Clinic Strategies to Reduce Burnout: 12 Actions to Create the Ideal Workplace

MAYO CLINIC SCIENTIFIC PRESS

Mayo Clinic Atlas of Regional Anesthesia and Ultrasound-Guided Nerve Blockade
Edited by James R. Hebl, MD, and Robert L. Lennon, DO

Mayo Clinic Preventive Medicine and Public Health Board Review
Edited by Prathibha Varkey, MBBS, MPH, MHPE

Mayo Clinic Infectious Diseases Board Review
Edited by Zelalem Temesgen, MD

Just Enough Physiology
By James R. Munis, MD, PhD

Mayo Clinic Cardiology: Concise Textbook, Fourth Edition
Edited by Joseph G. Murphy, MD, and Margaret A. Lloyd, MD

Mayo Clinic Electrophysiology Manual
Edited by Samuel J. Asirvatham, MD

Mayo Clinic Gastrointestinal Imaging Review, Second Edition
By C. Daniel Johnson, MD

Arrhythmias in Women: Diagnosis and Management
Edited by Yong-Mei Cha, MD, Margaret A. Lloyd, MD,
    and Ulrika M. Birgersdotter-Green, MD

Mayo Clinic Body MRI Case Review
By Christine U. Lee, MD, PhD, and James F. Glockner, MD, PhD

Mayo Clinic Gastroenterology and Hepatology Board Review, Fifth Edition
Edited by Stephen C. Hauser, MD

Mayo Clinic Guide to Cardiac Magnetic Resonance Imaging, Second Edition
Edited by Kiaran P. McGee, PhD, Eric E. Williamson, MD, and Matthew W. Martinez, MD

Mayo Clinic Neurology Board Review, First Edition [2 Volumes]
Edited by Kelly D. Flemming, MD, and Lyell K. Jones Jr, MD

Mayo Clinic Critical Care Case Review
Edited by Rahul Kashyap, MBBS, J. Christopher Farmer, MD, and John C. O'Horo, MD

Mayo Clinic Medical Neurosciences, Sixth Edition
Edited by Eduardo E. Benarroch, MD, Jeremy K. Cutsforth-Gregory, MD,
    and Kelly D. Flemming, MD

Mayo Clinic Principles of Shoulder Surgery
By Joaquin Sanchez-Sotelo, MD

Mayo Clinic Essential Neurology, Second Edition
By Andrea C. Adams, MD

Mayo Clinic Antimicrobial Handbook: Quick Guide, Third Edition
Edited by John W. Wilson, MD, and Lynn L. Estes, PharmD

Mayo Clinic Critical and Neurocritical Care Board Review
Edited by Eelco F. M. Wijdicks, MD, PhD, James Y. Findlay, MB, ChB,
    William D. Freeman, MD, and Ayan Sen, MD

Mayo Clinic Internal Medicine Board Review, Twelfth Edition
Edited by Christopher M. Wittich, MD, PharmD, Thomas J. Beckman, MD,
    Sara L. Bonnes, MD, Nerissa M. Collins, MD, Nina M. Schwenk, MD,
    Christopher R. Stephenson, MD, and Jason H. Szostek, MD

Mayo Clinic Strategies to Reduce Burnout: 12 Actions to Create the Ideal Workplace

Stephen J. Swensen, MD

Emeritus Professor of Radiology
Mayo Clinic College of Medicine and Science
Formerly, Medical Director
Leadership and Organization, Mayo Clinic
Senior Fellow, Institute for Healthcare Improvement

Tait D. Shanafelt, MD

Associate Dean and
Jeanie and Stew Ritchie Professor of Medicine
Stanford University School of Medicine
Director and Chief Wellness Officer,
Stanford Medicine WellMD Center

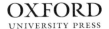

OXFORD
UNIVERSITY PRESS

MAYO CLINIC

OXFORD
UNIVERSITY PRESS

Oxford University Press Inc. is a department of the University of Oxford. It furthers the University's objective of excellence in research, scholarship, and education by publishing worldwide. Oxford is a registered trademark of Oxford University Press, Inc. in the UK and certain other countries.

Published in the United States of America by Oxford University Press, Inc. 198 Madison Avenue, New York, NY 10016, United States of America.

Names: Swensen, Stephen J., author. | Shanafelt, Tait D., author. | Mayo Clinic.
Title: Mayo Clinic strategies to reduce burnout : 12 actions to create the ideal workplace / Stephen J. Swensen, Tait D. Shanafelt.
Other titles: Strategies to reduce burnout | Mayo Clinic Scientific Press (Series)
Description: New York, NY : Oxford University Press, [2020] |
Series: Mayo Clinic Scientific Press | Includes bibliographical references and index.
Identifiers: LCCN 2019044695 (print) | LCCN 2019044696 (ebook) |
ISBN 9780190848965 (paperback) | ISBN 9780190848989 (epub) |
ISBN 9780190848996 (other)
Subjects: MESH: Burnout, Professional—prevention & control |
Personnel Management—methods | Organizational Culture
Classification: LCC RA785 (print) | LCC RA785 (ebook) | NLM WA 495 |
DDC 155.9/042—dc23
LC record available at https://lccn.loc.gov/2019044695
LC ebook record available at https://lccn.loc.gov/2019044696

Printed by Marquis, Canada

To the most important people in our lives:
Our beloved and trusted friends and wives, Lynn and Jaci . . .
Our incredible parents, for whom it was always about service to someone else . . .
And our sons and daughters: Scott, Callie, Kennedy, Grant, Evie, and Tyler—
we wish for each of you esprit de corps in your life's work.

CONTENTS

Section IV: The Journey

FOREWORD

In the dark and cold winter of my first year in medical school, I became burned out. Then, as too often occurs, I slipped into a depression. I was ready to quit, but with the thoughtful support of one of our deans, I was able to get the treatment I needed. Today, I look back on a fulfilling and decades-long career as a neuropsychiatrist, researcher, medical educator, and health care administrator.

Unfortunately, this experience of burnout, sometimes leading to anxiety, depression, and other illnesses, is far too common among health care professionals. Even more unfortunately, not every story ends as mine has—with success. In fact, all too many have tragic endings.

Through the pioneering work of Dr. Shanafelt and Dr. Swensen, we have learned much about the growing public health crisis of clinician burnout. And in the past two decades, we have experienced a groundswell of change in acknowledging the crisis for today's health care professionals and determining the need for action.

Despite recognizing the severity of the crisis and the negative effects of burnout on patient care, we have not had a comprehensive, validated compendium of evidence-based approaches to enhancing well-being of health care professionals.

Until now.

Brought to you by two of the world's foremost authorities on the subject, *Mayo Clinic Strategies to Reduce Burnout: 12 Actions to Create the Ideal Workplace* is a pragmatic plan for health care leaders and organizations to use in building professional fulfillment and esprit de corps—a combination of camaraderie, engagement, fulfillment, loyalty, passion, and meaning in work. Health care leaders have a moral obligation to build professional fulfillment and esprit de corps to ensure that their organizations are great places to work, but these characteristics are also key leading indicators of patient experience, outcomes, and costs.

This book is for all who aspire to create an environment that helps health care professionals take better care of patients while cultivating their own professional fulfillment in the process.

The Blueprint described for attaining the ideal workplace is based on a patient-centered moral imperative and a compelling business case. The authors define eight Ideal Work Elements and propose 12 organizational actions to cultivate the work elements.

At their core, the Ideal Work Elements provide for the fundamental needs of health care professionals, resulting in the positive culture that should be the goal of every health care organization. This book gives organizations a unified strategy for achieving that goal, along with a detailed road map for implementation and metrics for assessing progress.

The text is based on the experience of vanguard organizations and solid research published in peer-reviewed journals, including more than 140 articles published by the authors themselves. Many of the studies they draw from are rigorously controlled, including several randomized trials. The approach they describe can be applied in diverse settings, including ambulatory, inpatient, academic, and community-based practices. The methodology has been validated in medical organizations in the United States and abroad, and many of the strategies have also proven effective outside of health care.

The core of their approach focuses on:

1) Mitigating the drivers of burnout (decreasing negativity).
2) Cultivating a culture of wellness and leader behaviors that nurtures professional well-being (increasing positivity).
3) Bolstering individual and organizational resilience (increasing tolerance of negativity).

Drawing on their decades of experience, the authors propose the Intervention Triad, a set of evidence-based actions to address the drivers of professional burnout and promote the Ideal Work Elements. The Intervention Triad actions are grouped into the categories of:

- Agency—empowering individuals or teams to make decisions and optimize their local work environment.
- Coherence—an organizational state in which the parts fit together to form a coordinated and consistent whole.
- Camaraderie—the boundarylessness, social capital, mutual respect, and teamwork that organizations need to thrive.

We know enough about professional burnout and its adverse consequences for patients, providers, and the health care system. Now is the time for implementing an effective systems-based approach to address the problem. This requires appointing an empowered and accountable leader, establishing a formal structure, allocating resources, implementing effective processes and tactics, and longitudinally assessing outcomes. All of us in the health care professions can and should commit to the effort—with *Mayo Clinic Strategies to Reduce Burnout: 12 Actions to Create the Ideal Workplace* as our guide.

Darrell G. Kirch, M.D.
President Emeritus, Association of American Medical Colleges
Co-Chair, National Academy of Medicine Action Collaborative on Clinician
Well-Being and Resilience

ABOUT THE COVER

The cover illustration, *Teamwork*, by Björn Sjögren, is used with permission of the artist. Teamwork is an essential element in co-creating the ideal workplace.

PREFACE

In a way, we have both been writing this book about the well-being of health care professionals for two decades. The journey has been a labor of love for each of us. And it has been an experience like no other. Although we have published hundreds of peer-reviewed articles and a few textbooks, this experience was different. This work was profoundly unlike our research on leukemia (T.D.S.) and lung cancer (S.J.S.) or our clinical work. And yet it was done in the same spirit of helping patients . . . by helping professionals.

Mayo Clinic Strategies to Reduce Burnout: 12 Actions to Create the Ideal Workplace represents the current apex (we are not done yet . . .) of our decades of experience in health care leadership in many organizations. We were able to incorporate learning from our extensive research on well-being of health care professionals; from our deep experience in quality, department operations, leadership and organization development, management, safe havens, and care teams; and from our experiences in roles of president, chief wellness officer, chief quality officer, chair, principal investigator, senior fellow, and board director.

For us, the significance of this work is wrapped up in a sense of calling rather than in a career accomplishment. We are motivated by a desire to assist and serve the millions of health care professionals around the world who dedicate themselves and their talents to serving others. We have worked with and beside such professionals for many decades and have seen first hand the altruism, dedication, and commitment they bring to their work. We want the strategies in this book to reach and help as many people as possible—so much so that a matching donation to charity will be made each year equivalent to the collective author royalties received.

In the book, we tell the story of an evolving journey in our profession. We have chosen not to dwell on the story of burnout, distress, compassion fatigue, moral injury, and cognitive dissonance. Instead, we emphasize a narrative of hope for professional fulfillment, well-being, joy, and camaraderie. Achieving this aim requires health care professionals and administrative leaders to work together to co-create the ideal workplace—through nurturing positivity and pushing negativity aside. This requires identifying and embracing the Ideal Work Elements and developing strategies to achieve them.

The ultimate aspiration is esprit de corps—the common spirit existing in members of a group that inspires enthusiasm, devotion, loyalty, camaraderie, engagement, and strong regard for the welfare of the team and for shared interests and responsibilities. Esprit de corps engenders a team and organization with a common vision working together to realize something for patients and society that no one of us could do without the other.

In the following chapters, we provide a road map designed to help you create esprit de corps for your health care team and organization. The map is paved with information about reliable, patient-centered, and thoughtful systems embedded within psychologically safe and just cultures. In Section I ("Foundation"), we discuss the nature of the challenge before us and the principles we must apply to make progress. Section II ("Strategy") provides the Blueprint for success, including solutions for measurement, the eight Ideal Work Elements, and the business case to invest in pursuit of this objective. In Section III ("Execution"), we present 12 actions that organizations, leaders, and individuals can use to achieve the Ideal Work Elements and create an organizational practice environment that begets professional well-being with compassionate and superb patient care.

We included many case studies in the book to illustrate our findings related to burnout: Some were our experiences and some were experiences shared by colleagues inside and outside Mayo Clinic. Permission was obtained for use of all stories about real people, and we have provided attribution to colleagues who contributed case studies. The narratives at the beginning and end of select chapters were created to serve as examples of how individual health care professionals are impacted by the themes presented. The names, characters, and incidents they describe are fictitious. Any resemblance to actual health care professionals is coincidental.

Finally, this book is fruit from countless friendships, mentors, coaches, partners, and role models, especially:

Don Berwick—an advisor with vision, heart, and passion

Maureen Bisognano—a role model, advocate, and inspiration

James Dilling—a trusted administrative partner who got the job done

Morie Gertz—a leader and role model who always puts people first

Grace Gorringe—a teacher and partner whose focus is consistently patients and justice

Dan Johnson—no better friend and a root cause for so much of the success of others

Neil Kay—a mentor in the truest sense of the word

John Noseworthy—a thoughtful visionary

Carl Reading—a servant leader exemplar

We are deeply grateful for your support.

We are also indebted to the entire Oxford University Press and Mayo Clinic editorial team including Craig Panner, Joseph G. Murphy, M.D., LeAnn Stee, Kenna Atherton, Bev Pike, Angie Herron, and Marianne Mallia. Marianne would know a better way to communicate our sentiment, but we will say simply: editor *par excellence*.

Thank you!

SECTION I

Foundation

1

INTRODUCTION

The world as we have created it is a process of our thinking. It cannot be changed without changing our thinking.
—Albert Einstein

• • •

We need to change our thinking.
To have friends and colleagues abandon their dream profession in dismay—the
    one they gave two decades of their life to prepare for—
the one they were called to—
is both heartrending and tragic, and it happens every day . . .

In this book, we tell the story of burnout of health care professionals. Many believe burnout to be the result of individual weakness when, in fact, burnout is primarily the result of health care systems that take emotionally healthy, altruistic people and methodically squeeze the vitality and passion out of them. Burned-out professionals are exhausted, jaded, demoralized, and isolated, and they have lost their sense of meaning and purpose. Frequently, these individuals are shamed and blamed by leaders who suggest they should sleep longer, meditate, and become more resilient even as they expect them to work harder, see more patients, embrace rapidly changing technology, stay abreast of new medical advances, and provide quality health care.

We need to change our thinking.
So let's consider the ideal workplace.
Let's discuss professional fulfillment.
Let's talk about esprit de corps.

In this book, we will show you how the current vicious cycle of cognitive dissonance, moral injury, and shame-and-blame can be transformed into a virtuous cycle: a cycle where one beneficial change in the health care workplace leads to another and, ultimately, to esprit de corps—a common spirit existing in members of a group that inspires enthusiasm, devotion, loyalty, camaraderie, engagement, and strong regard for the welfare of the team. The road to esprit de corps for health care professionals is paved with reliable systems that are patient centered, considerate of the unique needs of health care professionals, and characterized by psychologically safe and just cultures.

This book provides a road map, a Blueprint, for creating esprit de corps among health care professionals and, in so doing, also provides the strategy to reduce burnout. In the first two sections, "Foundation" and "Strategy," we discuss the nature of the challenge before us and the principles we must apply to make progress. In the third section, "Execution," we describe the three validated Action Sets of the Intervention Triad (Agency, Coherence, and Camaraderie) that organizations, leaders, and individuals can use to create an ideal work environment. In the fourth section, "The Journey," we provide some final thoughts about creating esprit de corps in your organizations.

If you follow this Blueprint, you will be successful in the quest to transform your organization from a collection of cynical and discouraged individuals to a vibrant community of health care professionals working collaboratively to serve their patients and support each other.

If you are a family member or the concerned friend of a health care professional experiencing burnout, this book will help you understand the factors that are causing occupational burnout in health care professionals and know what can be done to decrease stress and mitigate burnout.

We hope that you will have enough information after reading this book to understand the pathway to esprit de corps!

THE INTERRELATED JOURNEYS OF QUALITY AND ESPRIT DE CORPS

The Quality Journey

The journey to esprit de corps can be better understood within the framework of the health care quality movement. In the 1980s, a few vanguard centers and organizations that truly wanted to improve care got serious and identified some metrics designed for organizations to measure and improve quality. Leaders in these institutions began to understand that providing quality health care was about far more than the knowledge, skill, and competency of the individual physicians, nurses, and other health care staff at their centers. They began to appreciate how team, culture, and psychological safety had a huge impact on what the professionals did for the patients they cared for. They sought to learn about a different type of science: one of process improvement and systems engineering, which can give users a powerful way to proactively identify, assess, and improve upon existing practices to affect change in quality of delivered services. They began to use this applied science to develop better hospital processes and systems. They identified better models of care delivery (the integrated, multidisciplinary team) and specific processes and tactics (e.g., checklists, huddles [short, daily meetings], guidelines, protocols, and reliable reporting of events and near misses) to profoundly improve patient outcomes. They uncovered new dimensions of leadership to achieve safety and quality, such as humility, Patient Safety Leadership WalkRounds, team focus, and working *across silos* to ensure communication among departments.

Leaders began to recognize the need to move beyond a focus on eliminating problems (i.e., safety issues) and instead to focus on creating systems and cultures that promoted the desired outcomes (i.e., quality). They began to understand that quality was a journey and not a destination. In keeping with that notion, they applied quality metrics in a comprehensive way that not only took horizontal slices across the institution to identify quality and safety shortfalls (e.g., team dynamics and interdepartmental connections) but also assessed them longitudinally (e.g., leader–direct report connections). They developed dedicated teams of professionals whose focus was to support the physicians, nurses, advanced practice providers, pharmacists, social workers, and leaders in the use of validated approaches as they took responsibility for improving quality in their own work units.

Chief quality officers were appointed in these institutions to lead efforts for regularly measuring quality, to coordinate the diverse improvement efforts, and to advocate and advance the quality strategy at the highest levels of their organizations. These efforts have led to profound improvements in quality and safety in the U.S. health care delivery system—and have saved countless patient lives.

It has taken decades and two Institute of Medicine reports to move our society and health care institutions closer to recognizing how to address the chasm between the health care that professionals actually deliver and the care that they aspire to provide.

The same discipline and planning must now be applied to the challenge of health care professional burnout. But how do we do this?

We need to change our thinking.

Toward Esprit de Corps

Because of the success of the quality movement, leaders in some of these same vanguard institutions have begun to recognize that the success of the organization is predicated on the well-being and professional fulfillment of health care workers. The alternative state to the burned-out individual is an engaged, fulfilled, and resilient individual who is connected to and supported by a network of similarly engaged colleagues with a shared purpose, working together in high-functioning teams to achieve a shared patient-centered mission. Individual teams must operate in a larger network of high-functioning teams toward a common goal: esprit de corps (Figure 1.1).

As with the quality movement, these ambitions must be recognized as a journey, not a destination. Metrics must be applied in a comprehensive way, evaluating both horizontal and vertical relationships within the institution. A dedicated network of collaborating leaders must be assembled (e.g., experts in organizational development, human resources, systems engineering, patient safety and experience, leadership development, communication, change management) whose focus is to help support professionals in their efforts to create a better work environment. Chief wellness officers are beginning to be appointed to coordinate such a diverse team and to advocate and advance the work at the highest levels of their organizations. We have begun to recognize that our aspiration is having not only engaged workers and high-functioning teams (Figure 1.2) but also resilient organizations.

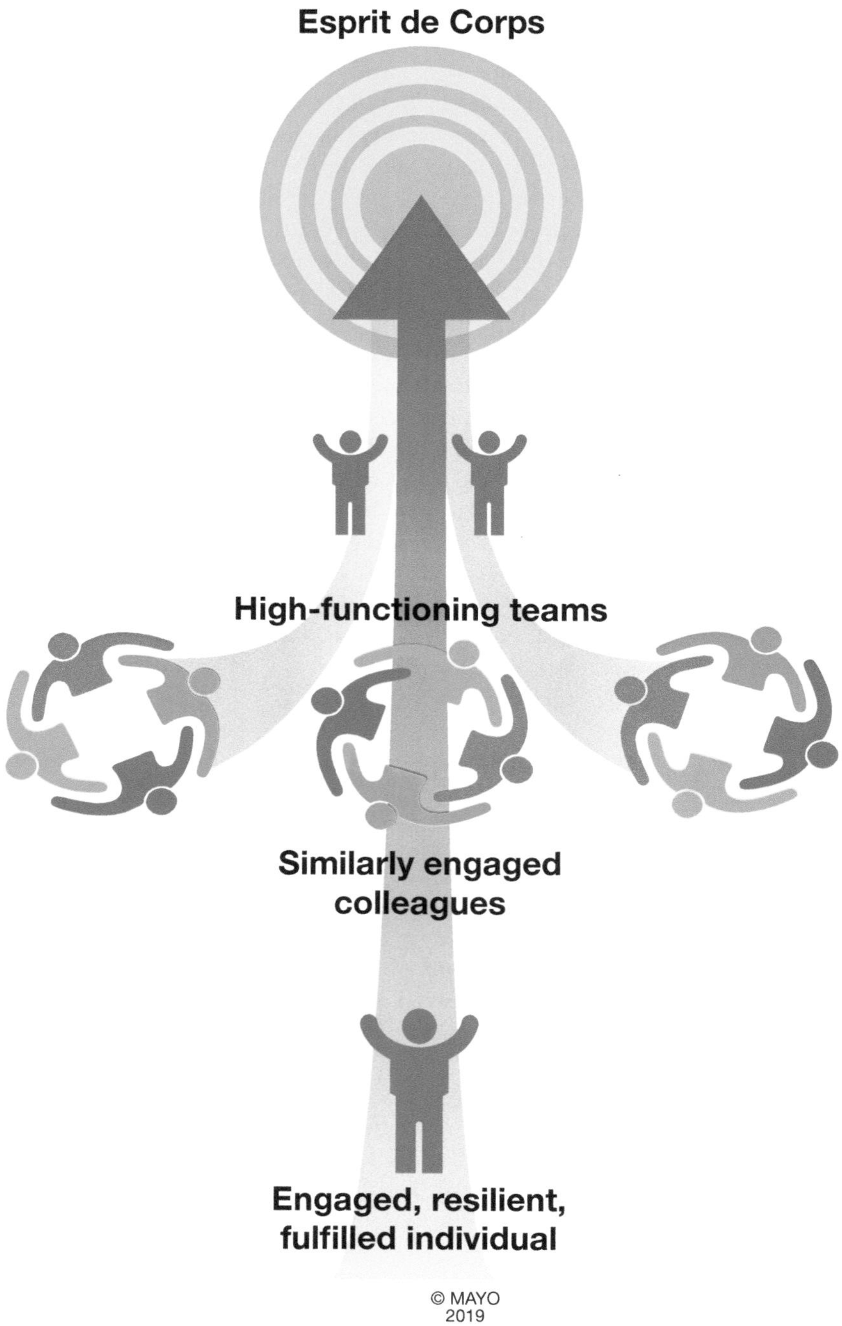

Esprit de Corps

High-functioning teams

Similarly engaged colleagues

Engaged, resilient, fulfilled individual

© MAYO
2019

Figure 1.1. Environment for Creating Esprit de Corps.

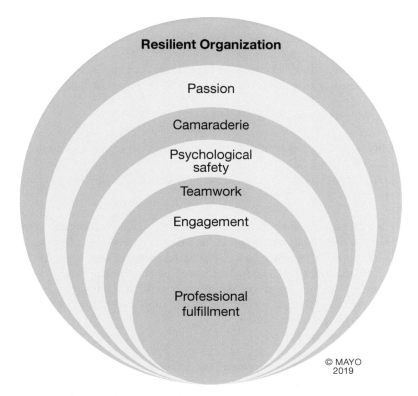

Figure 1.2. Qualities Leading to Esprit de Corps.

THE BIG PICTURE

We have chosen to frame the opportunity to create esprit de corps in health care organizations in a positive light. Although burnout is a problem that needs to be addressed, we believe the better approach is creating an environment that helps health care professionals take better care of patients and one that cultivates professional fulfillment in the process. We will make the case that cultivating esprit de corps is the strategy for solving the issue of burnout in all patient-centered medical organizations.

The approach we present for reducing burnout and creating esprit de corps is evidence based and has been validated in multiple business sectors from manufacturing to commercial aviation as well as in health care. Our Blueprint is a threefold process that addresses the core needs of health care professionals by:

1) Mitigating the drivers of burnout (decreasing negativity).
2) Cultivating a culture of wellness and leadership behavior that nurtures professional well-being (increasing positivity).
3) Bolstering individual and organizational resilience (increasing tolerance of negativity).

Today, the senior leaders of most U.S. medical centers frequently believe two fundamental misconceptions that will limit their success:

1) Quality is a necessary and important expense for the organization.
2) Esprit de corps is an expensive and thoughtful luxury for the organization.

In fact, what we believe is quite different:

1) Quality is a necessary and important business strategy for the organization (and the patient).
2) Esprit de corps is an indispensable business strategy for the organization (and the patient).

The big picture of esprit de corps includes the understanding that the best strategy is not really about fixing something that is broken (e.g., disengagement, burnout, turnover). That would be a deficit-based approach and limits the upside. Instead, the solution needs to be framed in a spirit of growth. Rather than asking what problem health care professionals must fix or what is enough to get by, the question should be what ideal state of vitality will allow health care professionals to flourish and experience esprit de corps?

Today we know . . .

- Enough about the drivers of professional fulfillment and engagement to recognize, measure, and foster them.
- Enough about professional burnout to recognize it, measure it, and begin to reduce its occurrence.
- That professional fulfillment and engagement form the bedrock of a high-functioning organization built upon esprit de corps.
- That implementing the strategy and tactics to create an organizational culture that cultivates esprit de corps does not require a large budget.
- Enough about the effect of burnout on quality of patient care that we cannot afford to wait any longer to address these problems.

◆ ◆ ◆

It is time to get serious about creating esprit de corps.
It is time to change our thinking.

(If you already have a thorough knowledge about the drivers of professional burnout and the business case, you may want to proceed directly to Chapter 6, "The Blueprint for Cultivating Esprit de Corps").

SUGGESTED READING

Swensen S, Pugh M, McMullan C, Kabcenell A. High-impact leadership: improve care, improve the health of populations, and reduce costs [Internet] [cited 2019 Jun 26]. IHI White Paper. Cambridge (MA): Institute for Healthcare Improvement; 2013. Available from: http://www.ihi.org/resources/Pages/IHIWhitePapers/HighImpactLeadership.aspx.

Swensen SJ, Dilling JA, Harper CM Jr, Noseworthy JH. The Mayo Clinic value creation system. Am J Med Qual. 2012 Jan-Feb;27(1):58–65.

2

CONSEQUENCES OF PROFESSIONAL BURNOUT

You can't give what you don't have.
—Maureen Bisognano

Work environments and interpersonal relationships often merge, eroding the passion and altruism of health care professionals and promoting burnout. Burnout has many consequences. We will discuss these in detail and offer solutions in the next two sections of the book. We want to start, however, by describing the problem.

THREE FAMILIAR STORIES

Mike, Sally, and Jennifer are three health care professionals whose stories describe a few of the consequences of burnout in the health care workplace today.

Mike

Mike is a general internist who has worked for a large medical center for the past 10 years. He views medicine as a calling, and although he works at least 60 hours a week, he has never minded putting in long hours to meet the needs of his patients.

Lately, however, things have been different. He routinely arrives at the clinic at 7:00 AM, catches up on inbox messages in the electronic health record and on emails, and starts seeing patients by 8:00 AM. Patients are scheduled every 20 minutes. Because it's impossible to provide what his patients need in that amount of time, Mike is behind schedule by his third patient and works nonstop through the rest of the day to catch up. He rarely has time to interact with colleagues.

The clinic workflow has also been a source of frustration for the nurses, advanced practice providers, and medical assistants on the care team. Turnover has been high, and Mike is orienting the third new nurse in the past four years. Every time it feels like the team is starting to work together well, someone else gets frustrated and leaves.

Mike usually finishes seeing patients by 5:30 PM, reviews laboratory and other test results for an hour, returns a few phone calls, and then races to get home. After he helps put his seven- and nine-year-old daughters to bed at 8:30 PM, Mike logs in to finish writing his notes for the day's patients, clear yet more inbox messages from the electronic health record, answer more emails, and review the patients scheduled for tomorrow. After a couple hours of work, he drops into bed. Weekends, he catches up on emails he couldn't answer during the week and on administrative work—all while trying to carve out some time for family.

This has been a particularly tough week. This morning, the clinic manager told him his production is 4% less than this time last year. She encouraged him to try and catch up. "Is this really what medicine is about?" Mike silently asks himself. He's running as fast as he can but is no longer sure that he is providing the best care for his patients, which weighs heavily on him. In addition, he doesn't have any time for himself or nearly enough time for his family.

If something doesn't change, Mike will leave the physician workforce.

Sally

Sally is a medical-surgical nurse who has worked at the same hospital for the past five years. She is passionate about nursing and considers caring for patients and supporting their families one of the most meaningful aspects of her life.

Other aspects of her work leave much to be desired, however. Her unit is perpetually understaffed, and she feels as if she is juggling too many tasks on every shift. She regularly worries that it's just a matter of time before something is missed and a patient harmed. The first two hours of each shift are particularly chaotic as Sally tries to understand her patients' issues and the care plans for the day. A dizzying number of physicians admit patients to the unit, and frequently, she doesn't even know or see them. All she has are orders. Although most of the physicians are professional and kind, they rarely inquire about what she has observed, ask for her insights, or provide an overview of the management plan.

The last few days have been especially discouraging. The oncology team recommended another round of chemotherapy for a patient who had a relapse of breast cancer. The patient told Sally she doesn't want the chemotherapy but agreed to appease her children. Sally knows from experience that the treatment will probably make the patient sick and offer little meaningful benefit. When she started the patient's intravenous chemotherapy this morning, Sally felt as though she was complicit in something she knew was wrong.

If something doesn't change, Sally's mental and physical exhaustion could affect patient safety.

Jennifer

Jennifer is the administrator for a small medical center, and she knows her job well. She wanted to work for a nonprofit patient care organization because she felt it would have more purpose than working at a for-profit company. She always wanted to help people, and as a hospital administrator, she thought she could interact with patients and learn what she personally could do to help the system function better.

Sadly, those dreams faded over the years. She feels as though she is running a business where volume overshadows value. Jennifer does not feel included in the camaraderie of the physicians or nurses. Her hours are just as long as theirs, and she basically is on call all the time responding to their needs, which are always categorized as "urgent." She can never catch up. Last month, the hospital started a program for clinician burnout. Jennifer thinks, "What about me?"

If something doesn't change, Jennifer will likely take her experience elsewhere at great cost to the hospital.

Mike, Sally, and Jennifer are all at risk for losing their compassion and concern for the patients they serve.

CONSEQUENCES FOR PROFESSIONALS AND PATIENTS

Burnout of health care professionals negatively impacts safety, team effectiveness, staff turnover, professional productivity, organizational effectiveness, and organizational brand. Professionals also experience personal consequences from burnout including higher rates of relationship issues, alcohol and substance use, clinical depression, and suicide (Figure 2.1). Evidence indicates that the excessive stress can make them angry, irritable, and vulnerable to developing illnesses, such as heart disease or high blood pressure.

Even more important, however, burnout has a profound, negative bearing on patient experience and outcomes. Patients perceive less empathy, compassion, and kindness and experience more unprofessional behavior when cared for by burned-out health care professionals. When patients believe that the professionals treating them don't really care about them personally, they have lower levels of trust and higher levels of anxiety and pain. Their length of hospital stay is often longer, and their readmission rate is higher. Incredibly, studies have shown that wounds actually heal faster when patients perceive their care team relationship as kind and empathetic (Doyle et al, 2013)!

Burned-out physicians and nurses also make more medical errors, appear less likely to adhere to standard procedures designed to increase quality, and have inferior patient outcomes reflected in higher infection and mortality rates. Burned-out physicians order more tests and procedures because doing so is often faster than having a discussion with a patient, and they are just trying to get through the day. They also spend less time listening to and talking with patients about their concerns. Ordering unnecessary tests and procedures creates cognitive dissonance for professionals (i.e., delivering care that one would not choose for family, friends, and loved ones). Other care team members recognize when unnecessary tests are ordered or treatment is inappropriate, but they may have little choice in carrying out the order or treatment. This situation can make the care team members feel complicit in inappropriate care, induce moral distress, predispose them to burnout— and erode esprit de corps.

CONSEQUENCES OF ENGAGEMENT

Throughout this book, we will talk about the importance of engagement for health care professionals. Engaged health care professionals have a heightened sense of emotional, behavioral, and psychological connection with their organizations and work, which shows in their dedication to patient care and professional fulfillment. Everyone should strive to have engaged health care professionals working in their organizations, and health professionals should strive to be engaged.

Paradoxically, without healthy boundaries, dedication and commitment can actually increase exhaustion. This is a real problem for dedicated health care professionals operating in a suboptimal system. When the system fails to provide adequate

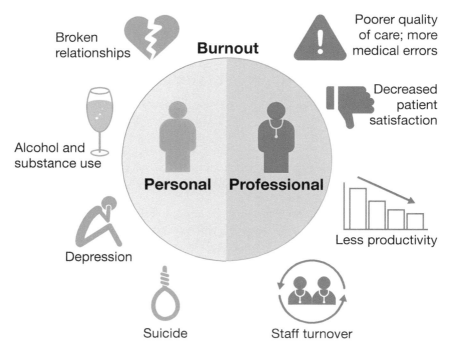

Figure 2.1. Personal and Professional Consequences of Burnout.
(Modified from Shanafelt TD, Noseworthy JH. Executive leadership and physician well-being: nine organizational strategies to promote engagement and reduce burnout. Mayo Clin Proc. 2017 Jan;92[1]:129-46; used with permission of Mayo Foundation for Medical Education and Research.)

professional time (e.g., the 15-minute clinic visit in primary care), these professionals often sacrifice themselves and their personal time to meet patient needs. Indeed, multiple studies have found that the most empathetic physicians and nurses and those with the highest patient satisfaction scores may be at greatest risk of experiencing burnout—if they are not in a highly supportive system.

CONCLUSION

The high prevalence of burnout among health care professionals has become a social epidemic that is spreading within and between care teams, departments, clinics, and hospitals. Health care professionals are suffering professionally and personally. The negative implications of burnout on health care are enormous. Addressing burnout and creating esprit de corps is an important opportunity for leaders and health care organizations.

Given the extensive consequences and implications, the issue of professional burnout must be reframed from an individual one (i.e., the professionals are at fault) to an organizational opportunity if patient care and organizational effectiveness are to improve. Stronger partnerships and professional fulfillment benefit the individual health care professional, as well as facilitate the organization's ability to deliver high-value, safe care. However, the effort to eliminate burnout, promote engagement, and nurture esprit de corps ultimately should be motivated by a genuine interest in the well-being of patients and health care professionals as well as in creating engaged and resilient teams operating in an environment of esprit de corps.

SUGGESTED READING

Barsade SG, O'Neill OA. What's love got to do with it? A longitudinal study of the culture of companionate love and employee and client outcomes in a long-term care setting. Adm Sci Q. 2014;59(4):551–98.

Cosley BJ, McCoy SK, Saslow LR, Epel ES. Is compassion for others stress buffering? Consequences of compassion and social support for physiological reactivity to stress. J Exp Soc Psychol. 2010;46:816–23.

Doyle C, Lennox L, Bell D. A systematic review of evidence on the links between patient experience and clinical safety and effectiveness. BMJ Open. 2013 Jan 3;3(1): e001570.

Dyrbye LN, West CP, Satele D, Boone S, Tan L, Sloan J, et al. Burnout among U.S. medical students, residents, and early career physicians relative to the general U.S. population. Acad Med. 2014 Mar;89(3):443–51.

Hibbard JH, Greene J, Overton V. Patients with lower activation associated with higher costs; delivery systems should know their patients' 'scores.' Health Aff (Millwood). 2013 Feb;32(2):216–22.

Hsu I, Saha S, Korthuis PT, Sharp V, Cohn J, Moore RD, et al. Providing support to patients in emotional encounters: a new perspective on missed empathic opportunities. Patient Educ Couns. 2012 Sep;88(3):436–42.

Maslach C, Jackson SE, Leiter MP. Maslach burnout inventory manual. 3rd ed: Consulting Psychologists Press; 1996.

Shanafelt TD, Hasan O, Dyrbye LN, Sinsky C, Satele D, Sloan J, et al. Changes in burnout and satisfaction with work-life balance in physicians and the general U.S. working population between 2011 and 2014. Mayo Clin Proc. 2015 Dec;90(12):1600–13.

Shanafelt TD, Noseworthy JH. Executive leadership and physician well-being: nine organizational strategies to promote engagement and reduce burnout. Mayo Clin Proc. 2017 Jan;92(1):129–46.

Swensen SJ. Esprit de corps and quality: making the case for eradicating burnout. J Healthc Manag. 2018 Jan/Feb;63(1):7–11.

Williams ES, Manwell LB, Konrad TR, Linzer M. The relationship of organizational culture, stress, satisfaction, and burnout with physician-reported error and suboptimal patient care: results from the MEMO study. Health Care Manage Rev. 2007 Jul-Sep;32(3):203–12.

3

DRIVERS OF BURNOUT AND ENGAGEMENT

A bad system will beat a good person every time.
—W. Edwards Deming

Many leaders in health care operate under the erroneous belief that burnout and professional satisfaction are primarily the responsibility of the individual professional. Studies of physicians throughout the course of their training strongly refute this premise (Brazeau et al, 2014; Dyrbye et al, 2014). Future physicians complete their undergraduate studies with excellent mental and emotional health. Once these students enter medical school, their enthusiasm, vitality, idealism, and engagement are systematically eroded by the training process. Within only a handful of years, approximately half of all medical students experience signs of burnout, a proportion that increases to 75% during residency, which we will discuss in detail in Chapter 33 ("Applying the Action Sets to Address the Unique Needs of Medical Students, Residents, and Fellows"). The situation improves modestly when residents enter practice. Similarly, more nurses also experience burnout during their early working years.

DRIVERS OF BURNOUT AND ENGAGEMENT

We believe a helpful way to look at burnout is to think about six characteristics of a health care system that, when working optimally, create engaged professionals and meaning and purpose in work. These are:

1) Workload and job demands
2) Efficiency and resources
3) Control and flexibility
4) Organizational culture and values
5) Social support and community at work
6) Work-life integration

When these six workplace dimensions do not function optimally, they become drivers of burnout (Figure 3.1).
Each of the six basic drivers and the overarching determinant, meaning and purpose in work, will be discussed in greater detail in subsequent chapters. However, we describe them below briefly to give you a cursory understanding of the categories and their importance.

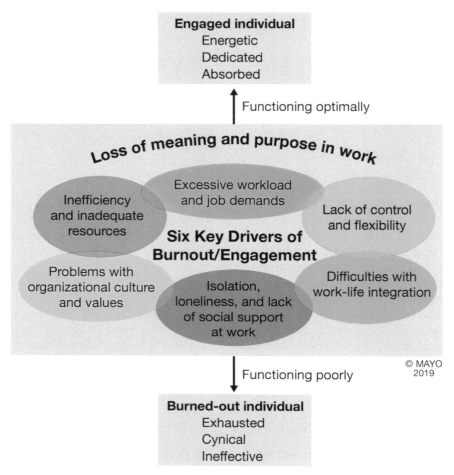

Figure 3.1. Key Drivers of Burnout and Engagement for Physicians.
(Modified from Shanafelt T, Noseworthy JH. Executive leadership and physician well-being: nine organizational strategies to promote engagement and reduce burnout. Mayo Clin Proc. Jan 2017;92[1]:129-46; used with permission of Mayo Foundation for Medical Education and Research.)

1) Excessive Workload and Job Demands

Workload and job demand issues boil down to some combination of too much work, not enough time to accomplish the expected output with the support provided, or both. Much of the productivity gains in health care over the past several decades have resulted from professionals working harder in the same systems. What does this mean for society?

The collective workload facing health care organizations is daunting. Every day for the next decade in the United States, approximately 10,000 citizens will reach the age of 65 years. This substantial demographic change will result in a large increase in the number of patients needing care and increased demands on the health care system. Most patients will be insured through Medicare rather than commercial insurance, which will make it difficult for organizations to maintain the same income level and profit margins. In addition, substantial shortfalls are forecast in the numbers of health care professionals available to treat these patients.

Unless new ways of working are implemented or massive reductions in operational cost structure made, the workload and job demands challenges faced by organizations and their professional workforce are likely to increase. The decisions about how these challenges will be addressed have tremendous implications for professional burnout among physicians, nurses, advanced practice providers (APPs), and other health care professionals.

When workload and job demands become unreasonable, professionals can suffer from burnout.

2) Inefficiency and Inadequate Resources

The optimal work environment is one that makes it easy to provide the best possible care for patients. That environment requires a team of individuals, all of whom operate at the top of their abilities and licenses. Unfortunately, in health care today, professionals are burdened with pervasive workflow inefficiencies such as unnecessary clerical work, poor triage systems, and cumbersome processes embedded in electronic health records. Without sufficient resources to correct the inefficiencies, patients suffer.

Workflow inefficiency and insufficient resources also affect health care professionals personally. Occupational stress results from an imbalance between demands on professionals and the resources they have to deal with those demands. Resources include the quality of the care team, staffing levels, the number of treatment rooms available per provider, sufficient time to accomplish required tasks, the quality and arrangement of the physical plant, and leadership support to navigate and simplify institutional, governmental, and reimbursement-related bureaucratic red tape.

When workflow inefficiency and insufficient resources hinder health care professionals from providing high-quality care, the resulting frustration contributes to burnout.

3) Lack of Control and Flexibility

High stress, high demand, and little control frequently characterize today's health care work environment. Health care professionals often believe they know the right thing to do for their patients, but their role, organizational limitations, support, or resources make it nearly impossible to deliver the best patient care. They feel like cogs in a rigid and inflexible system that requires them daily to work unreasonable hours and to ignore issues that they are not empowered to fix. Micromanagement, lack of influence, and accountability without authority result in moral distress and contribute to burnout.

For the best possible performance, care teams need to have some control and flexibility over their work lives. Physicians, nurses, APPs, pharmacists, and other health care professionals are highly trained and knowledgeable workers who want a voice in improving and co-creating efficient and effective care systems and work environments. Their voices should be trusted.

When their voices are ignored, health care professionals become subject to burnout.

4) Problems With Organizational Culture and Values

A positive, supportive organizational culture with strong and fair workplace values is a substantial determinant for professionals finding meaning in their work. Mayo Clinic is an excellent example of an organization that recognized a need a century ago and created a distinct culture to meet that need through a relentless focus on the patient, systems, and the team (Swensen et al, 2016). Section II ("Strategy") in this book describes in detail various strategies to change the organizational culture and values to create an environment that promotes esprit de corps. When culture and values are misaligned with those of professionals, burnout is common.

5) Isolation, Loneliness, and Lack of Social Support at Work

Social support and community at work are important to the welfare of professionals. Health care professionals frequently deal with patient suffering, the limited effectiveness of available treatments, and the emotional burdens of supporting patients and their family members; this can cause compassion fatigue. To preserve the ability to deal with these challenges over the course of their careers and to help prevent compassion fatigue, professionals must not only be personally resilient but they must also work within a community of colleagues who support each other.

When health care professionals experience social isolation, conflict, and disrespect, they become vulnerable to burnout.

6) Difficulties With Work-Life Integration

Although work-life integration is challenging in many professions, national studies of U.S. workers across all professions have shown that it is a more substantial issue for health care professionals than those in other disciplines (Shanafelt et al, 2018).

Work-life integration is challenging for all health care professionals in some way. For physicians, this is in part due to the extraordinarily long work hours most clock, along with frequent night and weekend call responsibilities. For nurses and other health care professionals, inflexible scheduling (including 10- to 12-hour shifts), the frequent need for night and weekend shifts, and the unpredictability of patient care and staffing needs (which often lead to unplanned overtime) all threaten work-life integration. Work-life integration for today's health care professionals is even more challenging for those in two-career relationships—often two careers in health care—and for women, for whom an inflexible work environment may be incongruent with their personal responsibilities and needs (Shanafelt et al, 2015).

Health care organizations must acknowledge the role they play in fostering or hindering work-life integration, recognize its impact on the well-being of health care professionals as well as on recruitment and retention, and consider organizational strategies to foster it. They also must acknowledge an evolving workplace that includes more millennials, who place greater value on work-life integration and attention to personal as well as professional ambitions.

If organizations ignore issues of work-life integration, they will fail health care professionals and contribute to their burnout.

Loss of Meaning and Purpose in Work

Meaning and purpose in work, overarching determinants of burnout, are fundamental for professional fulfillment and engagement. Health care seems the ideal field to provide for these important essentials of employee well-being because the work is inherently meaningful work.

Unfortunately, health care workers are often distracted from the altruistic reasons they chose their jobs by inefficient and poorly designed systems with insufficient resources and by co-workers functioning as a group of independent individuals rather than as a team. Meaning and purpose in work are also compromised by ethical conflicts that create cognitive dissonance, which results from the psychological stress of providing patient care that contradicts with their personal beliefs, ideals, or values. High-functioning organizations deliberately and intentionally develop strategies and tactics to manage these issues, which are described in detail in Section III ("Execution"). The best organizations help professionals recognize and reconnect with the meaning and purpose in their work.

When health care organizations do not recognize the importance of meaning and purpose in work, they subject their professional workforce to a higher risk of burnout.

RELATIVE IMPORTANCE OF THE STRESSORS

Burnout is not unique to one group of health care professionals. Such challenges as poorly functioning care teams, ineffective leadership, and incongruent values are highly relevant for all health care professionals and need to be corrected for esprit de corps to exist (Figure 3.2). The relative importance of other stressors may vary by occupation, specialty, and work setting (Figure 3.3). A nurse and a pharmacist have both shared and distinct professional challenges. A family physician, a radiologist, and a surgeon face different stressors. Optimal progress is not made by ignoring these differences but by recognizing them and addressing the unique needs of different professionals and the occupation in which they work.

CONCLUSION

The core work of addressing professional burnout requires identifying, mitigating, and eradicating the unique, local drivers of burnout in addition to creating an environment that fosters esprit de corps. Evidence-based solutions for each of the burnout drivers are included in Section III ("Execution").

Burnout	Esprit de Corps
High workload	Sustainable workload
Inefficient work environment	Well-organized work setting
Inadequate work-life integration	Work-life integration
Inflexible situation	Sense of control
Compassion fatigue	Empathy supported by trusted colleagues and team
Moral distress	Open discussion of optimal patient-centered care
Lack of psychological safety	Safe environment for voicing opinions
Hostile work environment	Respectful and inclusive work place
Practice inefficiency	Work flows without frustration
Excessive work unrelated to skill level	Necessary work performed by the most appropriate team member
Understaffed and undersupported team	Appropriately staffed and resourced team
Cognitive dissonance	Harmony between actions and values
Loss of meaning in work	Connection to core values
Culture of sleep deprivation	Healthy work and call schedules
Exposure to patient suffering and death	Team and professional safe haven support
Shame and blame response to medical errors	Fair and just culture
Malpractice suits	Organizational resource support for litigation
Gap between care desired and care delivered	Quality improvement culture
Culture of "cog in the wheel"	Culture of value and respect for each individual
Leaders who focus exclusively on productivity	Leaders who focus on engagement and unleashing the potential of individuals and the team to achieve objectives

© MAYO
2019

Figure 3.2. Factors Contributing to Burnout vs Esprit de Corps.

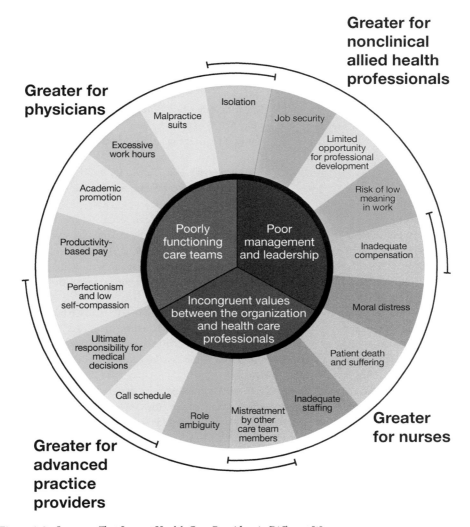

Figure 3.3. Stressors That Impact Health Care Providers in Different Ways.
(Modified from Shanafelt T, et al. Building a program on well-being: key design considerations to meet the unique needs of each organization. Acad Med. 2019 Feb;94[2]:156-61; used with permission.)

SUGGESTED READING

Brazeau CM, Shanafelt T, Durning SJ, Massie FS, Eacker A, Moutier C, et al. Distress among matriculating medical students relative to the general population. Acad Med. 2014 Nov;89(11)1520–5.

Dyrbye LN, Shanafelt TD, Balch CM, Satele D, Freischlag J. Physicians married or partnered to physicians: a comparative study in the American College of Surgeons. J Am Coll Surg. 2010 Nov;211(5):663–71.

Dyrbye LN, Shanafelt TD, Balch CM, Satele D, Sloan J, Freischlag J. Relationship between work-home conflicts and burnout among American surgeons: a comparison by sex. Arch Surg. 2011 Feb;146(2):211–7.

Dyrbye LN, West CP, Satele D, Boone S, Tan L, Sloan J, et al. Burnout among U.S. medical students, residents, and early career physicians relative to the general U.S. population. Acad Med. 2014 Mar;89(3):443–51.

Festinger L. Cognitive dissonance. Scientific American. 1962 Oct;207(4):93–106.

Shanafelt T, Trockel M, Ripp J, Murphy ML, Sandborg C, Bohman B. Building a program on well-being: key design considerations to meet the unique needs of each organization. Acad Med. 2019 Feb;94(2):156–61.

Shanafelt TD, Boone SL, Dyrbye LN, Oreskovich MR, Tan L, West CP, et al. The medical marriage: a national survey of the spouses/partners of U.S. physicians. Mayo Clinic Proceedings. 2013 Mar;88(3):216–25.

Shanafelt TD, Hasan O, Dyrbye LN, Sinsky C, Satele D, Sloan J, et al. Changes in burnout and satisfaction with work-life balance in physicians and the general U.S. working population between 2011 and 2014. Mayo Clin Proc. 2015 Dec;90(12):1600–13.

Shanafelt TD, Noseworthy JH. Executive leadership and physician well-being: nine organizational strategies to promote engagement and reduce burnout. Mayo Clin Proc. 2017 Jan;92(1):129–46.

Shanafelt TD, West CP, Sinsky C, Trockel M, Tutty M, Satele DV, et al. Changes in burnout and satisfaction with work life integration in physicians and the general U.S. working population between 2011–2017. Mayo Clin Proc. 2019 Sep;94(9):1681–94.

Swensen SJ. Esprit de corps and quality: making the case for eradicating burnout. J Healthc Manag. 2018 Jan/Feb;63(1):7–11.

Swensen SJ, Gorringe G, Caviness J, Peters D. Leadership by design: intentional organization development of physician leaders. J Manag Dev. 2016;35(4):549–70.

Zapf D, Seifert C, Schmutte B, Mertini H, Holz M. Emotion work and job stressors and their effects on burnout. Psychol Health. 2001 Sep;16(5):527–45.

4

THE BUSINESS CASE

You can do well by doing "good."
—Brent James, MD

DOING THE RIGHT THING

A few decades ago, in the early days of the quality movement, the business case for quality had to be made to health care leaders. Understanding the business case for quality allowed health care administrators to consider the topic through the lens of a mission-aligned business strategy. When the robust financial return on investment (ROI) for patient-centered quality improvement work was demonstrated (with an ROI in the range of 5:1), the possibilities to take on more major initiatives and make more substantive progress were realized (Swensen et al, 2013).

A similarly strong business case exists for organizations to invest in efforts to reduce professional burnout as well as to promote staff engagement and esprit de corps. Unfortunately, there is a widespread lack of awareness among health care organizations regarding the financial costs of professional burnout. There is also uncertainty regarding what organizational leaders can do to address the problem. This ambiguity and lack of awareness have been barriers to action.

The business case to address burnout is multifaceted and includes various issues for patients and health care professionals, such as direct costs from staff turnover, indirect costs from staff turnover (e.g., more adverse patient events with understaffing and newly onboarded nurses), lost revenue associated with decreased productivity, malpractice litigation risk, and other financial risks related to the organization's long-term viability (e.g., the relationship between burnout and lower quality of care, retention of talented professionals, brand, reputation, market share) (Figure 4.1). Health care organizations have used similar issues and analogous evidence to justify their investments to improve quality.

Thus, the financial ROI for decreasing burnout and promoting esprit de corps makes business sense. As with the quality movement, ROI calculations for addressing professional burnout must involve senior financial officers, and the calculations should distinguish hard-dollar from soft-dollar savings and dividends (Figure 4.2).

Three central observations are necessary for the business case:

1) Improvement is possible.
2) Investment is justified.
3) ROI is measurable.

With this backdrop, addressing professional burnout is a fiscally responsible decision.

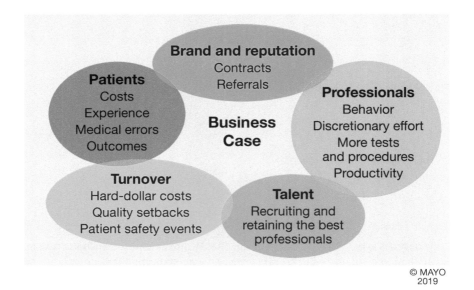

© MAYO
2019

Figure 4.1. The Business Case for Addressing Burnout and Cultivating Esprit de Corps.

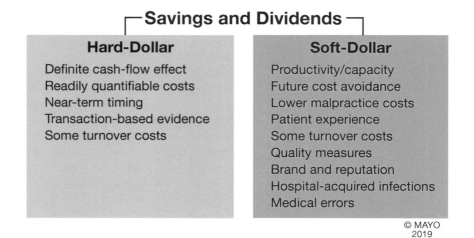

© MAYO
2019

Figure 4.2. Hard-Dollar and Soft-Dollar Considerations for Return on Investment.
(Data from Swensen SJ, Dilling JA, McCarty PM, Bolton JW, Harper CM Jr. The business case
for health-care quality improvement. J Patient Saf. 2013 Mar;9[1]:44-52.)

The Biggest Business Case Mistakes

Leaders make various mistakes when considering the business case for improving rates of burnout and cultivating esprit de corps, but two are common.

First, they incorrectly assume that addressing professional burnout is just an important expense. In fact, we will show you why addressing professional burnout is a stand-alone business strategy that makes financial sense.

Second, they incorrectly assume that employees are dispensable and easily replaced. In fact, we will show you that the costs associated with turnover and reduced productivity due to burnout are substantial, and replacing these professionals is becoming more challenging, given shortages of physicians, nurses, and advanced practice providers. Treating people with respect and dignity, as one would like their own family members to be treated, is a stand-alone business strategy that makes sense.

THE CURRENT FINANCIAL ECOSYSTEM IN HEALTH CARE

The only word to describe the current financial ecosystem in health care is *challenging*. Growing transparency and price competition, narrowing of insurance networks, a greater proportion of patients with noncommercial insurance (e.g., government payers), value-based purchasing, and risk sharing have changed the economics of health care. This shift has resulted in declining revenues for health care organizations and practices, efforts to reduce costs, and a focus on the more profitable areas of medical care under the current payment system, such as heart disease and cancer. For many medical organizations, market consolidation is another threat.

In the United States, the requirement for meaningful use of electronic health records has resulted in large expenditures for most organizations and substantially increased the clerical burden for health care professionals. These financial challenges have been addressed largely by increasing productivity expectations for professionals (i.e., caring for more patients with the same amount of time and resources), efforts to improve efficiency, and expense reductions to decrease the cost of care delivered. The actual strategy at most organizations can be described as "doing more with less." New quality metrics and requirements for public reporting also lead to increased clerical work for health care professionals, some of which does not appear to create value for patients.

These challenges and pressures typically cause leaders to focus on external economic threats to the organization and to have a blind spot for important internal threats, such as burnout of health care professionals. To accomplish the organization's mission, leaders must certainly traverse the external challenges, but they must also cultivate a committed, engaged, and productive staff working in partnership with leadership to adapt to the rapidly changing environment. This is esprit de corps.

Impact	Stage
Minor	Novice
	Issue identified
	Wellness committee
	Individual-focused interventions
	Mindfulness training
	Resources for exercise/nutrition
Moderate	Beginner
	Burnout drivers recognized
	Peer-support program
	Cross-sectional survey assessing well-being of health care professionals
	Struggling units identified
	Health care professionals' well-being considered when organizational decisions implemented
Major	Competent
	Business case to promote well-being of health care professionals
	Practice redesign based on dimensions of burnout drivers
	Coaching resources for physicians and other health care professionals to support career, work-life integration, and self-care
	Burnout/well-being measured to monitor trends
	Physicians given greater voice in decisions
	Work unit–level interventions designed but efficacy not objectively assessed
	Opportunity created for community building among professionals
Transformative	Proficient
	Impact of physician well-being known for organization objectives[a]
	Well-being considered in all operational decisions
	Program funded for well-being of health care professionals
	Clerical burden measured/reduced
	Training for leaders in participatory management
	System-level interventions with robust assessment of effectiveness
	Workflow improved by engaging and supporting local transformation
	Expert
	Well-being of health care professionals influences key operational decisions[b]
	Shared accountability for well-being among organizational leaders
	Chief well-being officer on executive leadership team
	Endowed program in well-being creates new knowledge that guides other organizations
	Strategic investment to promote well-being of health care professionals
	Culture of wellness

[a]Finances, turnover, safety/quality, patient satisfaction.
[b]Strategy, priorities, resource allocation, new initiatives.

Figure 4.3. Typical Stages in an Organization's Journey Toward Fulfilled Health Care Professionals.

(Data from Shanafelt T, Goh J, Sinsky C. The business case for investing in physician well-being. JAMA Intern Med. 2017 Dec 1;177[12]:1826-32.)

Stages

The journey to esprit de corps and the understanding of professional well-being as a business strategy takes time, and many organizations are still at the novice stage, implementing approaches that only have a minor impact (Figure 4.3).

To get beyond the novice stage, organizations need to realize that an exhausted and disillusioned professional workforce does not make for a good partner, and steps need to be taken to ensure their staff is engaged, resilient, and invested in partnering with the organization to improve quality and respond to external threats.

Intentional and wide-ranging efforts by leaders to reduce burnout and promote engagement can make a difference. Many effective interventions in the different stages of the journey are relatively inexpensive and primarily require the time and attention of staff. We will describe them in detail in Section III ("Execution"). Small investments in these areas can have a substantive impact. Other high-impact interventions (e.g., care team, practice redesign) take more time and investment but can pay large dividends, with a strongly positive ROI.

COST IMPLICATIONS FOR PATIENTS AND PROVIDERS

There are reasons that some of the most successful and enduring for-profit companies outside of health care focus on the well-being of their staff (Chapman and Sisodia, 2015): Engaged employees have higher levels of discretionary effort, collaboration, and productivity, which result in higher profits for the organization. These companies also experience lower levels of employee accidents and turnover (Harter et al, 2002; Swensen and Shanafelt, 2017). Similarly, clinics with higher teamwork ratings have higher nurse retention rates, lower operating costs, and better patient-experience scores (Jones and Gates, 2007) (Figure 4.4).

A critical (and arguably the most important) component of the business case for reducing professional burnout and promoting esprit de corps is, of course, better health for patients. Evidence indicates that physicians who feel appreciated and are professionally satisfied make diagnoses twice as fast and with higher accuracy rates, ultimately decreasing the cost of health care for patients and for providers. When patients perceive their relationship with professionals as trusting and empathetic, they are also far more likely to follow through on their care plans. Although the current system of reimbursement in the United States does not adequately reward low-cost, high-quality care, this is rapidly changing with the introduction of bundled payments, the value-based Medicare Access and CHIP Reauthorization Act, patient-centered medical homes, and risk-based contracting.

An established link also exists between burnout and unprofessional behavior among medical students, residents, and practicing physicians (Shanafelt et al, 2015). Depersonalization is associated with increased, unsolicited patient complaints and can cause patients to seek treatment elsewhere. Fewer patients mean less revenue for the organization. Physicians and medical students with burnout are more likely to exhibit less altruistic views regarding their responsibilities to society, such as providing care for the underserved (Dyrbye et al, 2010). None of this contributes to a robust business model for health care organizations.

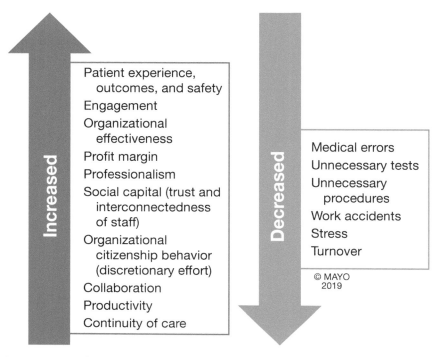

Figure 4.4. Benefits of Cultivating Esprit de Corps for Health Care Organizations.

Turnover

People talk with their feet. Stanford University (Hamidi et al, 2018) and the Cleveland Clinic (Windover et al, 2018) have reported a powerful link between burnout and turnover, which substantially impacts costs and the business case (Shanafelt et al, 2017). Physicians experiencing burnout are more than twice as likely as engaged physicians to leave their practices within two years. Approximately half of physicians intend to cut back on their practice time or seek other means of reducing work-related stress, often as a reaction to burnout. Similar challenges are experienced by nurses. One in seven nurses leaves their job every year.

Trust and patient-professional relationships deepen with continuity of care and are eroded by staff turnover. Turnover also increases the risk of errors associated with teamwork, communication, and hand offs of care among health care professionals. For example, a new primary care doctor working with a patient for the first time is more likely to order tests and unnecessarily initiate expensive workups to evaluate patient symptoms than a primary care provider who has an established relationship with the patient.

The Cost of Turnover

It is possible to estimate the financial ROI that health care organizations would achieve by reducing professional burnout (Appendixes 4.1 and 4.2). These estimates depend on whether both soft-dollar and hard-dollar costs are taken into account and on how conservative the assumptions used are.

Turnover of hospital staff accounts for at least 5% of total operating costs. Nursing turnover accounts for most of these costs and is an important aspect of the business case (Waldman et al, 2004). The turnover costs associated with the departure of a nurse are one to two times salary; the average turnover rate for nurses in the United States is about 15% (Jones and Gates, 2007; Allen, 2008; Willis Towers Watson, 2015/2016). Therefore, the approximate cost of nurse turnover is $7,000,000 to $8,000,000 each year for an average-sized hospital in the United States.

The costs of physician turnover are higher per capita, but their turnover rate is lower (approximately 7%-8% per year). The cost of turnover (recruitment, relocation, and replacement costs) per physician ranges from $500,000 to $1,000,000, depending on specialty. So, for example, the cost of physician turnover (assume a burnout rate of 50% and a turnover rate of 7.5% per year) to a U.S. hospital with 450 employed physicians is approximately $5,625,000 each year (Appendixes 4.1 and 4.2) (Shanafelt et al, 2017). These are real costs that are directly attributable to professional burnout.

To the U.S. health care system, turnover from burnout and reduced clinical hours costs about $4.5 billion per year (Han et al, 2019) or a staggering $7,600 per physician. That figure does not take into account the costs of turnover for other professionals or any of the other associated costs of burnout on quality, patient satisfaction, patient outcomes, or malpractice.

These extremely conservative estimates include loss of time related to malpractice suits and decreased productivity during recruitment of new physicians. But they do not include the costs of poor quality, adverse patient safety events, patient satisfaction, decreased academic output, and the potentially huge costs of prolonged vacancy of key revenue-stream professionals measured in lost revenue and opportunity costs (Atkinson et al, 2006).

Imagine, just a small improvement in these turnover rates could fund the annual budget of an amazing well-being program.

Malpractice Litigation

The risk of malpractice litigation is strongly linked to the well-being and professional fulfillment of health care workers, consistent with the relationship between burnout and medical errors and breakdowns in clinician-patient communications. Investigators at Stanford University showed a strong link between an individual physician's level of burnout and the physician's Patient Advocate and Reporting System score—a validated predictor of malpractice risk used by hospitals across the United States (Welle et al, 2017). Approximately three of four malpractice lawsuits have as their root cause miscommunication or poor clinician-patient relationships (Beckman et al, 1994). When researchers asked patients why they sued their physicians for malpractice, four issues surfaced. Each of these issues can be linked to burnout:

1) Patients believed they were deserted.
2) Patients felt devalued.
3) Patients believed information was communicated poorly.
4) Patients felt misunderstood by their physicians.

Thus, not only does burnout increase the risk of malpractice suits (and associated costs), but evidence indicates that malpractice suits and the litigious nature of society also increase professional burnout in a vicious cycle (Balch et al, 2011). A large proportion of physicians are sued for malpractice at least once during the course of their careers, including a majority of physicians in procedural specialties. Physicians who have a trusting, unrushed, and empathetic relationship with patients are less likely to be sued.

CONCLUSION

Enlightened health care leaders deliberately invest in and labor to create esprit de corps (Swensen, 2018) as a core component of their business strategy. They do this because esprit de corps makes a difference for patients and also their bottom line. Professionals with camaraderie, engagement, satisfaction, psychological safety, and resilience are not burned out and enable their organization to achieve its mission efficiently and effectively.

SUGGESTED READING

Allen DG. Retaining talent: a guide to analyzing and managing employee turnover. Foundation's Effective Practice Guideline Series [Internet]. 2008 [cited 2019 Feb 14]. Available from: https://www.shrm.org/hr-today/trends-and-forecasting/special-reports-and-expert-views/Documents/Retaining-Talent.pdf.

American Medical Group Association (AMGA). Physician turnover remains high as more physicians retire [Internet]. 2014 [cited 2019 Feb 15]. Available from: https://www.amga.org/wcm/AboutAMGA/News/2014/082114.aspx.

Atkinson W, Misra-Hebert A, Stoller JK. The impact on revenue of physician turnover: an assessment model and experience in a large healthcare center. J Med Pract Manage. 2006 May-Jun;21(6):351–5.

Balch CM, Oreskovich MR, Dyrbye LN, Colaiano JM, Satele DV, Sloan JA, et al. Personal consequences of malpractice lawsuits on American surgeons. J Am Coll Surg. 2011 Nov;213(5):657–67.

Beckman HB, Markakis KM, Suchman AL, Frankel RM. The doctor-patient relationship and malpractice: lessons from plaintiff depositions. Arch Intern Med. 1994 Jun 27;154(12):1365–70.

Chapman B, Sisodia R. Everybody matters: the extraordinary power of caring for your people life family. New York (NY): Portfolio/Penguin; 2015.

Dillard A. The writing life. New York (NY): HarperCollins; 1989.

Dyrbye LN, Massie FS Jr, Eacker A, Harper W, Power D, Durning SJ, et al. Relationship between burnout and professional conduct and attitudes among U.S. medical students. JAMA. 2010 Sep 15;304(11):1173–80.

Hamidi MS, Bohman B, Sandborg C, Smith-Coggins R, de Vries P, Albert MS, et al. Estimating institutional physician turnover attributable to self-reported burnout and associated financial burden: a case study. BMC Health Serv Res. 2018; 18:851.

Han S, Shanafelt TD, Sinsky CA, Awad KM, Dyrbye LN, Fiscus LC, et al. Estimating the attributable cost of physician burnout in the United States. Ann Intern Med. 2019;170:784–90.

Harter JK, Schmidt FL, Hayes TL. Business-unit-level relationship between employee satisfaction, employee engagement, and business outcomes: a meta-analysis. J Appl Psychol. 2002 Apr;87(2):268–79.

Hibbard JH, Greene J, Overton V. Patients with lower activation associated with higher costs: delivery systems should know their patients' "scores." Health Aff (Millwood). 2013 Feb;32(2):216–22.

Isen AM. An influence of positive affect on decision making in complex situations: theoretical issues with practical implications. J Consumer Psychol. 2001;11(2):75–85.

Jones CB, Gates M. The costs and benefits of nurse turnover: a business case for nurse retention. Online J Issues Nurs. 2007 Sep 30;12(3):4.

Nolin CE. Malpractice claims, patient communication, and critical paths: a lawyer's perspective. Qual Manag Health Care. 1995 Winter;3(2):65–70.

Roter DL, Hall JA, Merisca R, Nordstrom B, Cretin D, Svarstad B. Effectiveness of interventions to improve patient compliance: a meta-analysis. Med Care. 1998 Aug;36(8):1138–61.

Shanafelt T, Goh J, Sinsky C. The business case for investing in physician well-being. JAMA Intern Med. 2017 Dec 1;177(12):1826–32.

Shanafelt TD, Hasan O, Dyrbye LN, Sinsky C, Satele D, Sloan J, et al. Changes in burnout and satisfaction with work-life balance in physicians and the general U.S. working population between 2011 and 2014. Mayo Clin Proc. 2015 Dec;90(12):1600–13.

Swensen SJ. Esprit de corps and quality: making the case for eradicating burnout. J Healthc Manag. 2018 Jan/Feb;63(1):7–11.

Swensen SJ, Dilling JA, McCarty PM, Bolton JW, Harper CM Jr. The business case for health-care quality improvement. J Patient Saf. 2013 Mar;9(1):44–52.

Swensen SJ, Shanafelt T. An organizational framework to reduce professional burnout and bring back joy in practice. Jt Comm J Qual Patient Saf. 2017 Jun;43(6):308–13.

The Physicians Foundation. 2016 survey of America's physicians: practice patterns and perspectives [Internet]. 2016 [cited 2018 12 Sep]. Available from: https://physicians-foundation.org/wp-content/uploads/2018/01/Biennial_Physician_Survey_2016.pdf.

Virshup BB, Oppenberg AA, Coleman MM. Strategic risk management: reducing malpractice claims through more effective patient-doctor communication. Am J Med Qual. 1999 Jul-Aug;14(4):153–9.

Waldman JD, Kelly F, Arora S, Smith HL. The shocking cost of turnover in health care. Health Care Manage Rev. 2004 Jan-Mar;29(1):2–7.

Welle D, Trockel M, Hamidi M, Lesure SE, Hickson G, Cooper W. Physician wellness measures are associated with unsolicited patient complaints: a marker for increased liability risk. Abstract presented at: First American Conference on Physician Health; 2017 Oct 12-13; San Francisco, CA.

Willis Towers Watson. Improving workforce health and productivity. Connecting the elements of workplace culture: U.S. findings of Willis Towers Watson's 2015/2016 Staying@ Work Survey.

Windover AK, Martinez K, Mercer BM, Neuendorf K, Boissy A, Rothberg MB. Correlates and outcomes of physician burnout within a large academic medical center. JAMA Intern Med. 2018 Jun;178(6):856–8.

1. Input data   Enter values

N = No. of physicians at your center   _____

BO = Rate of burnout of physicians at your center   _____ a

TO = Current turnover rate per year   _____ b

C = Cost of turnover per physician   _____ c

2. Calculations

Estimated cost of physician turnover attributable to burnout

A. TO without burnout (solve for "TO without burnout"):

Formula[d]

TO = [TO without burnout × (1 − BO)] + [(2 × TO without burnout) × BO]

Simplified formula

TO without burnout = TO/(1 + BO)

B. Projected No. of physicians turning over per year due to burnout (solve using input variables and TO without burnout value from step A):

Formula

No. of physicians turning over due to burnout per year = (TO − TO without burnout) × N

C. Projected cost of physician turnover per year due to burnout (solve using input variables and No. of physicians turning over due to burnout per year from step B):

Formula

Esimated cost of turnover due to burnout = C × No. of physicians turning over due to burnout per year

---

Example using N = 450; BO = 50%; TO = 7.5%; C = $500,000

A. TO without burnout:
0.075 = [TO without burnout × (1 − 0.5)] + [(2 × TO without burnout) × 0.5] or 0.075/(1 + 0.5) = 5%

B. No. of physicians turning over due to burnout per year:
(0.075 − 0.05) × 450 = 11.25

C. Projected cost of physician turnover per year due to burnout:
$500,000 × 11.25 = $5,625,000

---

a National mean, approximately 54%.

b National mean, approximately 7%.

c Mean cost of $500,000 to $1,000,000 per physician.

d Assumes that burned–out physicians are approximately 2 times as likely to turn over as non–burned–out physicians.

Appendix 4.1. Worksheet for Projecting Organizational Cost of Physician Burnout. (From Shanafelt T, Goh J, Sinsky C. The business case for investing in physician well-being. JAMA Intern Med. 2017 Dec 1;177[12]:1826-32; used with permission.)

1. Input data   **Enter values**

   CB = Estimated cost of turnover due to   _____ [a]
      physician burnout (BO)

   CI = Cost of intervention per year   _____

   R = Relative reduction in BO   _____

2. Calculations

   Return on investment (ROI)

   A. Savings due to reduced BO:

      Formula

      Savings due to reduced BO = (CB × R)

   B. ROI:

      Formula:

      ROI = (Savings due to reduced BO − CI)/CI

Example using CB = $5,625,000; CI = $1,000,000; R = 20%

A. Savings due to reduced BO:
   $5,625,000 × 0.20 = $1,125,000

B. ROI:
   ($1,125,000 − $1,000,000)/$1,000,000 = 12.5%

---

[a] From Appendix 4.1.

Appendix 4.2. Worksheet for Determining Return on Investment From Reduced Turnover Costs After Interventions to Reduce Physician Burnout.
(From Shanafelt T, Goh J, Sinsky C. The business case for investing in physician well-being. JAMA Intern Med. 2017 Dec 1;177[12]:1826-32; used with permission.)

5

QUALITY SHORTFALLS FROM HEALTH CARE WASTE: A UNIFYING ROOT CAUSE OF BURNOUT

Every system is perfectly designed to get the results it gets.
—W. Edwards Deming

The current health care delivery system is perfectly designed to create high rates of professional burnout in physicians, nurses, advanced practice providers, and other health care professionals. In most organizations, a gap exists between the quality of care professionals aspire to deliver and the quality of care actually delivered, which creates burnout.

FIVE CATEGORIES OF WASTE

Poor quality health care is fundamentally about waste, and leaders in the health care industry have primary accountability and responsibility for system waste. Some experts have estimated that one-third of the approximately $3.2 trillion that the United States spends on health care is waste. According to the National Academy of Medicine, waste in health care systems can be found in:

1) Failures of care delivery and care coordination
2) Overtreatment
3) Administrative complexity
4) Pricing failures
5) Fraud and abuse

Each of these issues contributes substantially to decreased quality of care and impacts drivers and determinants of professional burnout. Excessive workload and job demands, inefficiency and inadequate resources, lack of control and flexibility, erosion of meaning and purpose in work, and unhealthy organizational culture all result from these categories of waste. Reducing waste in each category will improve the well-being of professionals, the wellness of patients, and the resilience of the organization (Figure 5.1).

1) Failures of Care Delivery and Care Coordination

Failures of care delivery and care coordination result in higher stress levels for health care professionals and expose patients to substantial health risks and, even, death. Adverse events, missed opportunities for recommended preventive or therapeutic

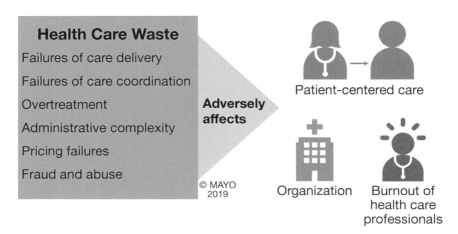

Figure 5.1. Effects of Reducing Waste in the Health Care System.

care, and preventable patient deaths also take a toll on professional well-being. This can come in the form of compassion fatigue, moral distress, or erosion of meaning and purpose in work. Quality shortfalls related to failures of care delivery and care coordination result in more work than care delivered flawlessly the first time. Reducing failures of care delivery and care coordination creates tremendous value for patients and organizations and diminishes professional burnout.

2) Overtreatment

A health care system that promotes overtreatment, including administration of ineffective or unnecessary management plans, creates incongruence between organizational and professional values by expecting or incentivizing professionals to administer medical care to patients that they would not want for themselves (Box 5.1).

Some of the roots of overtreatment are anchored in the litigious practice environment and flawed compensation models. The litigious practice environment creates waste by promulgating a mindset of defensive medicine that encourages excessive testing "to be on the safe side." In addition, most physicians in the United States have some element of productivity in the formula that determines their take-home pay, which encourages overtreatment. Production-based compensation models can also incentivize overwork and unsustainable practice patterns that undermine work-life integration and lead to burnout. Addressing overtreatment creates value for patients and reduces professional burnout.

3) Administrative Complexity

Inefficient and frustrating processes and workflow are causes of burnout for health care providers. Needless administrative complexity also increases the cost of overhead, which necessitates increased productivity expectations (i.e., less time for clinicians with patients) for the organization to stay in the black. Administrative

---

Box 5.1. Quality Shortfall From Overtreatment

Dr. Jones, a radiologist, is asked to perform and interpret a computed tomography (CT) head scan for a nine-year-old girl who had minor head trauma. The trauma episode did not meet the clinical prediction rule criteria suggesting a CT scan was necessary according to the Pediatric Emergency Care Applied Research Network (PECARN). Therefore, to order a head CT would be inappropriate. The physician who requested the CT didn't even bother to use the PECARN clinical prediction rule.

Should the radiology team perform and interpret the examination anyway? The test is unnecessary and exposes the child to needless ionizing radiation.

Should the radiologist intervene and stop the imaging study? Doing so would reduce the revenue generation for the group, and some of her colleagues in radiology may be unhappy.

Either choice creates stress from the intersection of overtreatment, unnecessary care, and a flawed compensation model. If the radiologist performs and completes the examination, cognitive dissonance develops between what the radiologist would do for her family and friends and what has actually happened. If she refuses to complete the study, she faces the ire of the ordering physician and, potentially, the disdain of colleagues in her group. The broken system has created an extremely complex situation—a true Gordian knot. This is just one example of how quality shortfalls can harm patients, professionals, and organizations.

---

complexity from national, state, local, and other regulatory organizations (or misinterpretation of them) results in a loss of control, flexibility, and autonomy for professionals. Administrative complexity ultimately erodes meaning and purpose of work and fuels cognitive dissonance because it requires health care professionals to spend time on tasks that do not appear to directly improve the care of patients. Mitigating the administrative complexity over which we have control reduces an important driver of burnout.

4) Pricing Failures

Medical centers have some control over pricing failures. Pricing failures occur when fees charged migrate far from the expected market rate, and the work of medicine becomes more about money than it does about patients. Pricing failures corrode the altruism of health care professionals, which can be compounded by the flawed compensation models previously discussed.

5) Fraud and Abuse

Fraud and abuse can unfortunately occur in health care organizations. When dedicated health care professionals are aware of organizational fraud and abuse, they experience cognitive dissonance and moral injury. They are predisposed to burnout.

GETTING RID OF WASTE

Waste often produces income for someone, which can make it a formidable barrier to remove. However, that cannot prevent health care professionals from living up to the core values they aspire to and the needs of their patients and the health care delivery system. Strategies for reducing waste will be presented in Chapter 16 ("Agency Action: Removing Pebbles") and Chapter 24 ("Coherence Action: Improving Practice Efficiency").

Each form of waste reduction has positive outcomes. For example, patients and their families benefit from fewer harm events (e.g., infection, falls, stroke, extended hospitalization, death) and decreased out-of-pocket and insurance costs. For health care professionals, moral distress and cognitive dissonance decrease as the care delivered approaches the care they aspire to give. These outcomes are even better when the professionals are part of the team that determines how to reduce waste.

The Result

The process improvement effort in and of itself is therapeutic. Camaraderie develops as teams engage in decreasing waste and improving processes, and work is given meaning and purpose. By supporting these efforts, leadership gives the message: "We trust you to be responsible and improve the systems of care." All of this bolsters esprit de corps and drives down burnout.

Beyond the merit for patients and professionals, eliminating waste improves quality and saves money for organizations, insurers, communities, and providers.

ALIGNED STRATEGIES: QUALITY AND ESPRIT DE CORPS

The aligned strategies of pursuing both quality and esprit de corps are central to the eradication of waste and burnout. Every driver of burnout has at its root an opportunity to improve outcomes, safety, or service to patients—or simply put, to improve quality. Shortfalls in quality, in turn, are a unifying cause of professional burnout.

To address the problems of quality shortfalls, health care delivery is evolving from a volume mindset to a value mindset, as seen through the eyes of the patient. In the new model, patients are seen as partners. The Institute for Healthcare Improvement's Triple Aim (i.e., better patient experience at lower cost with better outcomes) is the target. However, professional burnout makes achieving the Triple Aim a daunting and formidable task. It is hard to imagine attaining the Triple Aim with a workforce that has half of its key players impaired. It is now widely advocated that the Triple Aim be expanded to a Quadruple Aim, with the addition of a fourth objective: improving the work life of health care professionals. This framework illustrates the central role of esprit de corps and allows health care professionals to achieve the care they aspire to give.

In the new patient-centered model, health care professionals function as teams, clinicians are embraced as leaders, quality is embedded as a daily practice, and the finances are geared for creating value instead of creating revenue (Figure 5.2).

From Volume Mindset	To Value Mindset
Poor patient experience	Patients as partners
Dispensable employees	Colleagues caring for each other
Doctors as revenue centers	Physicians as leaders
Quality departments address only requirements	Quality in daily practice, efficiency, and teamwork
↑ Top-line revenue	↓ Unit cost + low-value work

© MAYO
2019

Figure 5.2. Changing the Model: Volume to Value.

The Value Equation

Value is a combination of appropriate care delivered in a patient-centered manner, resulting in the best outcomes at an appropriate price—quality without waste. The value equation is shown in Figure 5.3.

Unfortunately, value is not always created. For example, a coronary artery stent is flawlessly placed in a patient who has a superb experience; however, medical management (e.g., beta blockers, aspirin, statin therapy) was actually the most appropriate (and less expensive) therapy. In this situation, the value would be zero. The procedure was not appropriate. Anyone on the care team who understood the actual lack of value for the patient would have to deal with the attendant cognitive dissonance, which contributes to burnout. For optimal value delivery, a fully engaged workforce is needed—one with burnout rates as low as possible.

VIRTUOUS AND VICIOUS CYCLES

We have proposed that the fundamental culture of esprit de corps is inherently patient centered and inextricably linked with quality, waste reduction, and process

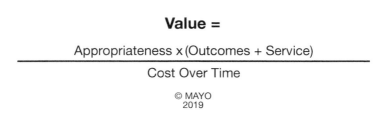

$$\text{Value} = \frac{\text{Appropriateness} \times (\text{Outcomes} + \text{Service})}{\text{Cost Over Time}}$$

© MAYO
2019

Figure 5.3. The Value Equation.

improvement in health care (Figure 5.4). This is a *virtuous cycle* (Figure 5.5) and can be readily explained with five assertions:

1) Quality improvement work enhances esprit de corps and repairs burnout because the work entails fellowship and requires health care professionals to connect to the meaning and purpose of their work.
2) Improved outcomes and safety result in patients having better health and paying less for their medical care.
3) When patients are treated with appropriate care, the system has reduced costs. For example, hypertension can be treated less expensively than can its complications.
4) If patients have a superlative experience and do well, the rate of professional fulfillment increases.
5) When esprit de corps improves and burnout dissipates, substantial soft-dollar and hard-dollar savings are realized from better staff engagement, retention rates, and patient outcomes. Staff teamwork and productivity increase, and work-related stress decreases.

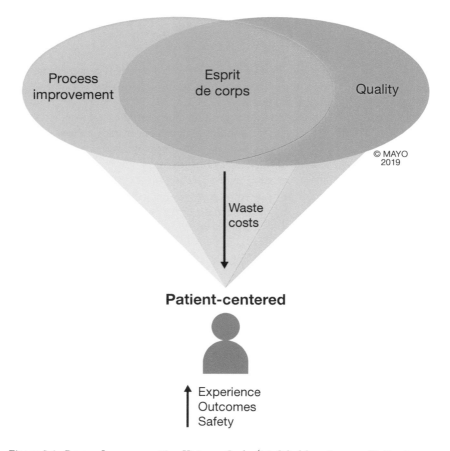

Figure 5.4. Process Improvement in a Virtuous Cycle. (Modified from Swensen SJ. Esprit de corps and quality: making the case for eradicating burnout. J Healthc Manag. 2018 Jan/Feb;63[1]:7-11; used with permission.)

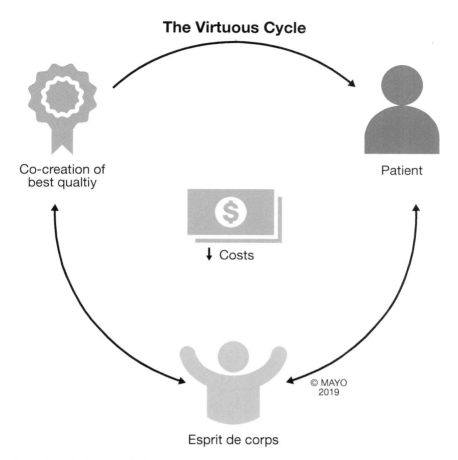

Figure 5.5. The Virtuous Cycle.

In contrast, poor quality care with systems waste creates a *vicious cycle* of cognitive dissonance and professional distress, which impacts patients and organizational costs and increases burnout (Figure 5.6).

Case Study: Intermountain Healthcare

The following example illustrates the benefit of reducing waste and eliminating the quality shortfall for all stakeholders.

Dr. Laurel Fedor is a hospitalist at Intermountain Healthcare in Utah. During their rounds in the intensive care unit (ICU), the entire multidisciplinary team reviews and discusses the care of individual patients. They came to understand that the rounds were terribly inefficient, including for patients. Dr. Fedor led a project to improve the process.

When she started the project, the average ICU rounding time was seven hours and 33 minutes! The structure varied substantially depending on the physician in charge. This inefficiency caused delays in care and also made managing care plans and patient

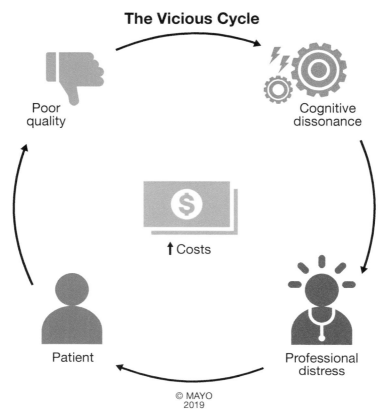

The Vicious Cycle

Poor quality

Cognitive dissonance

↑ Costs

Patient

Professional distress

© MAYO 2019

Figure 5.6. The Vicious Cycle.

and family interactions difficult for the other physicians and nurses. The system also caused profound patient and family frustration, leading to poor experiences. Imagine arriving hours earlier and waiting until 4:00 PM for a physician to make it to your room.

At the end of the improvement project, Dr. Fedor and the team of clinicians had created an elegant, standardized, multidisciplinary ICU rounding process that respected the time and responsibilities of all members of the critical care team. The average time for ICU rounds decreased to one hour and 41 minutes! With fewer interruptions, patient care was safer. The improved workflow greatly influenced the well-being and morale of the entire ICU team and the experiences of patients and families. The proportion of transfer orders written before 11:00 AM increased and length of stay in the ICU decreased. The reduced length of stay resulted in financial dividends for the organization and payers. The cost of care overall declined because of less waste and variation in procedures. Most important, patient experience scores on the unit changed from below average to excellent.

This is a wonderful example of the virtuous cycle. The work to co-create quality clearly had a positive impact on ICU patients and their families. The co-creating process and its result grew camaraderie, trust, and connectedness of the clinicians and managers. Costs were reduced and productivity gains realized.

CONCLUSION

Quality shortfalls from waste in the health care system are a unifying root cause of professional burnout. Organizations should embrace the aligned strategies of quality and esprit de corps on the road to building dynamic health care teams, eradicating burnout, and improving patient care.

SUGGESTED READING

Batalden M, Batalden P, Margolis P, Seid M, Armstrong G, Opipari-Arrigan L, et al. Coproduction of healthcare service. BMJ Qual Saf. 2016 Jul;25(7):509–17.

Berwick DM, Hackbarth AD. Eliminating waste in U.S. health care. JAMA. 2012 Apr 11;307(14):1513–6.

Berwick DM, Nolan TW, Whittington J. The triple aim: care, health, and cost. Health Aff (Millwood). 2008 May-Jun;27(3):759–69.

Bodenheimer T, Sinsky C. From triple to quadruple aim: care of the patient requires care of the provider. Ann Fam Med. 2014 Nov-Dec;12(6):573–6.

Chiappori PA, Levitt S, Groseclose T. Testing mixed-strategy equilibria when players are heterogeneous: the case of penalty kicks in soccer. Am Econ Rev. 2002;92(4):1138–51.

Swensen S, Pugh M, McMullan C, Kabcenell A. High-impact leadership: improve care, improve the health of populations, and reduce costs [Internet]. 2013 [cited 2019 Mar 20]. Available from: http://www.ihi.org/resources/Pages/IHIWhitePapers/HighImpactLeadership.aspx.

Swensen SJ. Esprit de corps and quality: making the case for eradicating burnout. J Healthc Manag. 2018 Jan/Feb;63(1):7–11.

Swensen SJ, Dilling JA, Harper CM Jr, Noseworthy JH. The Mayo Clinic value creation system. Am J Med Qual. 2012 Jan-Feb;27(1):58–65.

Swensen SJ, Dilling JA, McCarty PM, Bolton JW, Harper CM Jr. The business case for health-care quality improvement. J Patient Saf. 2013 Mar;9(1):44–52.

Swensen SJ, Kaplan GS, Meyer GS, Nelson EC, Hunt GC, Pryor DB, et al. Controlling healthcare costs by removing waste: what American doctors can do now. BMJ Qual Saf. 2011;20(6):534–7.

SECTION II

Strategy

6

THE BLUEPRINT FOR CULTIVATING ESPRIT DE CORPS

You have to act as if it were possible to radically transform the world. And you have to do it all the time.
—Angela Davis

THE BLUEPRINT

The Blueprint is an evidence-based framework for cultivating esprit de corps in an organization. It is grounded on a moral imperative and a business case, which is necessary to gain the support of senior leadership. The framework is aligned with the best interests of patients, health care professionals, and mission-driven organizations (Figure 6.1). The strategy within the Blueprint can help organizations create the ideal work environment through the Intervention Triad, which consists of Agency, Coherence, and Camaraderie Action Sets. The Actions Sets promote esprit de corps and use two validated indicators to measure progress. This chapter presents a brief overview of the components of the Blueprint.

IDEAL WORK ELEMENTS

The Blueprint aims to nurture the eight Ideal Work Elements. We believe these elements meet the psychological, social, and emotional needs necessary for health care professionals' well-being and for creating esprit de corps.

The eight Ideal Work Elements are community at work and camaraderie, control and flexibility, fairness and equity, intrinsic motivation and rewards, professional development and mentorship, partnership, safety, and, finally, trust and respect. In Section III ("Execution"), we will describe in detail these prerequisites to attaining esprit de corps and optimal organization performance.

The Losada Ratio

When professional burnout is considered from a systems perspective, the goal is to increase structural (e.g., policies, leader selection, decision-making processes) and functional (e.g., values alignment, leader behaviors, fair and just accountability) sources of positivity and decrease structural and functional sources of negativity in the work environment. This is achieved by cultivating the eight Ideal Work Elements.

Marcial Losada, Ph.D., an organizational psychologist, has studied positivity relative to the performance of teams. Fundamentally, high-performing teams have

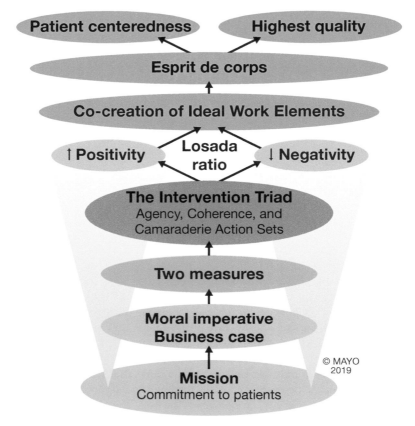

Figure 6.1. Overview of the Blueprint.

more positivity (Losada and Heaphy, 2004). The Losada ratio is the proportion of the positivity in a system (i.e., the number of comments or events that showed support, encouragement, or appreciation) relative to its negativity (i.e., the number of comments or events that showed sarcasm, disapproval, or cynicism). A Losada ratio of three positives for every negative event, comment, or relationship is the minimum ratio necessary for satisfactory team performance. A Losada ratio of approximately 6:1 is highly correlated with superior team performance. For example, decreasing clerical work or making work more efficient increases the Losada ratio by decreasing system negativity. Conversely, cultivating community, celebrating achievement, or telling the story of a gratifying patient outcome increases the Losada ratio by growing system positivity.

From a systems perspective, the Blueprint for creating esprit de corps is designed to increase positivity and decrease negativity in the workplace. How is this achieved? The Intervention Triad provides the formula. The Intervention Triad is specifically designed to mitigate or eliminate the known drivers of professional burnout, nurture supportive leaders, and foster all eight Ideal Work Elements.

THE INTERVENTION TRIAD

The imperative to improve clinician esprit de corps is a shared responsibility. Achieving it requires individuals and leaders across the organization working together to create the ideal work environment so that they can provide the best care for their patients. The Blueprint relies on the Intervention Triad, a proven set of tactics to increase positivity and decrease negativity within teams, work units, and organizations. The action components of the Intervention Triad, described briefly below, will be discussed in detail in Section III ("Execution") of this book.

Agency Action Set

Agency is the capacity of individuals or teams to act independently. The Agency Action Set comprises the following actions:

1) Measuring leader behaviors
   Develop leaders with five esprit de corps–nurturing behaviors.
2) Removing pebbles
   At the work-unit level, eliminate sources of frustration and inefficiency in collaboration with practicing professionals.
3) Introducing control and flexibility
   Design organizational systems and policies for optimal individual flexibility and local control as long as they support the patient-centered mission.
4) Creating a Values Alignment Compact
   Engage in conversations with staff to develop a mutual understanding for the shared responsibility of superlative patient care, professional well-being, and organizational effectiveness.

Coherence Action Set

Coherence is an organizational state in which all the parts fit together comfortably to form a united whole. The Coherence Action Set comprises the following actions:

1) Selecting and developing leaders
   Choose and develop leaders with high levels of emotional intelligence, integrity, and behaviors that will create esprit de corps.
2) Improving practice efficiency
   At the organizational level, reduce clerical burden, optimize workflows, and minimize the negative impact of the electronic environment.
3) Establishing fair and just accountability
   Instill fair and just accountability principles into the work culture (e.g., console professionals involved in adverse patient events caused by systems failure and expected human factor errors).
4) Forming safe havens
   Create a confidential, stigma-free refuge for emotional support of health care professionals experiencing burnout, compassion fatigue, moral injury, cognitive dissonance, and other forms of distress.

Camaraderie Action Set

Camaraderie includes nurturing social capital, mutual respect, and teamwork as well as eliminating internal boundaries to shared ownership of the organization's mission (i.e., *boundarylessness*). The Camaraderie Action Set comprises the following actions:

1) Cultivating community and offering commensality
   Build fellowship.
2) Optimizing rewards, recognition, and appreciation
   Embrace compensation and appreciation systems and practices grounded on intrinsic motivators.
3) Fostering boundarylessness
   Nurture and foster a culture of team-driven, psychologically safe, participative decision making with transparency to engage across all boundaries.

The methods in these Action Sets will enable leaders and organizations to meet the fundamental needs of health care professionals and to help create the Ideal Work Elements. The end result will be an environment of esprit de corps that provides support, cultivates resilience, enhances meaning in work, mitigates professional burnout, and optimizes quality of care.

TWO MEASURES

Accurate metrics allow us to determine whether aspirations are being achieved and where resources and attention need to be allocated to make continued progress. The Blueprint includes metrics for two critical dimensions: leader behaviors and esprit de corps. Optimal leader behaviors and esprit de corps among health care professionals will allow the organization to achieve the Quadruple Aim (i.e., improved patient experience and outcomes at lower cost with superior caregiver well-being).

Rather than a global assessment, the metric we propose for leadership assessment is the Leader Behavior Index. This instrument assesses the specific leader behaviors that cultivate engagement and professional fulfillment in health care professionals. A variety of survey instruments evaluating teamwork, burnout, values alignment, psychological safety, and professional fulfillment are recommended to assess dimensions of esprit de corps. Measurement of leader behaviors and esprit de corps should be assessed at the level of the work unit, the microcosm through which people experience the organization (Figure 6.2). A more detailed discussion of our recommended approach to assessment is provided in Chapter 9 ("Assessment").

SOFT SCIENCE

Finally, getting senior leaders on board is essential for cultivating esprit de corps in an organization (see Chapter 8, "Getting Senior Leadership on Board"). For this to happen, the case made to them must be evidence based and validated. Fortunately, the literature and organizational experience in this area is deep and broad, as you will see.

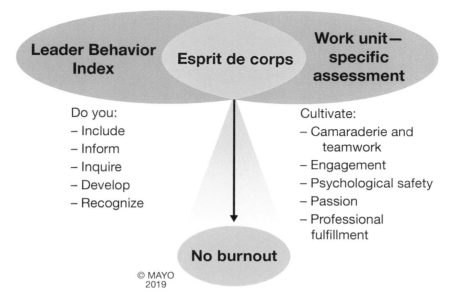

Figure 6.2. Two Measures. The Blueprint includes metrics in two critical dimensions: leadership and esprit de corps.

Between the two of us, we have spent five decades at some of the most elite health care institutions including over four decades at Mayo Clinic. We have separately served in multiple leadership roles, including chief wellness officer, chief quality officer, president of the staff, associate dean, chair of a large clinical department, and director of leadership and organization development. Our clinical and scientific work involved four different scientific approaches to improvement:

1) We ran randomized controlled studies to define the best approaches to treatment.
2) We led single-arm studies and conducted observational clinical research to improve patient care.
3) We used the applied sciences of systems engineering to redesign patient care and improve patient outcomes.
4) We leveraged the teachings of cultural anthropology, psychology, sociology, and organizational science to improve medical care.

Our Blueprint to create esprit de corps uses the best aspects of all four of these approaches.

Not too long ago, one of us made a public presentation regarding this evidence-based, validated approach to eradicating burnout and nurturing esprit de corps. A respected scientist and leader challenged the basis for our proposal. He labeled it soft science. He was coming from the perspective that physics, chemistry, medicine, and biology were hard sciences and therefore had objective results. He believed that the social sciences (e.g., sociology, psychology, anthropology, leadership, behavioral economics) and the applied sciences (e.g., systems and industrial engineering) were soft sciences and therefore less reliable.

His perspective was not only misguided but also inaccurate. The social and applied science disciplines have every bit as robust depth of knowledge to inform action. We have both spent much of our careers working in the hard sciences (i.e., research and treatment of leukemia, lung cancer, and diffuse lung disease) and have published more than 500 peer-reviewed scientific articles in respected scientific journals, as well as several books. We are obligated to ask ourselves the same questions for the social and applied sciences as we would for other areas of translational research:

- Was the science rigorous?
- Was the experimental design sound?
- Was the scientific method used?
- Were variables controlled?
- Did the proposal actually work when translated into real-life, clinical settings?

What we present in the following chapters is based on solid research published in peer-reviewed journals. Many of the studies we draw from are rigorous controlled studies, and several are randomized controlled trials. The approach we present has also been validated in medical organizations in the United States and other countries. The approach works for the many different settings of health care: ambulatory, inpatient, academic medical centers, and community practices. The strategies have proven effective outside of health care as well.

CONCLUSION

In this chapter, we have presented the initial overview of an evidence-based Blueprint to create esprit de corps for an organization. The foundation of the Blueprint is a patient-centered moral imperative in combination with a rational business case for action. The eight Ideal Work Elements are defined and the Intervention Triad proposed for organizations to cultivate these elements. Ultimately, the Ideal Work Elements provide for the fundamental needs of health care professionals, which results in esprit de corps. Metrics in two dimensions are used to assess progress: leader behaviors and esprit de corps. The remainder of this book will provide a detailed roadmap of how to implement this Blueprint.

SUGGESTED READING

Losada M, Heaphy E. The role of positivity and connectivity in the performance of business teams: a nonlinear dynamics model. Am Behav Sci. 2004;47(6):740–65.

Shanafelt TD, Noseworthy JH. Executive leadership and physician well-being: nine organizational strategies to promote engagement and reduce burnout. Mayo Clin Proc. 2017 Jan;92(1):129–46.

Swensen SJ, Shanafelt T. An organizational framework to reduce professional burnout and bring back joy in practice. Jt Comm J Qual Patient Saf. 2017 Jun;43(6):308–13.

7

IDEAL WORK ELEMENTS

In order to carry a positive action we must develop here a positive vision.
—Dalai Lama

If we could design our ideal work situation, what would it be like? *Just imagine.*

For starters, work would feel more like a calling than just a career or a job. Our work would make a difference. It would draw on our deeply held values, beliefs, and talents. It would demand our best but also support us so that we could deliver our best. Decisions would be made with the litmus test of what is best for patients. We would work for an organization that had integrity and that held values similar to our own.

- Our work would be filled with passion, meaning, and purpose.
- We would operate on highly functioning teams and have a sense of *community at work*. There would be *camaraderie*. Some of our best friends would be the fellow health care professionals we work with, and our behavior would demonstrate that we cared about and supported each other.
- Our leaders would recognize the values and purpose that inspire us, our *intrinsic motivation*; know that we thrive on *intrinsic rewards*; and treat us as unique, talented, and dedicated professionals—not dispensable, exchangeable parts in an impersonal health care delivery machine.
- There would be consistency, high ideals, and quality. Where standardization created quality and value for our patients, it would be vigorously pursued. In other areas, we would have *control and flexibility* over our work (with appropriate guidelines), without someone mandating that we adhere to a process that does not benefit patients.
- We would experience a culture of respect, as well as *fairness and equity*, even if our leader was of a different sex, skin color, or creed, or adhered to different politics.
- Our organization would genuinely care for its people and create a culture where health care professionals care for each other and help each other grow through *professional development and mentorship*.
- In authentic *partnership* with leaders, we would labor to accomplish the altruistic mission of a values-driven organization.
- We would have *psychological safety* to share our ideas and feelings. Because we would know that the organization cared about us, we would have *physical safety* as well.
- We would have the *trust and respect* of the organization and its leaders, most of whom would be practicing clinicians partnering with administrators. The administrators would be accountable for driving esprit de corps and quality as much as attending to financial measures such as relative value units, payer mix, and volumes.

Put simply: We would design a work environment where everyone in the organization was treated as a unique, talented, and dedicated professional working in partnership with co-workers to accomplish an aligned and worthy pursuit. *Just imagine the good we could do if we worked in such an environment. Imagine our esprit de corps...*

IDEAL WORK ELEMENTS

In the world of quality health care, processes are designed so the system performs perfectly even though those working within it will not. We recognize that individual error is part of human performance. In the world of esprit de corps, a group of resilient individuals is necessary but not sufficient to create a resilient organization. A resilient organization requires transformational leaders with aligned organizational values, policies, and infrastructure that support the health care professionals working in the institution. Thus, organizational resilience is the result of an optimal system and work environment.

The eight Ideal Work Elements create such a work environment by incorporating the spectrum of social, psychological, emotional, physical, intellectual, and spiritual needs of health care professionals (Figure 7.1). Such a work environment promotes meaning and purpose in work.

Individuals, leaders, and organizations share a mutual interest and responsibility for cultivating these eight elements:

1) Community at work and camaraderie
   Health care professionals will thrive within a supportive work group.
2) Intrinsic motivation and rewards
   Health care professionals are by nature internally motivated and should receive accolades, recognition, and appreciation that acknowledge their character and dedication—not superficial, ephemeral, and extrinsic rewards.

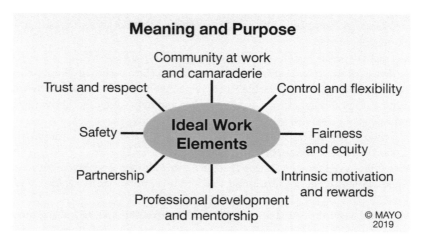

Figure 7.1. The Eight Ideal Work Elements. Organizations that promote the eight elements help health care professionals achieve meaning and purpose in work.

3) Control and flexibility
   Health care professionals need some degree of authority and jurisdiction over how they work, where they work, when they work, and how much they work (to the greatest extent that can be accommodated while advancing the organization's patient-centered mission). Professionals need Agency.

4) Fairness and equity
   Health care professionals need a fair and just culture that acknowledges human limitations and employs a framework of self-valuation and compassionate improvement—not shame and blame. They should be supported when they experience a patient's adverse event (whether the root cause was a systems failure or an anticipated human factor error).

5) Professional development and mentorship
   Health care professionals need to have others take an interest in their careers and feel that someone has their back when challenges arise.

6) Partnership
   Health care professionals should be led with the principles of participative management and embraced as allies and teammates involved in co-creation and continuous improvement of their work environments.

7) Safety
   Health care professionals need to feel psychologically and physically secure at work.

8) Trust and respect
   Health care professionals need to be considered reliable by the leaders of the organization and be included and regarded with dignity by all other team members, regardless of sex, race, discipline, orientation, creed, or tradition.

When these eight Ideal Work Elements are not adequately provided, organizations risk losing one of their most precious resources: engaged, loyal, and dedicated health care professionals. This loss may manifest as turnover, people working part time ("partial quitting"), or people staying full time but disengaging from work and simply collecting a paycheck. Organizations that do not nurture the eight Ideal Work Elements also put professionals at risk for occupational distress (e.g., burnout, posttraumatic stress disorder, depression, moral injury, compassion fatigue), with their patients the ultimate victims.

In contrast, organizations that develop the eight Ideal Work Elements produce meaning and purpose in work, promote engagement and discretionary effort, and cultivate esprit de corps. Such organizations flourish because they have professional staffs who come to work with passion and who do not limit their work to what is in their job description. They do whatever is necessary to support each other and to get the job done.

A JOB, A CAREER, OR A CALLING

Several decades ago, Professor Robert Bellah at the University of California, Berkeley (Bellah et al, 1987), described three relationships that people have with their work. Some see their work as a job, others view it as a career, and still others pursue their work with the passion of a calling. Approximately one-third of workers are in each category.

Job

Those who connect to work as a job see it as a means to an end. It is a paycheck that opens doors for what is really meaningful to them. The reward is extrinsic to their work (e.g., money that allows them to achieve other goals such as buying a new car or putting the kids through college).

Career

For those who relate to their work as a career, the predominant focus is on advancement, titles, recognition, and achievement within their organization.

Calling

Those who view their work as a calling experience work as an end rather than as a means. Their work is their purpose, and it's largely focused on making a difference in an arena that matters to them. They want to make the world a better place. The reward is intrinsic. People who relate to work as a calling still need a paycheck, but they get up in the morning for a different reason. People who engage in work as a calling are seldom absent.

The goal of leaders is to connect or, more often, reconnect professionals with the sense of calling in their work. This is achieved by helping to promote meaning and purpose in work.

Meaning and Purpose

A large Gallup poll conducted in 155 countries asked people what made them happy. Results showed that a top determinant of happiness was meaningful work. In our Blueprint, the eight Ideal Work Elements are the building blocks of meaning and purpose in work. For optimal meaning and purpose, professionals need to work in an organization with values that align with their own (e.g., providing healing and the best possible care to their patients).

Meaning in work is also strongly related to the risk of burnout. In a large study, approximately 500 physicians were asked what aspect of their work was most meaningful to them (Shanafelt et al, 2009). For some, it was teaching medical students. For others, it was doing research or working with patients. No matter what activity was specifically meaningful to respondents, the amount of their work week focused on that activity had a strong, inverse relationship to burnout. In fact, physicians who spent 20% or more of their time in their most meaningful activity had half the burnout rate as those who did not. Remarkably, a threshold effect occurred at approximately 20%. Once physicians spent at least 20% of their time dedicated to the most personally fulfilling professional activity, burnout was maximally reduced (Shanafelt et al, 2009). Although everyone would like to spend 100% of their professional life on the things that they care about most, the critical amount needed is just 20%.

Health care professionals who are connected to the meaning and purpose of their work do not study their job descriptions to make sure they do just enough to get by. They don't watch the clock or stand by the time clock at the end of their shift so that they can disappear when the hands hit the precise end of their official work time. They don't just show up and put in their time. They care for each other, and they care for patients. They care about their meaning and purpose.

Case Study: Call Center

In an elegant controlled study, Grant and colleagues (2007) showed that connection to meaning and purpose in work has very positive results. The researchers studied call-center operators at a public university who solicited scholarship donations for students from people they did not know. The operators did not get paid much, and their requests were frequently rejected by the alumni they contacted. For the study, the researchers arranged for half of the operators to have simple, five-minute interactions with students who had received scholarships. The other operators carried on with business as usual. Among the intervention group, the brief connection with students dramatically increased the operators' productivity. The operators who met with students who had received scholarships spent twice as much time on the telephone and raised three times more money than operators who had not met with students. Meeting the students changed how these operators viewed their work: It connected them to meaning and purpose. They were helping students pursue their dreams. The operators who had not met the students were just making phone calls for money.

CONCLUSION

The evidence clearly indicates that satisfying the human need for meaning and purpose leads to lower burnout rates and greater clinician engagement. Meaningful work is a byproduct of creating the Ideal Work Elements and is fostered when individual and organizational values are aligned. As health care professionals connect to meaning and purpose through their daily work, they are more likely to experience their work as a calling, a means for self-fulfillment, an integral part of their identity, and a cause worthy of discretionary effort and pursuit of excellence. Their work will not be just a job, a paycheck to support other needs and interests, or a career focused on titles, upward mobility, success, or social standing. Their work will be a professional calling that fuels meaning in both their personal and professional lives.

Just imagine.

SUGGESTED READING

Bellah RN, Madsen R, Sullivan WM, Swidler A, Tipton SM. Habits of the heart: individualism and commitment in American life. Berkeley (CA): University of California Press; 1987.

Gallup. Work and workplace [Internet] [cited 2019 Feb 27]. Available from: https://news.gallup.com/poll/1720/work-work-place.aspx.

Grant AM, Campbell EM, Chen G, Cottone K, Lapedis D, Lee K. Impact and the art of motivation maintenance: the effect of contact with beneficiaries on persistence behavior. Organ Behav Hum Decis Process. 2007 May;103(1):53–67.

Reker GT, Peacock EJ, Wong PT. Meaning and purpose in life and well-being: a life-span perspective. J Gerontol. 1987 Jan;42(1):44–9.

Shanafelt T, Goh J, Sinsky C. The business case for investing in physician well-being. JAMA Intern Med. 2017 Dec 1;177(12):1826–32.

Shanafelt TD, West CP, Sloan JA, Novotny PJ, Poland GA, Menaker R, et al. Career fit and burnout among academic faculty. Arch Intern Med. 2009 May 25;169(10):990–5.

Steptoe A, Deaton A, Stone AA. Subjective wellbeing, health, and ageing. Lancet. 2015 Feb 14;385(9968):640–8.

Swensen S, Kabcenell A, Shanafelt T. Physician-organization collaboration reduces physician burnout and promotes engagement: the Mayo Clinic experience. J Healthc Manag. 2016 Mar-Apr;61(2):105–27.

Wrzesniewski A, McCauley C, Rozin P, Schwartz B. Jobs, careers, and callings: people's relations to their work. J Res Pers. 1997;31:21–33.

8

GETTING SENIOR LEADERSHIP ON BOARD

Leadership is a potent combination of strategy and character.
But if you must be without one, be without the strategy.
—General Norman Schwarzkopf

Many improvements in esprit de corps can be realized at the unit level with directed efforts. Most of the Intervention Triad can be successfully deployed in patient care work units by departmental leaders without executive-level support. However, optimizing the organizational environment to promote esprit de corps can't happen without senior leadership prioritizing the issues and dedicating time, attention, and other resources to address them. For meaningful and sustainable results, the commitment by leadership must be authentic. In other words, leaders must embrace this quest because they genuinely care, not just because they believe it is a good business strategy.

THE FOUR MOTIVATIONS FOR LEADERS

In our experience, there are four reasons why senior leaders become committed to the well-being of the health care professionals in their organization (Figure 8.1).

1) Moral/Ethical Case

Many senior leaders sincerely care about the welfare of their people and believe that preserving and promoting their well-being is one of the fundamental reasons their organization exists. We refer to this as the *moral/ethical case.* The leaders recognize

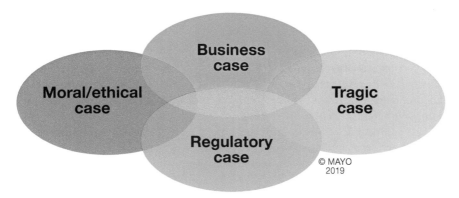

Figure 8.1. Four Reasons Executives Act.

the personal consequences of burnout and accept responsibility for creating a work environment that supports professional fulfillment. They view cultivating esprit de corps as central to a healthy organizational culture and fundamental to its mission.

2) Business Case

A second group of leaders is primarily motivated by the mounting evidence demonstrating the effects of burnout on quality of care, patient satisfaction, and financial performance, which we have described as the *business case* (Chapter 4, "The Business Case"). Such leaders recognize that they must attend to the well-being of professionals because neglecting to do so is a threat to the organization's achieving its mission. They view the welfare of their people as a strategy to achieve the mission rather than as part of the mission.

3) Regulatory Case

The third group of leaders acts because their organization trains medical residents and is therefore governed by the Common Program Requirements of the Accreditation Council for Graduate Medical Education (ACGME), and the ACGME is increasingly placing more attention on the well-being of learners. The Joint Commission and the American Association of Medical Colleges (AAMC) have also heightened their focus on trainee and clinician well-being (AAMC, 2019). Collectively, these forces comprise the *regulatory case.*

These national organizations are focusing on multiple important dimensions including work hours, fatigue management, decreasing the stigma associated with seeking help, and providing resources, education, and support to those experiencing distress. The ACGME imposed these regulations because some organizations were not doing the right things on their own and, according to Tim Brigham, M.D., Ph.D., of the ACGME, "We need to protect the workforce that protects our patients." Many organizations have decided to parlay the ACGME's regulations governing trainees into a more comprehensive approach for all clinical staff (see Chapter 33, "Applying the Action Sets to Address the Unique Needs of Medical Students, Residents, and Fellows").

4) Tragic Case

A fourth group of leaders is motivated to act to improve well-being because something terrible has either happened (e.g., a suicide of someone in the organization) or is likely, they believe, to happen (e.g., a spike in turnover, difficulty recruiting health care professionals). This is the *tragic case.* For these leaders, the risk-avoidance motivation is inherently reactive.

This approach is reminiscent of the early days of the health care safety movement, when a preventable patient injury or death was an all too common tragic motivator for hospital executives or boards to ask:

- How could this happen here?
- How can we prevent it from ever happening again?

Motivating Leaders

Ideally, most organizations should be motivated by the moral-ethical case; however, that is not reality. The best approach is to meet leaders where they are, provide the information and evidence that builds the case that motivates them, and then work toward getting them to believe in the moral/ethical case.

Case Study: Reducing Burnout at Mayo Clinic

John Noseworthy, M.D., is an expert neurologist who cared for patients with multiple sclerosis for decades. He is also the former president and chief executive officer of Mayo Clinic. He cares as deeply about the well-being of his colleagues and staff as he does about his patients. He understands that to achieve Mayo Clinic's primary value, *the needs of the patient come first,* Mayo Clinic must care for its health care professionals.

Dr. Noseworthy identified mitigating professional burnout and promoting professional fulfillment as top priorities for Mayo Clinic on the basis of the moral/ethical case. Of course, he also understood the business case for these goals, but he was authentically motivated to help his colleagues.

In 2015, he prioritized reducing burnout and improving professional fulfillment as one of three metrics on his CEO scorecard with the Board of Trustees, and he took personal responsibility for improving this metric. He was a fully committed executive leader who made a bold statement and move.

Dr. Noseworthy used the existing organizational structure as a tool to drive this change. Specifically, he targeted departments, divisions, and work units performing below external benchmarks for their specialty. His goal was to work with the leaders of those units to have at least 50% improve enough so that, within one year, the unit would no longer be below external benchmarks. He met with the leaders involved and supported the time and resources needed to understand and address the unique department drivers of burnout for which there was a remedy.

He didn't hit this goal.

He surpassed it.

In fact, 80% of the high-risk units were at or above benchmarks within 12 months. He spent the next year working on the remaining 20%. This is an example of a committed executive publicly leading from the front and taking personal responsibility for something that really mattered to him and to the people of his institution.

HEART TO HEAD

In Chapter 4 ("The Business Case"), we presented a compelling business case for organizations to improve the well-being of health care professionals. If senior leadership promotes esprit de corps and quality, the organization will be on course toward solid financial performance. If its people are well, its product and services for patients are high quality, and needless variation, waste, and defects are substantially reduced, the organization is positioned to flourish.

But that data alone is often not enough to convince senior leaders to embrace a strategy not yet widely pursued. Leaders and colleagues must be engaged to face and overcome challenges as part of their motivation to change. One way to motivate leaders is to create stories that evoke emotion. Leaders are humans, and most humans make decisions first with their hearts and then rationalize them with selected, supportive evidence. Thus, for leaders to make the journey from the heart to the head, they need evidence ("no stories without data, no data without stories") (Neylon, 2015).

If you want to change your organization, become a *change agent.* Identify stories that show the ravages of burnout and the effects on patients. Strengthen those anecdotes with evidence about the prevalence of burnout among health care professionals and its impact on quality of care, patient satisfaction, productivity, professional fulfillment, and turnover. Evaluate psychological safety, hostile work environments, camaraderie, leadership behaviors, and esprit de corps for the entire care team. Use or collect evidence from your own institution if possible (see Chapter 9, "Assessment"). If that is not possible, use national data. Present the aspirational state of an engaged team coming to work with purpose and meaning, waking up in the morning to serve, not just trying to collect a paycheck.

CULTURE CHANGE

Ultimately, creating an environment of well-being for health care professionals is about culture change. Professor Edgar Schein, a world authority on organizational culture for the last 50 years, suggested that culture change is usually stimulated and opposed by predictable forces. He refers to the notion that "something bad will happen" if change doesn't occur as *survival anxiety.* Survival anxiety is the catalyst that makes leaders consider making a change; it is the realization that the only way to survive is to evolve. The business case, regulatory case, and tragic case are forms of survival anxiety. The moment survival anxiety is experienced, however, a second force that Schein coined *learning anxiety* becomes manifest. People recognizing the need for change don't necessarily make a change because of fear (What will I give up or lose? Can we change?) or indecision (I don't know what to do.). This can often result in a number of predictable behaviors including denial, minimizing the problem, ignoring evidence, scape goating, or waiting for others to go first.

Amidst these competing forces, Schein posits that the way to tip the scale in favor of change is not to further increase survival anxiety but to decrease learning anxiety. This requires identifying specific areas where change is possible, articulating a compelling vision of a better future state, creating psychological safety for the people who must try things a new way, identifying strategies and tactics to facilitate new ways of working, and providing training and support to those who go first.

Without intentionality and a plan, learning anxiety may increase and create a barrier to transformation. With intentionality and a plan, health care professionals should be able to recognize the need for change, see the path, and link the future vision with the organization's mission (Shanafelt et al, 2019b).

Will, Ideas, and Execution

The Institute for Healthcare Improvement has an elegant approach to creating culture change. The methodology involves three tactics:

1) Garner the *will* to improve (create survival anxiety).
2) Generate *ideas* for change (decrease learning anxiety).
3) *Execute*—get the job done.

Garner the Will to Improve

Successful organizational change requires building will at all levels. Senior leaders must be fully committed to achieve results at the systems level. Change agents and senior leaders need to create urgency for change by making a new way of working attractive and the status quo uncomfortable. Change agents and leaders must repeatedly articulate a clear and compelling vision for a future with highly engaged health care professionals experiencing esprit de corps with the attendant benefits to the organization. The messaging and talking points of leaders articulating the need for change must be clear, authentic, and congruent with the actions initiated.

Generate Ideas for Change

In Section III ("Execution"), we present tangible steps to drive improvement, create the eight Ideal Work Elements, and implement the Intervention Triad. These interventions can be used as a framework that can serve as a starting point to create ideas for change and lessen learning anxiety (i.e., using proven tactics to make progress). Although specific, the actions are best adapted to each organizational culture and norms for optimal impact. The health care professionals at each organization should be involved in adapting, customizing, sequencing, and deploying the action plans. If properly customized and adapted, the approach should feel as if it is a unique plan, not a cookbook recipe.

Get the Job Done

Execution is where many of the best ideas and plans die. Senior leaders must lead visibly and unambiguously from the front. They should appoint an executive-level leader who is accountable and leads a deployment team on their behalf. Execution can be assisted by connecting identified concerns to systematic, organizational-level interventions to drive improvement. Survey results and feedback from focus groups should inform major initiatives, such as driving practice improvement, professional fulfillment, and esprit de corps.

HIGH-IMPACT EXECUTIVE PRACTICES

Five high-impact executive leadership practices can help the organization build will, generate ideas, and enable execution of plans:

1) Person-centeredness: Be consistently focused on the individual in word and deed.
2) Frontline engagement: Be a regular, authentic presence in the forefront and a visible champion of improvement.

3) Relentless focus: Remain centered on the vision and strategy.
4) Transparency: Be candid and honest about aims, results, and progress.
5) Boundarylessness: Encourage and practice comprehensive systems thinking and collaboration across boundaries (Swensen et al, 2013).

Case Study: Patient Safety Leadership WalkRounds

The Institute for Healthcare Improvement Patient Safety Leadership WalkRounds is a tangible example of frontline engagement that exhibits all of the five high-impact senior leadership practices. For WalkRounds, senior leaders visit clinical areas weekly to discuss safety issues and concerns with clinicians, both in groups and individually. They also meet at least weekly with nonphysician health care professionals.

Leadership WalkRounds achieve four desired outcomes:

1) Relationships are built with point-of-care professionals.
2) Patient safety is shown to be a top priority.
3) Awareness of safety and quality issues increases.
4) Information is obtained from staff and acted upon by senior leaders.

WalkRounds are associated with an improved safety climate (Frankel et al, 2008). Safety climate and esprit de corps share common cultural attributes associated with teams (e.g., teamwork, psychological safety, engagement). Achieving these attributes drives progress for both end points. Communication to staff about the actions taken after Leadership WalkRounds, along with closing the feedback loop to the individuals who raised the concerns, substantially lowers feelings of burnout (Sexton et al, 2018; Singer, 2018). WalkRounds have one risk: If leaders ask for input but don't follow up on issues identified and communicated, WalkRounds can increase cynicism and worsen morale (Tucker and Singer, 2014).

Case Study: Leadership Prioritizing Improvement, Atrius Health (Personal Communication, Steve Strongwater, M.D., Chief Executive Officer)

Atrius Health is the largest not-for-profit independent medical group in the Northeast, with 900 physicians in 36 locations treating 740,000 patients. The practice has committed to dramatically improve efficiency in order to create a culture of wellness and personal resilience for their health care professionals.

With a relentless focus to improve employee well-being, they enacted two initiatives. The first was their "returning joy to the practice of medicine" initiative, a pillar of their strategic plan. As a proxy for measuring joy in work, administration used "returning time to clinicians" by reducing clerical and administrative burden. Efforts to improve efficiency of practice were assigned to the executive leaders and departmental chairs. A department of clinical affairs was established to focus on professional development, leadership development, and professional affairs (maintenance of a professional practice standard). Two leading indicator questions were tracked quarterly to measure progress:

1) Would you recommend working here to a peer?
2) Do you feel the amount of time spent interfacing with the electronic health record is appropriate?

The second initiative Atrius developed and deployed was empathy training for over 4,000 physicians and other staff. The training, designed to improve teamwork, included a three-hour program that involved 1) training site-based leaders to co-facilitate empathy forums with an organizational development leader (train the trainer); 2) prework empathy reading materials distributed to participants two weeks before training; 3) a 90-minute, in-person empathy forum for all participants; and 4) postwork guidelines and leadership development opportunities. Health care professionals who participated in the interdisciplinary program bonded with each other and felt they now had an empathy lexicon to use when talking with colleagues and struggling patients. In the months after this relatively brief intervention, patient satisfaction scores improved across the organization.

These two initiatives show how leaders can prioritize professional well-being, with impressive results.

CRITICAL SUCCESS FACTORS

Although senior leadership must be on board to mobilize the necessary resources to implement a plan for organizational change, a large budget is not required. Most of the work involves prioritization along with the time and attention of leaders in partnership with all members of every team. Senior leaders should assess whether the critical success factors are in place before initiating the three Action Sets (Box 8.1).

It is critical to establish the organizational infrastructure and a specific operational leader who will lead the improvement effort. To be successful, this infrastructure must include a formal functional unit devoted to this process (office or program center) rather than an ad hoc wellness committee that is composed of individuals whose primary duties and focus lie elsewhere and that does not have sufficient resources or authority to drive change. Once in place, a formal, functional team can establish goals and targets, determine the metrics to evaluate progress, develop a change management plan, and oversee execution.

Chief Wellness Officer

To drive change at the organizational level, it is paramount to have an officer and an office responsible for leading this effort. Having a chief wellness officer (CWO), or equivalent, as part of the executive team is an excellent strategy. The CWO can help organizations accelerate change. The CWO and their team are responsible for assessing and benchmarking the current health of the organization with respect to well-being and professional fulfillment and for helping to operationalize the organizational

Box 8.1. Critical Success Factors Worksheet

Using the scale below, assess your organization against the critical success factors identified at the senior leader and organizational levels.

Rating Scale: 5, Achieved/Completed; 4, In process; 3, Just starting; 2, Discussing; 1, No action

Rating (1-5)

1. Identify well-being as a key strategic priority
2. Establish an accountability entity (center, program, or office)
3. Appoint operational leadership oversight (chief wellness officer, vice president, associate dean)
   o Engage and empower physician, nurse, and team champions
   o Define roles, responsibilities, resources needed, and timeline
4. Create goals and targets
5. Implement a regular schedule of measurement
   • Measure well-being and esprit de corps
   • Measure Leader Behavior Index
   • Identify and collect data on practice efficiency metrics
     o Leverage organizational engagement/satisfaction survey data or identify other organizational markers for success
     o Create a visible dashboard for the executive team and hospital board of trustees
6. Establish a change management plan
   • Engage and define the senior leader sponsor role
   • Assess health care professional readiness to change
     o Do they have awareness, desire, knowledge, capacity, and capability for this change?
     o Does operational readiness exist—technical, financial, human resources?
     o Does psychological readiness exist—understanding of the barriers for change, including assumptions and beliefs?
   • Create a resistance management plan
7. Develop a communication plan
8. Celebrate and acknowledge progress toward goals

strategy and tactics to drive change (i.e., the Intervention Triad). The CWO should also have a sophisticated understanding of organizational culture and the science of culture change as well as the ability to work in partnership with other leaders and build coalitions to catalyze progress (Kishore et al, 2018; Shanafelt et al, 2019).

The initial task for this officer is to build a coalition of leaders from across the institution to drive the internal wellness journey—just as was done in the quality movement (Chapter 5, "Quality Shortfalls From Health Care Waste: A Unifying Root Cause of Burnout"). The CWO and their team should have a thorough understanding of improvement science and develop expertise in the tactics and processes to promote well-being and esprit de corps for health care professionals. This includes building a robust safety net for individuals who are struggling as well as developing proactive approaches to improve the work environment for all. Organizations will flourish if they engage individual work units and provide the support, expertise, and framework to embed the improvement process at the local point of care.

Case Study: Stanford Medicine and the CWO

In 2017, the Stanford School of Medicine became the first academic medical center to appoint a CWO. Informed by the national data demonstrating the high prevalence of burnout among health care professionals and mounting evidence of its effects on quality of care, Stanford leaders believed it was necessary to have an officer on the executive team coordinating and overseeing the enterprise-wide effort to cultivate well-being for its health care professionals. Longitudinal studies of its own physicians that measured burnout and its relationship to actual turnover showed that the incremental turnover attributable to burnout among Stanford faculty physicians was costing the school of medicine between $15 million and $55 million each year (Hamidi et al, 2018). That estimate did not include other costs associated with burnout: its effects on quality, patient satisfaction, risk of malpractice litigation, and productivity. Lloyd B. Minor, M.D., the dean of the Stanford School of Medicine, took action. In collaboration with the chief executive officers of Stanford Health Care and the Lucille Packard Children's Hospital, Stanford created its WellMD Center and appointed a CWO.

Following Stanford's lead, within 24 months, approximately 20 vanguard health care institutions had appointed a CWO. The presidents of the American Association of Medical Colleges, American College of Graduate Medical Education, and the National Academy of Medicine have now recommended that all medical centers appoint a CWO to their executive team with the "authority, budget, staff, and mandate to implement an ambitious agenda" to improve health care professional well-being (Kishore et al, 2018). In January 2019, the Massachusetts Medical Society released its report "A Crisis in Health Care: A Call to Action on Physician Burnout" and also recommended that all health care organizations appoint a CWO as one of its three foundational recommendations (Jha et al, 2019).

CONCLUSION

Engaged senior leaders are critical to achieving esprit de corps and to changing the world of health care. They set the tone and drive progress. The factors that engage senior leaders and motivate them to improve the well-being of health care professionals tend to aggregate in predictable domains (i.e., moral/ethical case, business case, regulatory case, and tragic case). Once leadership is engaged, assessing the organization's current state and establishing the structure and leadership group that will drive change is necessary for progress.

Although a CWO should be appointed to lead this group, it remains critical for other senior leaders to remain visible and demonstrate their commitment to improve well-being. Successful senior leaders are a regular, authentic presence at the frontline and visible champions of improvement. They are consistently person centered in word and deed, use transparency to catalyze action, and encourage systems thinking and collaboration across boundaries to get results. They relentlessly focus on creating esprit de corps.

SUGGESTED READING

Association of American Medical Colleges. AAMC statement on commitment to clinician well-being and resilience [Internet]. 2019 [cited 2019 Feb 28]. Available from: https://www.aamc.org/download/482732/data/aamc-statement-on-commitment-to-clinicianwell-beingandresilience.pdf.

Coutu D. The anxiety of learning [Internet]. 2002 [cited 2019 Apr 2]. Available from: https://hbr.org/2002/03/the-anxiety-of-learning.

Frankel A, Grillo SP, Pittman M, Thomas EJ, Horowitz L, Page M, et al. Revealing and resolving patient safety defects: the impact of leadership WalkRounds on frontline caregiver assessments of patient safety. Health Serv Res. 2008 Dec;43(6):2050–66.

Hamidi MS, Bohman B, Sandborg C, Smith-Coggins R, de Vries P, Albert MS, et al. Estimating institutional physician turnover attributable to self-reported burnout and associated financial burden: a case study. BMC Health Serv Res. 2018 Nov 27;18(1):851.

Jha AK, Iliff AR, Chaoui AA, Defossez S, Bombaugh MC, Miller YR. A crisis in health care: a call to action on physician burnout [Internet]. 2019 [cited 2019 Feb 28]. Available from: http://www.massmed.org/News-and-Publications/MMS-News-Releases/Physician-Burnout-Report-2018/.

Kishore S, Ripp J, Shanafelt T, Melnyk B, Rogers D, Brigham T, et al. Making the case for the chief wellness officer in America's health systems: a call to action [Internet]. 2018 [cited 2019 Feb 28]. Available from: https://www.healthaffairs.org/do/10.1377/hblog20181025.308059/full/.

Neylon, C. No evidence without stories, no stories without evidence [Internet]. 2015 [cited 2019 Jul 2]. Available from: https://www.slideshare.net/CameronNeylon/no-stories-without-evidence-no-evidence-without-stories.

Nolan TW. Execution of strategic improvement initiatives to produce system-level results. IHI white papers. Cambridge (MA): Institute for Healthcare Improvement; 2007.

Sexton JB, Adair KC, Leonard MW, Frankel TC, Proulx J, Watson SR, et al. Providing feedback following Leadership WalkRounds is associated with better patient safety culture, higher employee engagement and lower burnout. BMJ Qual Saf. 2018 Apr;27(4):261–70.

Shanafelt T, Swensen S. Leadership and physician burnout: using the annual review to reduce burnout and promote engagement. Am J Med Qual. 2017 Sep/Oct;32(5):563–5.

Shanafelt T, Trockel M, Ripp J, Murphy ML, Sandborg C, Bohman B. Building a program on well-being: key design considerations to meet the unique needs of each organization. Acad Med. 2019a Feb;94(2):156–61.

Shanafelt TD, Gorringe G, Menaker R, Storz KA, Reeves D, Buskirk SJ, et al. Impact of organizational leadership on physician burnout and satisfaction. Mayo Clin Proc. 2015 Apr;90(4):432–40.

Shanafelt TD, Schein E, Trockel M, Schein P, Minor L, Kirch D. Healing the professional culture of medicine. Mayo Clin Proc. 2019b Aug;94(8):1556–66.

Singer SJ. Successfully implementing Safety WalkRounds: secret sauce more than a magic bullet. BMJ Qual Saf. 2018 Apr;27(4):251–3.

Swensen S, Pugh M, McMullan C, Kabcenell A. High-impact leadership: improve care, improve the health of populations, and reduce costs. IHI white paper. Cambridge (MA): Institute for Healthcare Improvement; 2013.

Thomas EJ, Sexton JB, Neilands TB, Frankel A, Helmreich RL. The effect of executive walk rounds on nurse safety climate attitudes: a randomized trial of clinical units[ISRCTN85147255]. BMC Health Serv Res. 2005 Apr 11;5(1):28.

Tucker AL, Singer SJ. The effectiveness of management-by-walking-around: a randomized field study. Prod Oper Manag. 2015 Feb;24(2):253–71.

9

ASSESSMENT

Every line is the perfect length if you don't measure it.
—Marty Rubin

SOCIAL CAPITAL

The most important determinant of value in a health care organization is an intangible asset called *social capital*. Social capital comprises the talent, knowledge, goodwill, trust, skill, and interconnectedness of people. Social capital is a critical characteristic of organizations and the ingredient that allows people to work together for a common purpose. In health care, social capital produces what we need to best serve patients: diffusion of ideas, teamwork, learning, ability to change, and discretionary effort. Esprit de corps is predicated on a high degree of social capital.

Measuring Social Capital

How well an organization performs on the *pronoun test* (discussed in more detail in Chapter 12, "Agency Ideal Work Element: Partnership") is a qualitative measure of social capital. Organizations whose staff use the pronouns "we" and "us" are more likely to have a culture of cooperation and collaboration (i.e., one of high social capital). More than qualitative measures are needed, however, to obtain meaningful data about the social capital and esprit de corps in health care organizations. So we need to survey!

THE SURVEY PROCESS

Why Measure?

Organizations need objective data to understand the experience and well-being of their health care professionals. A baseline measurement is necessary to assess the current state and to evaluate progress toward an ideal future state.

One of the most prevalent mistakes by health care administrators is to assume that a baseline assessment of their organizations is unnecessary because national benchmarks are available. In our work with organizations, we typically hear, "Why do we need to conduct a baseline survey? We already know from national studies that burnout rates among health care professionals are high. We are ready to act." Although well intentioned, this mindset neglects three important principles:

1) The local experience may not match the national experience.
2) The attention, energy, and financial capital to address burnout (or any issue) are finite resources and cannot be optimally deployed in a targeted manner that maximizes impact without organization-specific information.
3) Metrics are necessary to evaluate the effectiveness of interventions intended to drive improvement.

We have worked with large medical centers in which one of the specialty disciplines at highest risk of burnout in national studies had the most favorable burnout scores of all the specialties at that organization. We have also consulted with organizations where the specialty disciplines at lowest risk for burnout nationally had the highest rates of burnout. The notion that we can jump to action without assessment would be the equivalent of using national averages for relative value unit (RVU) generation, payer mix, and net operating income to guide the financial actions of an organization.

What Is the Best Approach?

Health care professionals are overwhelmed with surveys and requests for information. Therefore, organizations must develop a comprehensive and coordinated approach to collect feedback that is efficient, not redundant, and minimizes *survey fatigue*. Most organizations assess quality, safety, and measures of engagement annually. Measures of burnout, leadership, and esprit de corps can easily be incorporated into the same instrument.

To achieve the best outcomes, a robust communication plan and survey execution process must be used, which involves:

1) Having experts design the survey process, including the instrument to be used, content included, and benchmarks.
2) Choosing only questions that leadership is fully committed to managing.
3) Clearly communicating the purpose of the survey and how data will be used to help the organization and the health care professionals being surveyed.
4) Administering the survey.
5) Communicating results to all health care professionals transparently (at the work-unit level by the unit leader).
6) Strategizing how results will be used at both the executive and work-unit levels.
7) Using the data collected to co-generate ideas and solutions for improvement at the work-unit level.
8) Co-creating action plans at the work-unit level in parallel with organization-wide action plans for improvement in appropriate domains.
9) Approving action plans at the reporting level.
10) Executing work-unit plans with the support of administration.
11) Reassessing annually to evaluate progress.

In addition to survey data, objective operational efficiency of practice measures should be made available to relevant leaders. These include leading performance indicators from the electronic health record (e.g., "work after work," "click counts" for common workflow tasks, ratio of staff-entered to physician-entered data and orders) (DiAngi et al, 2017). These objective measures of the efficiency of the practice environment (i.e., important burnout drivers) can serve as improvement targets and often provide continuous real-time data on progress without burdening staff with repeated surveys.

What Dimensions Should Be Assessed?

Leaders should measure what matters most to their organizations, which must include what matters to their health care professionals. They should also only measure what they are committed to improving, nothing more and nothing less.

What leaders choose to measure and focus on sends a message to their employees. For example, when leaders focus primarily on financial dimensions (e.g., RVUs, net operating income, payer mix, patient volumes), it should be no surprise that professionals observe that behavior, interpret it as what leaders and the organization value and, enthusiastically or begrudgingly, act accordingly. If, however, esprit de corps, teamwork, professional fulfillment, and participative management behaviors are measured, health care professionals are more likely to develop and embody these behaviors.

An organization committed to achieving esprit de corps should measure the Ideal Work Elements they are committed to improving, as well as the following: leadership behavior; teamwork and team dynamics; professional fulfillment, burnout, and personal well-being; psychological safety; and alignment with the mission of the organization. Without these measurements, it is impossible to know if health care professionals are in a community rich in support and social capital, and with the necessary resources to achieve their goals.

Whom to Survey

We believe that surveys should include everyone in the organization: those caring directly for patients and those whose jobs support those caring for patients. All health care professionals and employees should be invited to share their perceptions of the organization, work unit, unit leader, and their own well-being. If cost is a barrier to initial implementation of an organization-wide survey, focusing on frontline care providers (i.e., physicians, advanced practice providers [APPs], and nurses) is a reasonable place to start.

How to Survey

All health care professionals must understand that the survey is absolutely confidential and that the survey is grounded in a deep-seated interest of leadership to improve the work life of staff and the health of the organization.

A robust electronic survey tool that can disseminate a web link to a secure site via email is the most efficient approach to conduct the survey. We favor independent survey administration by external vendors to create psychological safety and preserve employee anonymity. Reports at all levels of the organization are important and provide complementary information that can help guide action throughout the organization, as well as for each type of health care professional (e.g., physician, APP, nurse, pharmacist).

How Often to Measure

Representatives of professional survey organizations that consult for large institutions in the United States have shared with us that approximately 75% to 80% of organizations survey their employees annually, 15% to 20% survey more frequently than once a year, and 5% to 10% survey every two years. We believe annual measurement is a good place to start. The expectation should be set that all health care professionals will be formally asked for their ideas and perceptions at least annually and that the organization will commit to working with work-unit leaders and teams to address issues that are raised.

An annual frequency is the survey sweet spot for most organizations—as long as plans are acted upon continuously throughout the year. In one large organization with more than 60,000 health care workers, we experimented with adding pulse surveys to a representative subset of the organization every three months to supplement annual surveys. This approach required substantial energy and investment, and we found little change from quarter to quarter. In addition, the quarterly results at the organization level were not actionable. However, pulse surveys can be helpful in a targeted manner for units implementing interventions that require frequent assessment (e.g., implementation of an electronic health record).

How to Share Results

Once available, survey results should be shared with all staff as soon as possible. This should happen within several weeks of the survey closure date. Senior leaders should share high-level results with the organization as a whole. Work-unit leaders should share their local results with all professionals on their teams.

In contrast to the group-level findings (i.e., teamwork and team dynamics; professional fulfillment, burnout, and personal well-being; psychological safety; and engagement with the mission of the organization), Leader Behavior Index scores, which are a person-level result, should not be discussed publicaly (See Chapter 15, "Agency Action: Measuring Leader Behaviors" for a description of the Leader Behavior Index). Leader Behavior Index score results should be provided as feedback in a confidential manner by supervisors, with a comparison to anonymous Leader Behavior Index data from across the organization for the scored categories.

All data should ideally be benchmarked with national health care and internal work-unit results.

Unit Readiness for Action

Before sharing data with a work unit, senior leaders should assess the ability of unit leadership to communicate the survey results in an appropriate manner. If unit leaders cannot communicate the results effectively, their supervisors should step in or provide training and resources to assist them (e.g., a standard presentation slide deck or report).

The work unit also needs to be ready to embrace the opportunities identified by survey findings. Readiness of the leader as well as readiness of the unit team members must be assessed. Appropriate dialogue and communication before survey administration can help increase readiness. In some cases, the leadership team may need to address an ongoing issue before they can effectively deal with survey results. When this is the case, the issue should, ideally, be dealt with during the several-month interval between survey launch and the time results are received.

THREE ACTION SESSIONS

Once survey results are available, leaders should plan three separate sessions for sharing survey results, identifying and prioritizing opportunities, and developing an action plan. During these sessions, some individuals may not feel comfortable raising certain topics in public. Other individuals may not feel comfortable speaking at all. Often, people share additional ideas after a meeting when they have had time to process what was discussed. Therefore, other options for giving feedback should be offered (e.g., group, one-on-one, email follow-up).

Session One: Sharing Survey Results

The focus of the first session is to transparently share and confirm the accuracy of the survey results. The results are about feelings and perceptions, and the process should be participatory.

Actions for Leaders to Use in Sharing Results

1) Begin by thanking everyone for participating in the survey. Overtly state that this is the first of three sessions to act on the results. Communicate that sharing the results is just the start of a dialogue and that the work group will begin to devise an action plan to improve over the following sessions. Sharing this information will allow you to redirect the group if people try to identify opportunities or solutions in the first session.
2) Acknowledge, appreciate, and affirm the positive results. Express appreciation for honest feedback about areas that need to improve, and never imply that you know any individual's response to items on the survey.
3) Ask for perspective on whether the results accurately reflect the health care professionals' experiences.
4) Remember to listen. The health care professionals should do most of the talking. Use reflective listening to ensure that you hear correctly.
5) Keep the meeting constructive.
6) Take special care regarding sensitive issues.
7) Be willing to say you don't know or don't have all the answers but are committed to working with the group to find the answers.

Session Two: Identifying and Prioritizing Opportunities

We recommend beginning this session by introducing the six key drivers of burnout and professional fulfillment (i.e., workload and job demands, efficiency and resources, control and flexibility, organizational culture and values, social support and community at work, and work-life integration) (Shanafelt and Noseworthy, 2017) as a framework for root-cause analysis (Swensen et al, 2009) and improvement planning.

It is also helpful to introduce the concepts of the sphere of control, sphere of influence, and sphere of concern (Covey, 1992) (Figure 9.1). In the sphere of control are opportunities for improvement that can be addressed without permission or support of others (e.g., unit workflow, team communication). These opportunities should be addressed as they are prioritized, based on impact and feasibility. In the sphere of influence are opportunities for improvement that require collaboration, conversations, and partnership (e.g., interdepartmental hand offs, service-line protocols spanning department boundaries). A coalition can be built with other interested parties who have shared influence to move forward on these opportunities. In the sphere of concern are opportunities for improvement that are of interest to

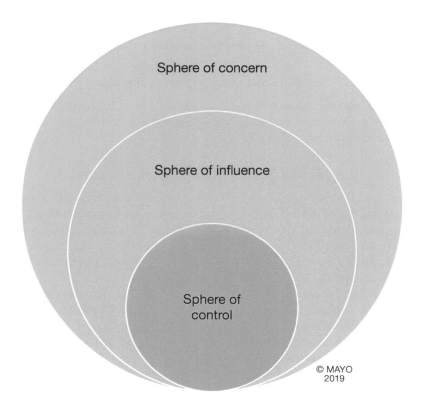

Figure 9.1. Spheres of Influence. Focusing on factors that can be controlled will yield the greatest benefit for improving the well-being of health care professionals.
(Modified from Covey SR. The 7 habits of highly effective people. London: Simon & Schuster; 1992; used with permission.)

individuals and teams but that can't be directly remediated (e.g., decisions about the electronic health record, organization part-time policies).

State that the focus of this session is to identify what is under the sphere of control of the work unit that can be acted on most rapidly (next three to four months). Acknowledge that there are also at least six contexts that influence these dimensions and improvement planning (i.e., factors external to the organization, organization-level factors, work-unit factors, the unit leader, team factors, and individual factors).

Actions for Leaders to Use in Identifying and Prioritizing Opportunities

1) Overtly state that the purpose of this session is to identify the greatest opportunities for improvement under the control of the work unit. Remind the group that the third session will focus on developing solutions to take advantage of the opportunities identified in the second session.

2) Introduce the six driver dimensions. Ask the group to identify the one or two dimensions of greatest challenge to their work unit and get consensus. The nominal group process is one technique you can use for gaining group consensus (Box 9.1).

3) Introduce the concept of the sphere of control, sphere of influence, and sphere of concern once there is consensus. Ask participants to identify key factors in the sphere of control and sphere of influence of the work unit that are the root causes contributing to the one or two driver dimensions identified as the greatest challenges in step two.

4) Engage staff in discussion. Seek to understand the factors contributing to the challenge without drifting too deeply into possible solutions (reserved for session three).

Box 9.1. Nominal Group Technique

The nominal group technique is a participative management process for problem identification and solution generation.

1) Create six posters, one for each of the driver dimensions, and post them on the walls of the meeting room.

2) Write the description of the driver dimension at the top of each poster: workload and job demands, efficiency and resources, control and flexibility, organizational culture and values, social support and community at work, and work-life integration.

3) Distribute a sheet of five sticky dots to each team member and have them place the sticky dots on the posters to identify the ideas they would prioritize for the first round of action. Allow them to place a maximum of three dots on the dimension most important to them.

4) Use the posters with the largest number of dots as the focus for discussion.

5) For the remainder of the session, write discussion notes on the poster regarding the factors contributing to the challenge in that driver dimension.

This process of participative management engages the whole team as partners.

5) Commit to communicating the ideas outside of the sphere of influence to the next level of leadership.

6) Share and gain clinician support for key priorities under local control for improvement.

Session Three: Developing an Action Plan

Action plans must be generated and executed through participative management with collaborative planning. This is often best accomplished by launching a task force with a leader appointed by unit leadership to focus on areas for improvement. The focus areas should be overtly specified when the task force is launched and should be determined on the basis of the areas prioritized in session two. All members of the unit who are interested in developing potential interventions to drive improvement in the focus area should be invited to join the task force.

Actions for Leaders to Use in Developing an Action Plan

1) Engage the team in co-creating solutions.

2) Follow through on action plans and communicating progress.

3) Serve as a role model to others in embracing change, and reinforce positive impacts you see occurring.

4) Discuss and determine which factors are and are not within the control of the group or within their sphere of influence.

5) Emphasize that those factors not in the group's sphere of influence will be logged and communicated to the appropriate senior leader or team but that the focus of the task force is to develop interventions under the work unit's sphere of control to bring about improvement (even if only incremental) over the next three to four months.

6) Finalize the action plan draft.

7) Take the action plan draft to senior leaders for their input and revisions.

8) Implement action plans:
   - Assign responsibility for action plans/action plan steps.
   - Determine and address any quick wins.
   - Establish milestones and timelines for each goal.
   - Develop a new way of working and pilot test in a limited way (e.g., one clinic, section, ward, hospital) or for a defined period of time before evaluating impact, refining, and scaling.
   - Report progress on an ongoing basis to senior leaders.

9) Use the next annual resurvey (or a pulse survey, if indicated) to evaluate progress and identify new ways to enhance satisfaction, engagement, and partnership.

Actions to Avoid

In all three sessions, avoid the following actions:

1) Reacting defensively to questions and comments

2) Allowing one individual to dominate the conversation

3) Accepting any one individual's comments as the sentiment of the group too quickly. Confirm with the entire team.

4) Spending too much time on any one issue
5) Promising too much, too soon
6) Suggesting that you or the leadership team already have the solution or action plan

CONCLUSION

Leaders should measure and manage what matters to their employees and to their organizations. Time, attention, and resources cannot be optimally deployed to decrease burnout and engender esprit de corps without gathering organization-specific data regarding elements of their social capital including leadership behavior, teamwork and team dynamics, professional fulfillment and personal well-being, psychological safety, and engagement with the mission of the organization. Attention to the appropriate steps of survey design and execution, communication of results, co-creation of action plans, and longitudinal measurement are keys to harnessing the power of assessment to drive organizational progress (Box 9.2).

Box 9.2. The Playbook

- Commit to an annual staff survey with timely and transparent sharing of results with all staff.
- Include only topics that senior leadership is fully committed to improving.
- Include professional fulfillment, burnout, leader behaviors, psychological safety, engagement, and teamwork in assessments.
- Provide confidential or anonymous surveys at the individual level.
- Use validated instruments with external benchmarks to provide context to the extent possible.
- Engage health care professionals in selecting the targets for improvement.
- Provide opportunities for health care professionals to participate in designing potential solutions.
- Provide sufficient time and attention from organizational leaders to support unit and leader improvement, which is critical for success.

SUGGESTED READING

Barrington L, Silvert H. CEO challenge: the conference board. New York (NY): Brookings Institute; 2004.

Covey SR. The 7 habits of highly effective people. London: Simon & Schuster; 1992.

DiAngi YT, Lee TC, Sinsky CA, Bohman BD, Sharp CD. Novel metrics for improving professional fulfillment. Ann Intern Med. 2017 Nov 21;167(10):740–1.

Shanafelt TD, Noseworthy JH. Executive leadership and physician well-being: nine organizational strategies to promote engagement and reduce burnout. Mayo Clin Proc. 2017 Jan;92(1):129–46.

Swensen SJ, Dilling JA, Milliner DS, Zimmerman RS, Maples WJ, Lindsay ME, et al. Quality: the Mayo Clinic approach. Am J Med Qual. 2009 Sep-Oct;24(5):428–40.

SECTION III

Execution

10

THE THREE ACTION SETS OF THE INTERVENTION TRIAD: EVIDENCE-BASED STRATEGIES FOR REDUCING BURNOUT AND PROMOTING ESPRIT DE CORPS

I'm always doing that which I cannot do,
in order that I may learn how to do it.
—Pablo Picasso

THREE ACTION SETS

In the next three sections, we present the substance of this book: a new model composed of the Action Sets of the Intervention Triad (Agency, Coherence, and Camaraderie)—specific tactics for executing the strategies for reducing burnout and promoting esprit de corps. The model is evidence based and has been proven to work.

Each of the specific tactics in the Action Sets accomplishes one or more of the following three objectives:

1) Mitigates the drivers of burnout to decrease negativity.
2) Cultivates leadership behaviors and processes that increase positivity.
3) Strengthens individual and team resilience to increase tolerance of negativity.

By using the three Action Sets, leaders can create systems and nurture behaviors that promote the eight Ideal Work Elements, address the drivers of burnout, and build esprit de corps (Figure 10.1). Collectively, the Action Sets are designed to foster all of the Ideal Work Elements. For example, successfully accomplishing the Agency Action Set positively influences three of the Ideal Work Elements (i.e., trust and respect, control and flexibility, and partnership) (Figure 10.2).

SHARED RESPONSIBILITY FOR THE ACTION SETS

Addressing burnout and promoting esprit de corps are a shared responsibility. The actions are focused on what individuals, work-unit leaders, and organizational leaders can refine within their spheres of influence. For example, in order to optimize efficiency and resources:

- Individuals must learn how to use the electronic health record efficiently and collaborate with and empower other members of the care team to work to the scope of their licensure.

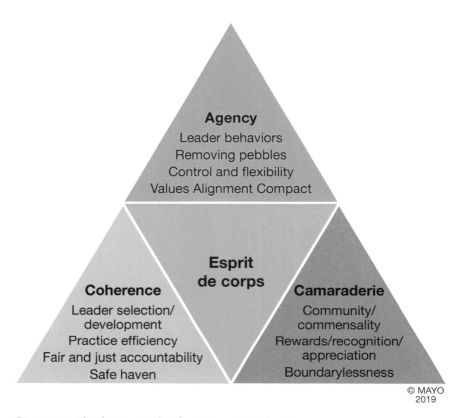

Figure 10.1. The Three Action Sets for Creating Esprit de Corps.

- Work-unit leaders must co-create and implement optimal workflows for patients and professionals in each practice environment (e.g., triage, scheduling, rooming, team-based care, order entry, follow-up care).
- Organizational leaders must support appropriate staffing, identify the best care-team professional to perform each task, foster teamwork, develop leaders and hold them accountable, and avoid misinterpreting regulations in a manner that needlessly increases clerical burden for the care team.

Only by co-creating in partnership is it possible to optimize esprit de corps. Collaborative engagement between medical and administrative staff is a prerequisite for effective improvement work and consistently delivering the best outcomes. The evidence-based Action Sets work to improve the well-being of patients by fostering the well-being of health care professionals. In a virtuous cycle, improved patient outcomes and experience, in turn, increase the professional satisfaction of health care professionals on the care delivery team. Efforts to promote esprit de corps advance quality of care and the suitable use of institutional assets.

How to achieve these organizational attributes will be presented in detail in the following chapters. Health care organizations should use this framework to organize and implement their institutional approach to promoting provider well-being, including for trainees.

Action Sets of the Intervention Triad	Community at Work and Camaraderie	Intrinsic Motivation and Rewards	Control and Flexibility	Fairness and Equity	Professional Development and Mentorship	Partnership	Safety	Trust and Respect
Agency			★			★		★
Measuring leader behaviors					X	X		X
Removing pebbles	X		X			X		X
Introducing control and flexibility		X	X			X		X
Creating a Values Alignment Compact		X		X		X		X
Coherence				★	★		★	
Selecting and developing leaders			X	X				X
Improving practice efficiency			X		X			X
Establishing fair and just accountability		X					X	X
Forming safe havens				X			X	
Camaraderie	★	★						
Cultivating community and commensality	X	X				X		
Optimizing rewards, recognition, and appreciation		X		X				X
Fostering boundary-lessness	X		X			X	X	

© MAYO 2019

★ Primary objective of the Action Set

X Ideal Work Element impacted by the action

Figure 10.2. Association of Ideal Work Elements and Action Sets.

CONCLUSION

Experience and research show that the evidence-based Action Sets of the Intervention Triad (Agency, Coherence, and Camaraderie) are an effective means to reduce burnout and cultivate professional fulfillment. They transform individual behavior and organizational culture to provide the Ideal Work Elements and mitigate the drivers of burnout. In doing so, they create esprit de corps. The Elements and Action Sets are described in the remainder of this section.

SUGGESTED READING

Fowler JH, Christakis NA. Dynamic spread of happiness in a large social network: longitudinal analysis over 20 years in the Framingham Heart Study. BMJ. 2008 Dec 4;337:a2338.

11

AGENCY ACTION SET: INTRODUCTION

Never tell people how to do things.
Tell them what to do and they will surprise you with their ingenuity.
—General George Patton

Agency is the capacity of individuals or teams to act independently.

For professionals to flourish and patients to receive the best care, attention to organizational culture and a balance between independence and standardization in work must be achieved. The Agency Action Set has been designed to mitigate or eliminate specific drivers of professional burnout and to develop leaders and systems that foster the related Ideal Work Elements.

Primary burnout drivers addressed by Agency Actions:

1) Lack of control and flexibility
2) Problems with organizational culture and values

Ideal Work Elements cultivated by Agency Actions:

1) Partnership (Chapter 12)
2) Trust and respect (Chapter 13)
3) Control and flexibility (Chapter 14)

Agency Actions:

1) Measuring leader behaviors (Chapter 15)
2) Removing pebbles (Chapter 16)
3) Introducing control and flexibility (Chapter 17)
4) Creating a Values Alignment Compact (Chapter 18)

In this section, we discuss the three germane Ideal Work Elements followed directly by the four aligned Agency Actions.

12

AGENCY IDEAL WORK ELEMENT: PARTNERSHIP

Individual commitment to a group effort . . . that is what makes a team work, a company work, a society work, a civilization work.
—Vince Lombardi

Partnerships are an inherent attribute of esprit de corps, and partnership is one of the three Ideal Work Elements fostered by Agency Actions. Partners have a shared vision, invest discretionary effort, and look to accomplish a vision together. Health care professionals should be treated as partners, never as employees (Schein, 2013).

There are different types of partnerships. For example, horizontal partnerships occur on the same level of a process (e.g., a multidisciplinary team of health care professionals in the emergency department treating a trauma victim). Vertical integration partnerships involve distinct, sequentially related processes linked to the same final service (e.g., the relationship of affiliated physicians with the organization where they have privileges).

When there is maximal trust and connectedness in horizontal and vertical organizational partnerships, social capital is optimized, and the organization is poised to deliver on its mission and vision.

THE PRONOUN TEST AND SOCIAL CAPITAL

Robert Reich, the former U.S. Secretary of Labor, uses a simple method for assessing the health of an organization. When he visits companies and talks with employees, he listens carefully for the pronouns people use. Do they refer to their organization and its leaders as *we/us* or *they/them* and *I*? Healthier organizations have employees who use first-person plural.

The pronoun test is easy to apply to health care organizations. If you hear more of *they/them* or *I*, it's likely that there is some degree of disengagement and distancing between leaders and practicing professionals, whereas more of *we/us* suggests the opposite: an ideal culture where health care professionals feel they are a valued part of something special, meaningful, and larger than self or discipline (Figure 12.1). The use of first-person plural pronouns signals a spirit of cooperation with higher levels of trust and interconnectedness (i.e., social capital). Without social capital, there will be more competition and mistrust within the organization, neither of which are in the best interests of health care professionals or the patients they serve (Bezrukova et al, 2012).

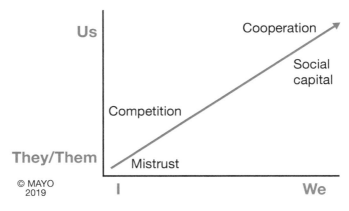

Figure 12.1. The Pronoun Test. Organizations with employees that use first-person plural (we/us) are less competitive and more cooperative. They have high social capital.

ORGANIZATIONAL PARTNERSHIP IN HEALTH CARE ORGANIZATIONS

How organizations are designed determines the level of partnership fostered. The following two analogies explain the different partnership models in health care organizations.

The Farmers Market

Many hospitals take a noncollaborative farmers market approach to partnering with their physicians. The farmers market offers a location for independent merchants to sell their products for the mutual benefit of the market and the farmers—but the arrangement is not aligned toward any type of shared mission (e.g., helping customers eat healthier). The organizer of the market has little control over those who sell products or the quality of those products. The organizer often just wants as many merchants as possible to gain the largest share of the market and fill all the stalls (Figure 12.2).

Like a vendor in a farmers market, physicians in open-staff hospitals are affiliated but have independent practices. This arrangement has some benefits for hospitals because, for example, their overhead may be lower (i.e., no physician salaries) and advantageous for physicians because they have more independence and often have more income from owning their practice. But this relationship does not optimize and coordinate the best care and results for patients and, ultimately, is not in the best interest of the organization or the well-being of the organization's health care professionals.

With the farmers market model, it is difficult to build high-trust multidisciplinary teams and to standardize care processes for safety and efficiency. The culture is by design not one of collaboration, cooperation, and consistency (Swensen et al, 2010). The farmers market model treats physicians as revenue centers, not partners, and the physicians most commonly use the words *they* and *them*, not *we* and *us*.

Physicians' actions and behaviors under this approach are not necessarily aligned with the mission, strategy, and vision of the organization with whom they

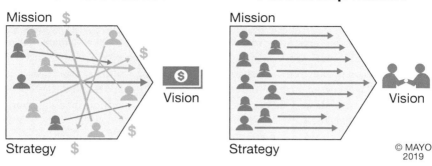

Figure 12.2. Farmers Market Model vs. Partnership Market Model. (Data from Swensen, et al. Cottage industry to postindustrial care: the revolution in health care delivery. N Engl J Med. 2010 Feb 4;362[5]:e12.)

are affiliated. Rather, physician-hospital relationships are based on volume, with dedicated but independent practitioners focused on personal needs and preferences, not necessarily a patient's best interest. Independent practitioners often shun standardization, which, for the most part, yields the most reliable, high-quality care. In the farmers market model, hospital culture is often one of competition rather than coordinated care.

Partnership Market

Medical centers may be designed as partnership markets instead of farmers markets. In a partnership market arrangement, the culture is intentionally one of collaboration and cooperation. There is standard work instead of "market-driven" variation. Partnership market cultures have high levels of social capital because they function with higher levels of trust and interconnectedness. When physicians in the partnership market culture talk about the organization, they most commonly use the words *we* and *us*, not *they* and *them*.

In a partnership market culture, physicians are hired, selected, and developed so that their behaviors and actions are aligned with the mission strategy and vision of the organization. Physicians are more likely to feel as though they are an important part of the organization, and they are dedicated and work together to promote the organization's mission, which is in contrast to the farmers market with its independent, competitive practitioners.

To thrive, health care professionals need to feel a sense of *ownership* of the mission, vision, and values of the organization. They should view their relationship as a partnership, with the express goal of achieving the shared mission (Atkinson et al, 2011). We believe an organizational partnership structure is the most patient centered and addresses the well-being of health care professionals. A true partnership between professionals and leadership is a primary mitigating strategy for professional burnout. In a true *we/us* partnership, health care professionals have choices and *own* the organizational mission and values.

BURNOUT AND THE FARMERS MARKET MODEL

Hospitals organized like noncollaborative farmers markets are systems designed to fuel burnout. They are characterized by greater social isolation, less integration, and higher variation—resulting in poorer quality and safety. In a farmers market model, clinicians must work harder to increase productivity. Compensation is strictly based on production—a situation that burns out health care professionals. Physicians experiencing burnout order more tests and procedures, and they spend less time with patients and colleagues. There is more competition than collaboration (Swensen et al, 2010).

In contrast, professionals in an integrated system (i.e., the partnership market model) partner with the organization and its leaders to improve productivity by streamlining systems and driving out needless variation and defective processes (D'Innocenzo et al, 2014).

CONCLUSION

Partnership is an important element of the ideal work environment for health care professionals. Organizational design that promotes partnership should be embedded into the infrastructure and culture of any health care organization. The noncollaborative farmers market model should be avoided because its independent nature predisposes to burnout and does not engender esprit de corps.

Health care professionals need a culture of collaboration, cooperation, and consistency—one that promotes embracing the mission and vision of the organization and the strategy to achieve those goals—a *we/us* partnership. This type of partnership occurs when leaders and professionals work together for the benefit of patients. Such a true partnership between professionals and leadership is a primary mitigating strategy for professional burnout.

SUGGESTED READING

Atkinson S, Spurgeon P, Clark J, Armit K. Engaging doctors: what can we learn from trusts with high levels of medical engagement? Coventry (United Kingdom): NHS Institute for Innovation and Improvement; 2011.

Bezrukova K, Thatcher SM, Jehn KA, Spell CS. The effects of alignments: examining group faultlines, organizational cultures, and performance. J Appl Psychol. 2012 Jan;97(1):77–92.

D'Innocenzo L, Mathieu JE, Kukenberger MR. A meta-analysis of different forms of shared leadership-team performance relations. J Manag. 2016;42(7):1964–91.

Pink DH. Drive: the surprising truth about what motivates us. New York (NY): Riverhead Books; 2009.

Schein EH. Humble inquiry: the gentle art of asking instead of telling. San Francisco (CA): Berrett-Koehler Publishers, Inc; 2013.

Swensen SJ, Meyer GS, Nelson EC, Hunt GC Jr, Pryor DB, Weissberg JI, et al. Cottage industry to postindustrial care: the revolution in health care delivery. N Engl J Med. 2010 Feb 4;362(5):e12.

13

AGENCY IDEAL WORK ELEMENT: TRUST AND RESPECT

The glue that holds all relationships together—including between the leader and the led—is trust, and trust is based on integrity.
—Brian Tracy

Trust and respect, an Ideal Work Element, is also related to Agency. Health care professionals need to feel trusted by the leaders of their organization, regardless of their sex, race, orientation, creed, tradition, or discipline (LoCurto and Berg, 2016; Rohman, 2016). Micromanagement and unnecessary adherence to process without justification are the antithesis of trust and respect. Without trust and the supportive, respectful environment it creates, health care professionals will be less likely to do their best or be invested in the organizational mission.

TRUST: THE ROOT OF THE TREE

Michael Bush is the president and chief executive officer of Great Place to Work for All, an organization that analyzes workplace culture. In one sentence, he summarized decades of research by the company: "The root of the tree is trust." The key to having people feel trusted is respect. They must believe that their leaders are authentic and equitable in their treatment of all team members. These qualities transcend across industries and directly impact organizational performance. The top companies in the annual Great Place to Work for All survey, which includes health care, are characterized by (Rohman, 2016):

- Threefold higher stock market returns
- Fourfold higher employee productivity
- Ninety percent lower employee turnover

Other research has confirmed that people who work in high-trust organizations remain with the organization longer (Rohman, 2016). Employees are happier, and happier employees are more likely to maintain their employment and be more innovative and productive (Ray et al, 2017)—critical advantages in a competitive marketplace.

Too Many Metrics

Excessive metrics are a manifestation of lack of trust. Today's physicians are frequently measured by patient satisfaction scores, relative value units, patient volumes, minutes per visit, speed of clearing inbox messages, and countless other things. In some cases, these metrics are needed, but to the extent a metric does not create value, it falls into the category of *waste*. Worse, it communicates a lack of trust. Such metrics contribute to cognitive dissonance because of the disconnect between how health care professionals should spend time with patients and what they are often being asked to do (e.g., low-value clerical work).

Whenever possible, metrics should be eliminated and professionals trusted to do the right thing, the right way. The act of eliminating unnecessary metrics is a powerful way to reduce cognitive dissonance and raise respect levels.

RESPECT

Respect is a basic human need. Unfortunately, respect is all too often absent or compromised in today's workplace. Extensive conscious and unconscious biases result in feelings of disrespect. Health care is not immune to these biases, including overt racism and inequality of the sexes, as expressed by co-workers, patients, and policies that adversely or disproportionally impact persons of a specific sex. More subtle slights include assumptions that women in scrubs are nurses rather than physicians and women being introduced by their first names in professional settings when it is appropriate to use their title or academic rank (Wyatt et al, 2016; Files et al, 2017). If health care professionals are to flourish, environments must be created that recognize and reduce these biased behaviors and that create teams who support and advocate for all team members. Health care professionals must grow and earn respect.

Organizations build trust and respect by making every attempt to treat all staff fairly. All team members must work together to make sure an inclusive and respectful work environment is created and maintained. This includes recognizing and addressing implicit bias as best as possible. For example, at Mayo Clinic, leader selection search committees discuss unconscious bias as part of their introduction and before the interview process occurs to acknowledge and attempt to mitigate its effect on their work. Over the last decade, the diversity in senior leaders and department chairs has increased in part due to raised awareness and these selection committee discussions.

Respect has implications for patients, too. In the World Health Organization Surgical Safety Checklist, team members are required to introduce themselves by role and name (World Health Organization, 2008; Haynes et al, 2009). This briefing helps create a sense of familiarity and respect among the team, which allows members to work together more efficiently during a procedure, with improved patient safety as the result.

When people feel respected and supported, productivity and effectiveness increase. Their work becomes more fulfilling. Cohesive teams develop, opening the door to improve interactions and workflows of the unit for the benefit of both patients and team members (Ray et al, 2017). To seriously address burnout and achieve esprit de corps, mutual respect must be a core value.

Case Study: Barry-Wehmiller

Barry-Wehmiller is a manufacturing company that has been built for long-term sustainability and success. Bob Chapman has been its chairman and chief executive officer (CEO) for over 40 years. He is the type of boss everyone wants to have. Chapman, a servant leader, focuses on enriching the lives of his employees, operating more as a father figure than a boss. When Chapman became CEO, Barry-Wehmiller had only one factory and a very weak financial position. The company now has 80 manufacturing plants with annual revenues of $2.4 billion.

How did Chapman accomplish this feat? The core philosophical principle of building trust and respect is at the heart of Barry-Wehmiller's success. In Chapman's words, "The machinery we build is just the economic engine that enables us to touch lives." He is referring to the lives of the company employees and team members, not just the customers.

Most of his 11,000 employees are blue-collar union workers. Early on, Chapman observed that the executives at Barry-Wehmiller had no time clocks, but the workers did. To Chapman, that meant the workers weren't trusted in the same manner as executives. The executive team agreed, and with that, the time clocks were turned off. Chapman then noticed that the executive supply cabinets weren't locked, but the supply cabinets of the blue-collar workers *were* locked. Pretty soon, all of the locks were gone. You get the idea. Chapman and his leadership team created a workplace where they demonstrated that they trusted their people, and, in return, everyone trusted them. Unions aside, the employees felt that Barry-Wehmiller was their company, their family. They felt that way because they had been treated that way.

At Barry-Wehmiller, this core value runs much deeper than just time clocks and supply cabinets. In the serious recession in the late 2000s, Chapman's team succeeded in their aspiration not to lay off a single person. To make this happen, they deployed a rolling wave of furloughs and delayed retirement fund payments. As the nation transitioned out of the recession, the Barry-Wehmiller company outperformed its peers, in part because they passed the pronoun test—they always thought of themselves as *we* and *us* (Reich, 1993). How they handled the recession proved this.

Many experts have studied the success of this employee-supportive organization. In a recent survey by business school scholars described in a book by Chapman and Sisodia (2015), four of five workers at Barry-Wehmiller said that they believed their company actually cared about them. This is completely opposite of how most employees feel, including health care professionals. To best serve patients, their families, and our communities, health care professionals need to have this level of trust in their organization.

The Needs of Patients and Employees

Five years ago, one of us (S.J.S.) engaged in a public discussion with Bob Chapman at the National Press Club. His fundamental premise was *employee well-being is paramount for organizational success.* Our contention (Mayo Clinic's primary value) was *the needs of the patient come first.* We learned a lot more from him than he learned from us. The lesson: In order to best serve our patients, families, and communities, we should not be ashamed to place a high priority on taking care of each other. As a health care organization, we can't take care of the needs of the patient if we don't trust and take care of the needs of our people. The fundamental job of the organization and its leaders is to create such an environment so that health care professionals can do what most are naturally driven to do—give their best to meet the needs of their patients.

CONCLUSION

Trust and respect are important elements of the ideal work environment for health care professionals. Behaviors and actions that cultivate these qualities should be embedded into leadership development and organizational infrastructure. Creating an environment characterized by trust and respect requires recognition and understanding of conscious and unconscious biases and taking action to address them. The goal is for everyone to feel respected and for diversity to exist in the workplace.

SUGGESTED READING

Chapman B, Sisodia R. Everybody matters: the extraordinary power of caring for your people like family. New York (NY): Penguin Random House LLC; 2015.

Files JA, Mayer AP, Ko MG, Friedrich P, Jenkins M, Bryan MJ, et al. Speaker introductions at internal medicine grand rounds: forms of address reveal gender bias. J Womens Health (Larchmt). 2017 May;26(5):413–9.

Goldin C, Rouse C. Orchestrating impartiality: the impact of "blind" auditions on female musicians. Am Econ Rev. 2000;90(4):715–41.

Haynes AB, Weiser TG, Berry WR, Lipsitz SR, Breizat AH, Dellinger EP, et al. A surgical safety checklist to reduce morbidity and mortality in a global population. N Engl J Med. 2009 Jan 29;360(5):491–9.

LoCurto J, Berg GM. Trust in healthcare settings: scale development, methods, and preliminary determinants. SAGE Open Med. 2016;4:2050312116664224.

Ray RL, Aparicio R, Hyland P, Dye DA, Simco J, Caputo A. DNA of engagement: how organizations can foster employee ownership of engagement [Internet]. 2017 [cited 2019 Mar 7]. Available from: https://www.conference-board.org/publications/publicationdetail.cfm?publicationid=7424.

Reich RB. The 'pronoun test' for success [Internet]. 1993 [cited 2019 Mar 28]. Available from: https://www.washingtonpost.com/archive/opinions/1993/07/28/the-pronoun-test-for-success/e45f3343-8b9b-444c-b7c2-2afa235c53e3/?noredirect=on&utm_term=.a0007d272687.

Rohman J. Great place to work: the business case for a high-trust culture [Internet]. 2016 [cited 2019 Mar 7]. Available from: https://s3.amazonaws.com/media.greatplacetowork.com/pdfs/Business+Case+for+a+High-Trust+Culture_081816.pdf.

World Health Organization. Surgical safety checklist [Internet]. 2008 [cited 2019 Mar 7]. Available from: https://www.who.int/patientsafety/safesurgery/tools_resources/SSSL_Checklist_finalJun08.pdf?ua=1.

Wyatt R, Laderman M, Botwinick L, Mate K, Whittington J. Achieving health equity: a guide for health care organizations [Internet]. IHI White Papers. 2016 [cited 2019 Mar 7]. Available from: http://www.ihi.org/resources/Pages/IHIWhitePapers/Achieving-Health-Equity.aspx.

14

AGENCY IDEAL WORK ELEMENT: CONTROL AND FLEXIBILITY

Nothing is better learned than that which is discovered.
—Socrates

BALANCING CONTROL AND FLEXIBILITY

Question: What cost-neutral organizational actions can improve well-being, decrease burnout, and promote esprit de corps?

Answer: Increasing control and flexibility.

Control and flexibility are strong moderators of work pressures and an important work element to balance. Control gives health care professionals permission to change their work lives, and flexibility gives them the capacity to manage the circumstances of their work lives. Health care professionals function optimally when they have greater ability to determine when they work, how they work, where they work, and how much they work (to the extent that control and flexibility help advance an organization's patient-centered mission). The ideal is a balance of personal control and flexibility coupled with standard processes and work flows that maximize patient safety and organizational efficiency. This situation represents the healthy tension between Agency and Coherence.

The safest and best care is team based, wherein all members sacrifice some individual control and flexibility for the benefit of the patient and the team. But whenever possible, teams of health care professionals should be granted control and flexibility to co-create workflow and interteam dynamics. This does not mean professionals are free to ignore standardized care pathways when they are appropriate or do whatever they want to care for patients when evidenced-based standards exist.

Being able to make choices also affects physical health. Employees who have less control over their work life have higher blood pressure, more back pain, greater clinical depression, more absenteeism, and higher levels of burnout than those who have greater control. Those with greater control also live longer (Marmot et al, 1991)!

Partnerships between health care professionals and organizations that give professionals control and flexibility over their work lives improve employee health and reduce burnout (Freeborn, 1998). Businesses based on greater employee self-determination have been reported to grow faster and have markedly lower turnover than command-and-control–oriented organizations (Baard et al, 2004).

Implications of Control and Flexibility

Consider the implications of the above studies for health care professionals. People need to be able to exercise choice in their lives to flourish. In today's health care environment, most professionals work for someone else (e.g., hospitals and academic medical centers, health maintenance organizations, large practice groups). This working environment makes achieving the optimal balance of control and flexibility more challenging without the support of organizational leaders.

The leadership of Kaiser Permanente surveyed their physicians to determine what contributed the most to their professional satisfaction and what would make them most committed to the organization. Control over their practice environment (including participating in decision making and scheduling flexibility) emerged as the dominant factor (Freeborn, 1998).

The 20% Threshold

Two relevant research studies related to control and flexibility centered on a 20% threshold:

1) First: Nearly half of employees would forgo a 20% raise for greater control over how they work (Citigroup Inc., 2014).
   The lesson: *Give people discretion in how their work is done.*
2) Second: Physicians who spend at least 20% of their time focused on the aspect of work they find most personally meaningful have burnout rates that are about half that of those who spent less than 20% of their time doing what is most meaningful to them (Shanafelt et al, 2009).
   The lesson: *Give people at least some discretion in what type of work is done.*

Case Study: Arden House

The Arden House retirement home in Hamden, Connecticut, empirically evaluated the principle of balancing control and flexibility by providing residents on one of the floors more control over their lives than residents on another floor (Langer and Rodin, 1976). On the first floor, residents were given a choice of staying in their rooms or going to a movie. They were also invited to choose a plant and take care of it if they so desired. On the second floor, residents were given a plant for their room and told that staff would take care of it for them. They were also told that on Thursdays they would go to a movie.

The residents of the first floor, who had more control over their daily lives, had more happiness, less dementia, and more social interactions. They also lived longer! There was an actual difference in mortality rates between the two floors.

The importance of the Arden House study is not in whether residents watched a movie or watered a plant. Rather, the story reveals that humans afforded even small amounts of control and flexibility have greater happiness, more social interactions, and longer lives. The lessons learned from this study have relevance to improving well-being among health care professionals.

OPPORTUNITIES TO IMPROVE
CONTROL AND FLEXIBILITY

Control and flexibility are evidence-based opportunities (Carayon and Zijlstra, 1999) to address burnout and improve the care of patients. A disturbing finding of numerous studies is that health care professionals who devote more time to clinical work (the fundamental work of the health care system) are at greater risk for burnout. Indeed, many report pursuing research, education, and administrative work to "escape" the clinic and have greater control—not because they have a passion for these activities. A holistic strategy to make the clinical environment as fulfilling and desirable as possible is long overdue. The following are three areas in which introducing control and flexibility can improve not only the clinical environment but also the organization as a whole.

Work-Life Integration

Control and flexibility help to reduce difficulties with work-life integration, a driver of burnout, by allowing integration of work and home responsibilities. Each health care professional has a unique set of personal and professional responsibilities, desires, and commitments (e.g., work hours, specialty, call schedule, family commitments, personal priorities), and integrating them is necessary for well-being.

Studies suggest it is often not personal or professional characteristics on their own that lead to burnout, but it is the unique way personal and professional responsibilities interact that creates problems. Work-family conflicts and tensions between personal and professional responsibilities appear to be one of the primary mechanisms that cause work characteristics to contribute to burnout. Providing flexibility can often relieve tensions and decrease the likelihood of work responsibilities resulting in burnout.

Standard Work

Standard procedures and processes are necessary in health care to improve consistency for better safety and quality. For example, preoperative checklists have reduced surgical errors and improved patient outcomes, and use of standard procedures has reduced line- and catheter-associated infections. However, standard work in and of itself is not a virtue. Processes should be standardized and streamlined when they create value for patients or free up time for professionals. Health care professionals should be an integral part of team-making decisions about standard work.

Professionals as Part of a Collective

Many health care professionals are transitioning from solo or small group practices to being employed by large organizations. This shift is often particularly hard for physicians. To become part of the larger organization, physicians must change the way they have always worked. The changes in human and team dynamics can be substantial. If organizational leaders do not handle such changes properly and provide appropriate control and flexibility, they are likely to see burnout and poor performance from their new employees. If health care professionals are treated as dispensable revenue centers, they behave differently, are cynical, and are more likely to burn out.

Orpheus Chamber Orchestra

Orpheus Chamber Orchestra is a renowned classical music ensemble in New York City. Unlike most others, this chamber orchestra does not have a conductor, so no one person is in control. The musicians rotate that responsibility (i.e., the "conductors" are leaders among peers). Orpheus musicians are collaborators who have an opportunity for voice and input. When they speak of their chamber orchestra, they use the pronouns *we* and *us* because they are all part of a team working together in a flexible system.

In an Orpheus-type health care organization, leaders and other health care professionals would view each other as colleagues and peers. For example, the leader of each nursing unit would be a practicing nurse, and the leader of each physician unit would be a practicing physician. Assuming they are doing a good job, these leaders would rotate control after a defined term (e.g., 7-10 years).

Health care organizations are, of course, larger than a chamber orchestra. The best balance would be an integration of the Orpheus model (where musicians co-create the music production in a flexible system) and a symphonic orchestra (where the conductor primarily interprets and directs the music in a more controlled system). This type of organization, with both control and flexibility, will flourish. In this situation, health care professionals would describe the organization as their organization. They would understand that, working together and supporting one another, they could achieve something bigger and more beautiful than even the best of them could do alone.

CONCLUSION

Control and flexibility are important elements of the ideal work environment for health care professionals. Balance must be found between patient-centered, clinician-friendly individualism and collectivism—between Agency and Coherence. Behaviors and actions that promote and grow control and flexibility should be embedded into leadership behavior and the organization's functional infrastructure, as described in Chapter 17 ("Agency Action: Introducing Control and Flexibility").

SUGGESTED READING

Baard PP, Deci EL, Ryan RM. Intrinsic need satisfaction: a motivational basis of performance and well-being in two work settings. J Appl Soc Psychol. 2004;34(10):2045–68.

Carayon P, Zijlstra F. Relationship between job control, work pressure and strain: studies in the U.S.A. and in The Netherlands. Work Stress. 1999;13(1):32–48.

Citigroup Inc. New Citi/LinkedIn survey reveals men struggle with work-life balance, but may not be telling women their concerns [Internet]. 2014 [cited 2019 Mar 12]. Available from: https://www.citigroup.com/citi/news/2014/141028a.htm.

Freeborn DK. Satisfaction, commitment, and psychological well-being among HMO physicians. Perm J. 1998;2(2):22–30.

Langer EJ, Rodin J. The effects of choice and enhanced personal responsibility for the aged: a field experiment in an institutional setting. J Pers Soc Psychol. 1976 Aug;34(2):191–8.

Marmot MG, Smith GD, Stansfeld S, Patel C, North F, Head J, et al. Health inequalities among British civil servants: the Whitehall II study. Lancet. 1991 Jun 8;337(8754):1387–93.

Schein EH. Humble inquiry: the gentle art of asking instead of telling. Oakland (CA): Berrett-Koehler Publishers; 2013.

Shanafelt TD, West CP, Sloan JA, Novotny PJ, Poland GA, Menaker R, et al. Career fit and burnout among academic faculty. Arch Intern Med. 2009 May 25;169(10):990–5.

15

AGENCY ACTION: MEASURING LEADER BEHAVIORS

TODAY: DISTRESS

Angela, a cardiologist, always dreamed of belonging to a team that worked together to deliver the best possible care to patients. In her current position, her team leader seems to have all the answers and is interested only in communicating what needs to be done. Most of her colleagues are not comfortable speaking up, and most of them do not appear to be interested in the careers of the women physicians or the unique challenges they face. Angela has started to wonder if there is a more nurturing and congenial place for her to work, but she decides to talk first to her team leader about how she feels and give her team leader a chance.

◆ ◆ ◆

Measuring Leader Behaviors is the first of four Agency Actions. These four actions are validated means to create the Ideal Work Elements of partnership, trust and respect, and control and flexibility. The first action is principally focused on cultivating the leader behaviors that promote professional fulfillment ("Coherence Action: Selecting and Developing Leaders" is discussed in Chapter 23).

CHARACTERISTICS OF GOOD LEADERS

Signature Size

Nick Seybert, M.S., Ph.D., of the Robert H. Smith School of Business at the University of Maryland measured the signature size of 605 chief executive officers (CEOs) from Standard & Poor's 500 companies over 10 years of annual reports (Seybert, 2013). He found an interesting relationship between the size of their signatures and the success of their companies.

What was it?

It turns out that the businesses led by CEOs who had large signatures performed worse than those with leaders who had small signatures. Large signatures correlated to lower return on assets, fewer patent citations (i.e., lack of innovation), lower sales growth, and overspending (i.e., underperformance by both leaders and their organizations). The CEOs with larger signatures also had higher compensation than their industry peers. It is tempting to speculate that an association between increased signature size and arrogance may explain these findings.

The most effective CEOs concentrate more on their organization and its people than on themselves. They know that, collectively, the leadership team has greater wisdom than they do individually and that they will perform at a higher level if they draw on the expertise of the team (Box 15.1). These are the behaviors of

---

Box 15.1. A Secret to Success

A gifted and successful leader likes to tell the story about a senior leadership meeting early in his tenure as chief executive officer (CEO). After the weekly executive meeting, another senior leader pulled him aside and asked, "When someone asks you a question, why do you always answer it?"

He replied, "What *should* I do?"

The other leader replied, "You should ask what they think and then ask the rest of group for their ideas and perspectives."

The CEO took the advice to heart, and it became a signature of his leadership approach. When he retired, after a luminous term as CEO, he credited it as part of the secret to his success.

"small-signature" leaders (Seybert, 2013; Mintz and Stoller, 2014). CEOs who lead businesses with the best financial performance stand out in three ways. They have:

1) A sense of purpose and mission.
2) A keen sense of urgency.
3) A passion that drives them.

Of course we don't measure the actual signature sizes of leaders. But we should measure the behaviors that lead to staff well-being and reduce professional distress.

The Mayo Leader Behavior Index

Studies we led at Mayo Clinic demonstrated a relationship between leader behaviors and esprit de corps (Shanafelt et al, 2015; Swensen et al, 2016; Shanafelt and Swensen, 2017; Swensen and Shanafelt, 2017). We asked health care professionals to evaluate the behaviors of their leaders (not whether they liked the leaders) on a 12-item Leader Behavior Index that we developed (Box 15.2).

Each item was scored on a 5-point scale (1=strongly disagree; 5= strongly agree). The scores for the 12 individual items were summed to yield a total leader behavior score from 12 to 60 (unless a question was answered "NA"). We subsequently evaluated how this composite Leader Behavior Index score related to esprit de corps outcomes. What did we find? For every 1-point increase in composite leadership score on the 60-point scale, there was a statistically significant 3.3% decrease in the likelihood of burnout and a 9.0% increase in the likelihood of satisfaction of the health care professionals completing the evaluations, after adjusting for age, sex, specialty area, and length of service.

At the work-unit level, the aggregate Leader Behavior Index score (i.e., the average score on the 60-point scale determined by the mean rating of the leader by all reports) was strongly related to the aggregate burnout and professional fulfillment scores within the unit. The aggregate Leader Behavior Index score of the unit leader explained approximately 11% of the variation in burnout and 50% of the variation in satisfaction across approximately 130 work units.

Box 15.2. Mayo Clinic Leader Behavior Index

To what extent do you agree or disagree with each of the following statements about (*name of immediate supervisor*)?

Response options for items 1-11: 5=strongly agree; 4=agree; 3=neither agree nor disagree; 2=disagree; 1=strongly disagree; NA=don't know/not applicable

1	Holds career development conversations with me
2	Inspires me to do my best
3	Empowers me to do my job
4	Is interested in my opinion
5	Encourages employees to suggest ideas for improvement
6	Treats me with respect and dignity
7	Provides helpful feedback and coaching on my performance
8	Recognizes me for a job well done
9	Keeps me informed about changes taking place at (*my organization*)
10	Encourages me to develop my talents and skills
11	I would recommend working for (*name of immediate supervisor*)
12	Overall, how satisfied are you with (*name of immediate supervisor*)
	Total Score[a]

[a] To score, sum 1 to 5 for each of the 12 items to generate a total score (range, 12-60 [unless some questions answered with NA]).

Modified from Shanafelt TD, Gorringe G, Menaker R, Storz KA, Reeves D, Buskirk SJ, Swensen SJ. Impact of organizational leadership on physician burnout and satisfaction. Mayo Clin Proc. 2015 Apr;90(4):432-40; used with permission.

Amidst all the qualities of the organization—its culture, high-level organizational strategy, salaries, benefits, efficiency of the practice environment, and the impact of the electronic health record—the single biggest driver of professional satisfaction was the behavior of each individual's immediate supervisor. Nothing else even came close. These findings demonstrate the importance of good frontline leadership on the well-being and satisfaction of health care professionals as well as the success of the health care organization.

Frontline leaders are not the leaders organizations typically focus on developing. Armed with these results, we readily convinced senior leadership at Mayo Clinic to invest in the development of frontline leaders—especially those with lower scores. After de-identifying data, senior leadership shared average leadership scores from the Leader Behavior Index and benchmarking data with frontline leaders (see below). All leaders were thanked for their service, provided feedback on their leader behavior score, and offered development opportunities, including executive coaching, to improve their leadership skills. This type of sharing should always be done in the spirit of helping individuals become better leaders. In our experience, leaders who improved their leader behaviors were happier and had happier and more engaged staff. Mayo Clinic and numerous other organizations now use this Leader Behavior Index to help leaders improve their leader behaviors.

FIVE LEADER BEHAVIORS

When we provide leaders their scores and explain how their behaviors impact the burnout, engagement, and professional fulfillment of those they lead, their first (and correct) impulse is almost always to ask for the questions in the index so that they can know what behaviors are being evaluated. There are five general categories of behavior evaluated by the 12 items of the Leader Behavior Index. All five behaviors build esprit de corps of the team and the well-being of the individuals:

1) Include: Treat everyone with respect and nurture a culture where all are welcome and are psychologically safe.
2) Inform: Transparently share what they know with the team.
3) Inquire: Consistently solicit input of those they lead (participatory management).
4) Develop: Nurture and support the professional development and aspirations of staff.
5) Recognize: Express appreciation and gratitude in an authentic way to those they lead.

The most successful organizations select and develop leaders for these behaviors. We have frequently seen substantive morale turnarounds in a unit facilitated solely by a change in the behavior of the unit leader. When a supervisor employs all five behaviors, there will be a trusting environment—one of the most valuable characteristics of high-functioning companies.

The behaviors in the Leader Behavior Index are common sense but not common practice. Exemplifying these behaviors requires leaders to be confident in their position, willing to tackle difficult problems, and bold enough to explore diverse views regarding new approaches and solutions.

Although not every leader can be charismatic, almost every leader can be inspirational. The need for leaders to inspire those they lead has never been more important than in today's volatile, uncertain, challenging, and ambiguous health care world. The formula for each leader is to learn and live these five behaviors in a manner authentic to their leadership style.

Evaluating Leader Behavior

Historically, frontline leaders at Mayo Clinic were evaluated each year by senior leaders, who rated them on their effectiveness at delivering expected results of the operational plan on a 1-to-5 scale. After our research demonstrated the importance of leadership behavior, we added the composite Leader Behavior Index score as a second dimension in their evaluation. We learned that some leaders scored high on delivering results but poorly on leader behaviors. They were task masters without much regard for their employees. Others scored well on leader behaviors but poorly on the evaluation by senior leaders. They were well liked but couldn't deliver results for the operational plan.

Effective leaders must perform well from both perspectives. We subsequently began measuring Leader Behavior Index scores for all of the approximately 3,300 organizational leaders across Mayo Clinic (Figure 15.1). This allowed executive leadership to have a more balanced and accurate assessment of the leadership capabilities of the organization and insight into which dimensions of professional development would be most helpful to each leader.

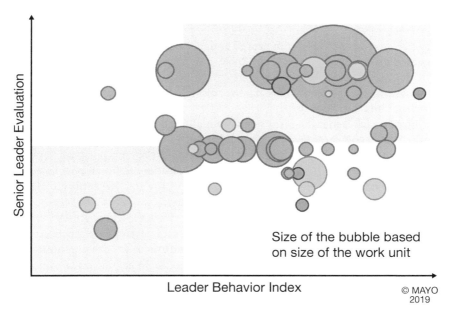

Figure 15.1. Leader Behavior Index Heat Map. The map shows overall performance of a subset of clinician leaders.

Y-axis = senior leadership rating of department/division leader's performance in executing their portion of the organizational operational plan based on "live-360" interviews.

X-axis = staff ratings of their leader on the annual survey, using Leader Behavior Index questions.

Size of bubble = size of department/division.

Color of bubble = succession-pool rating of leader readiness as well as ethnic and gender diversity. Green bubbles denote leaders who met all three performance criteria.

Surveys of Health Care Professionals

All-staff surveys are intended to measure the critical elements of organizational health:

- Quality of care
- Organizational culture (e.g., values, teamwork, psychological safety)
- Individual engagement/professional fulfillment

We believe that the behaviors of a leader (as assessed by those they lead) are one of the most important drivers of these outcomes. Accordingly, Mayo Clinic includes the Leader Behavior Index questions in the annual staff survey sent to the 65,000 employees at Mayo Clinic.

We believe the behaviors evaluated by the Leader Behavior Index should be assessed by all organizations trying to cultivate esprit de corps. The objective is to assess the organization's current leadership capacity, give feedback to leaders, provide support for leadership development, and see Leader Behavior Index scores improve over time. The intent is to help each leader be the best they can be, not to remove and replace.

DRIVING IMPROVEMENT

How can organizations foster improved and more consistent leader behaviors? We suggest a six-step process.

1) Obtain a baseline score for each leader by including the Leader Behavior Index in the annual staff survey.
2) Provide each leader the results confidentially, along with information for how their score compares to those of other leaders in the organization (e.g., percentile score). Results should be provided by the supervisor in a personal conversation. For credibility, the scores should compare leaders in similar positions (e.g., nurse managers should receive their leadership score and percentile rank [25th, 50th, and 75th] relative to other nurse managers).
3) Ask leaders to commit to improving in one or two areas where scores were not optimal and provide support and opportunities for development, such as workshops, seminars, online modules, mentoring, and executive coaching. Strategies, tactics, and conversation aids for supervisors to use in helping leaders improve their behaviors are provided in Appendix 15.1.
4) Let leaders know that their score will be reassessed annually. Those who have made progress at the time of the second assessment should be encouraged and complimented. At this meeting, leaders should be informed that the Leader Behavior Index score will be used as part of their annual performance assessment, beginning at the next evaluation (two years from baseline). Set realistic targets for improvement of weak areas.
5) Set performance targets at individual and organizational levels. For example, as an individual target, leaders could be asked to improve their personal Leader Behavior Index score by 10% in the next 12 months, and resources to help them improve should be provided. As an initial organizational target, the current 20th percentile for the overall Leader Behavior Index should be determined from baseline data. All leaders should be informed that the organizational expectation is for all leaders to have scores above that threshold at the next annual assessment. In subsequent years, the goal may be to maintain the previous goal and improve the median score within the organization by 10%. This multistep process should be used for two to three years to allow existing leaders, who may not have been selected for the specific skills being evaluated, to improve. In addition, when new responsibilities are assigned,

leaders may need training, time, and support to become proficient in the skill or responsibility.

6) Incorporate accountability for the Leader Behavior Index score into performance evaluations. If leader compensation includes an incentive component, the Leader Behavior Index score may be one component of the formula used to determine the incentive.

The obvious resulting question is how an organization should respond if a leader has an inferior score (i.e., below the established threshold of the 20th percentile of the peer group of leaders) that does not improve despite opportunities for leadership development, mentorship, and coaching. This situation may mean that an individual is not interested in improving and is unwilling to be accountable for the behaviors being evaluated, or they may not be able to develop these behaviors for various reasons. In such cases, ineffective frontline leaders should not be allowed to derail the organization's commitment to improving leader behavior, upholding a standard, and, ultimately, creating esprit de corps. When such leaders are retained, the organization sends the message to those they supervise that their opinion and well-being are not important. The result will be cynicism, distrust, burnout, and turnover. Therefore, organizations must compassionately and respectfully help such leaders find a role in the organization where they can create value. Some people may have excellent professional skills but may not be cut out to be leaders.

Annual Leader-Professional Conversations

The best relationship health care professionals can have with the person to whom they report is not one characterized just by a yearly meeting with an annual performance review. The best relationship is one with ongoing weekly, monthly, and quarterly dialogues that include appreciation, feedback, and support in addition to an annual review.

The annual review is, however, one natural place for leaders to demonstrate the five leader behaviors. The annual review conversation is often an underutilized tool leaders can use to reduce burnout and cultivate esprit de corps. All too often, annual leader-professional conversations are hollow exercises comprising a review of productivity metrics (e.g., relative value units) and business outcomes that are not meaningful to health care professionals. Such meetings fail to nurture a partnership between the professional, the work-unit leader, and the organization. They are a missed opportunity.

During the annual review conversation, areas that are important to employees should be identified and a plan developed for them to do more meaningful work. Consider asking questions like the following:

- What brings you the most meaning (or professional fulfillment) at work right now?
- How do you see that interest developing over the next several years?
- What next steps do you want to pursue to help you develop your interest?
- How can I help?

We have found that few work-unit leaders know what the most meaningful area of work is for each of the health care professionals on their team. Leaders frequently make basic and incorrect assumptions and often project them to all members broadly. Before the annual review, we have found it helpful to have health care professionals complete a brief reflection to facilitate introspection and a discussion of values and motivators. Informed by this discussion, leaders can then work collaboratively with the team member to explore how that interest may be developed (e.g., training, coaching, mentorship, building new skills, taking on new duties, postgraduate courses), how interest may be harnessed to serve the needs of the unit, and whether there are opportunities to expand the proportion of time dedicated to the area of interest—all of which decrease the chance of burnout.

With deliberate intention and, in the context of a year-long, leader-clinician dialogue and relationship, the annual leader-professional conversation can be a compelling way for leaders to demonstrate the five critical leader behaviors, build alignment, nurture esprit de corps, and reduce burnout.

CONCLUSION

Leaders matter. The leader behaviors of frontline supervisors are one of the single biggest drivers of health care professionals' satisfaction with their organization. Measuring Leader Behaviors is the first of four Agency Actions. The five leader behaviors of the Leader Behavior Index (include, inform, inquire, develop, and recognize) increase positivity by creating the Ideal Work Elements of partnership, trust and respect, and control and flexibility.

By increasing positivity, these five leader behaviors cultivate team building and enable professional fulfillment. Long-term leader behaviors are very important to organizational success. Accordingly, senior leaders should systematically measure leader effectiveness in specific behaviors, provide feedback, give leaders opportunities for development, reassess performance, and incorporate accountability to build skill and drive organizational progress. The goal is to support and help all leaders improve so that esprit de corps and superior patient outcomes can be realized (Box 15.3).

TOMORROW: FULFILLMENT

Angela's team leader appreciated her openness. After their discussion, he realized that he was not measuring up. He surveyed and met with the entire team, vowing to lead in a way that would make everyone on the team feel included and respected. The team leader now meets with everyone individually to understand what their career aspirations are and what really matters to them. He is interested in everyone's ideas and has asked Angela to help lead the group to make decisions together. Even though everyone does not always get their way, they always feel respected and listened to. The members of the group feel appreciated and valued. Angela now loves her work and so do her colleagues.

Box 15.3. The Playbook

- The single biggest driver of staff satisfaction is the behavior of each individual's immediate supervisor.
- The five paramount leader behaviors are: include, inform, inquire, develop, recognize.
- The Leader Behavior Index score of each supervisor should be evaluated as part of an annual staff survey.
- The intent of measurement is to help each leader develop and improve.
- Leadership scores should be shared with each leader in a supportive, confidential conversation along with an offer to support the leader's development and improvement.
- It is possible to improve leader behaviors with awareness, mentorship, coaching, and training.

SUGGESTED READING

Mintz LJ, Stoller JK. A systematic review of physician leadership and emotional intelligence. J Grad Med Educ. 2014 Mar;6(1):21–31.

Seybert N. Size does matter (in signatures). Harv Bus Rev. 2013;May. Available from: https://hbr.org/2013/05/size-does-matter-in-signatures.

Shanafelt T, Swensen S. Leadership and physician burnout: using the annual review to reduce burnout and promote engagement. Am J Med Qual. 2017 Sep/Oct;32(5):563–5.

Shanafelt TD, Gorringe G, Menaker R, Storz KA, Reeves D, Buskirk SJ, Swensen, SJ. Impact of organizational leadership on physician burnout and satisfaction. Mayo Clin Proc. 2015 Apr;90(4):432–40.

Swensen S, Gorringe G, Caviness J, Peters D. Leadership by design: intentional organization development of physician leaders. J Manag Dev. 2016;35(4):549–70.

Swensen SJ, Shanafelt T. An organizational framework to reduce professional burnout and bring back joy in practice. Jt Comm J Qual Patient Saf. 2017 Jun;43(6):308–13.

Appendix 15.1. Cultivating Optimal Leader Behaviors

The tactics that follow can be used to develop conversations with point-of-care leaders, with the goal of improving their behaviors with the health care professionals they support. Each section is related to one of the survey questions in the Leader Behavior Index and links to desired leader behaviors.

1) My Work-Unit Leader Holds Career Development Conversations With Me

A large part of satisfaction with work depends on health care professionals' perceptions regarding:

- The degree of *fit* between their day-to-day work and their skills, abilities, interests, and experience.
- The degree to which they feel they can grow and develop within their work.
- The degree to which they generate a sense of purpose from their work.

(continued)

Appendix 15.1. (*Continued*)

When health care professionals have good feelings about these issues, they are likely to be motivated and engaged, and perform well. They support their leaders and are loyal to the organization. Leaders can do a great deal to facilitate the perception of fit between work tasks and abilities and the opportunity for health care professionals to develop and derive a sense of purpose from work.

Leader Action Plan

✓ Schedule one-on-one time to meet with health care professionals to discuss personal development plans.
✓ Identify strengths and weaknesses.
✓ Coach and support health care professionals to identify specific short-term and long-term learning opportunities.
✓ Identify appropriate and meaningful goals for the next one to two years, and coach health care professionals in identifying specific formal and informal opportunities to build skills and achieve those goals.
✓ Track progress and development.
✓ Share information about career opportunities within the organization.
✓ Recognize efforts and accomplishments related to learning and professional development.
✓ Encourage a realistic self-assessment in which health care professionals identify strengths as well as limitations in skills and abilities.
✓ Identify formal and informal (on the job) learning opportunities that target competencies for the current role as well as for possible future roles.
✓ Match health care professionals with mentors and discuss leadership opportunities, if appropriate.
✓ Encourage health care professionals to take on *stretch* assignments (expanded job roles and responsibilities) or expose them to assignments across the organization (expand skills and benefit from multiple areas of the organization), or both.

2) My Work-Unit Leader Empowers Me To Do My Job

Empowerment is a form of control in the workplace that has substantial impact on health care professionals' motivation, satisfaction, and engagement. Empowerment enables health care professionals to take ownership of their work, to feel accountable, to be creative, to take calculated risks as part of their work, and to find meaning in their work. In addition, empowered health care professionals feel trusted by their leaders. Lack of empowerment and decision-making authority are associated with stress, dissatisfaction, lack of motivation, and disengagement.

Leader Action Plan

✓ Hold team meetings and share information with team members about organizational goals, unit goals, challenges, and strategy.
✓ Know health care professionals' areas of expertise and interests so that their skills are best utilized and they feel engaged.

Appendix 15.1. *(Continued)*

✓ Design processes and structures for upward communication and information sharing from all directions (i.e., lower levels, peers, and outside the organization).

✓ Ask staff for feedback and take appropriate action.

✓ Support, enable, and empower health care professionals as they do their work.

✓ Help people connect to meaning and purpose in their work.

✓ Create a safe environment whereby health care professionals feel free to speak up without fear and can demonstrate a questioning and receptive attitude.

✓ Allow health care professionals to explore new ways or processes to accomplish work goals.

✓ Involve health care professionals in the decision-making process. Have them identify problems, possible solutions, and take ownership/take lead on action plans.

✓ Genuinely appreciate the work others do. A sincere *thank you* can go a long way.

3) My Work-Unit Leader Encourages Me To Suggest Ideas for Improvement

It has been shown time and time again that health care professionals have great ideas to improve the work environment. Involving staff in the improvement process creates a culture of engagement, co-creation, and service excellence, as well as fosters a growth mindset. Good leaders are able to solicit suggestions and lead discussions on the merits of potential improvements and impact to the team and organization.

Fostering trust of health care professionals can be facilitated by transparent communication and collaborative team planning. Leaders who intentionally involve health care professionals in decision making reap benefits long term. Health care professionals who feel invested in decisions are much more likely to accept the new direction—whether or not they agree with it. If they see the process as fair and transparent, they feel respected.

Leader Action Plan

✓ Elicit more frequent and honest responses through one-on-one conversations, small group discussions, or anonymous methods of sharing.

✓ Create a process for ideas to be communicated often or via multiple venues as the ideas arise.

✓ If a particular issue or problem occurs, share this with your team, and request that they share feedback or specific ideas and solutions in a particular timeframe.

✓ When suggestions result in improvement, publicize the results so that all team members understand the importance of sharing their ideas.

✓ Communicate that *all* ideas are considered, even though they may not be practical or feasible to implement and may not all work.

✓ When someone comes to you with an idea, give feedback promptly to support and encourage the culture of sharing ideas.

✓ Encourage people to share specific solutions/better process ideas as part of improvement suggestions.

✓ Design processes and structures for suggestions and information sharing from all directions (i.e., lower levels, peers, and outside the organization).

✓ Have team members meet with the senior executive team to share ideas for improving organizational processes, services, or products.

Appendix 15.1. *(Continued)*

✓ Actively bring in new ideas by sending health care professionals from your team to external workshops and conferences in related fields. Invite guest speakers to share information/ideas/new perspectives. Follow-up to ensure learning, cross-fertilization of ideas, and pursuit of new projects/ideas.

4) My Work-Unit Leader Treats Me With Respect and Dignity

The extent to which health care professionals are treated with respect and their dignity maintained is an essential component of perceived fairness, equity, and inclusion in the workplace. Fairness, in turn, is linked to many important organizational outcomes, including cooperation, performance, feelings of belonging to the group, satisfaction, and motivation.

Health care professionals who do not feel respected are likely to withdraw from their work, not support their leaders, and even seek employment elsewhere. Respect can greatly enhance relationships and create a more enjoyable and more productive work environment. Respect should be conveyed through day-to-day practices, such as through communication (e.g., style, frequency, method, timeliness), information sharing, and decision making.

Leader Action Plan

✓ Treat health care professionals equitably and fairly; check in with them to ensure fair and equitable treatment is their perception as well.

✓ Recognize health care professionals for their contributions and achievements. Give credit where it is due.

✓ Create an environment of safety, respect, and comfort for health care professionals to speak their minds without fear. This type of environment shows a commitment to safety initiatives and to creating a culture of respect.

✓ Be open, honest, and transparent towards health care professionals. Treat them as partners. Follow through on commitments.

✓ Support, enable, and empower health care professionals as they do their work. Make resources available and empower them to take initiative, communicate upward, and share concerns in an open and supportive climate.

✓ Support the interests of health care professionals and advocate on their behalf. Make sure their voices are collectively heard, and help them resolve challenges within and between groups.

✓ Ask for feedback from others (e.g., leader, colleagues, staff) to identify behaviors that could be perceived as disrespectful and create a plan for working on the issue (e.g., someone may embrace every recommended practice but have a communication style that makes people feel disrespected; working with a mentor would help this situation).

5) My Work-Unit Leader Provides Helpful Feedback and Coaching on My Performance

Coaching is an excellent leadership approach to use with most health care professionals because it draws on their training, experience, and desire to solve problems. Coaching is not about giving advice but rather about asking the proper questions so that individuals

Appendix 15.1. (*Continued*)

can discover the answer for themselves. Ongoing coaching can help employees build skills, confidence, and independence; increase productivity, quality of work, and effectiveness of the work group; encourage initiative in professional development; and support creativity, innovation, and problem solving.

Leader Action Plan

✓ Be descriptive and not judgmental in giving feedback. Effective feedback is focused on behavior rather than personal characteristics. Ask open-ended questions. Be mindful of tone and body language. Know and stick to the facts.

✓ If a conversation is escalating with emotion or defensiveness, pause and suggest a future date to continue.

✓ Talk with health care professionals to identify specific learning opportunities. Identify strengths and weaknesses and help them track their personal development plans.

✓ Coach health care professionals by ensuring that they are learning from their actions (i.e., discuss and reflect on learning points). Learning should build on current and future competencies.

✓ Take a life-long learner perspective. Be open to coaching yourself.

✓ When asking questions, use the words of journalists: who, what, when, where, why, and how.

✓ Invite health care professionals to visualize and describe success in achieving the goal.

✓ Offer resources or encourage networking, or both.

✓ Check back with the individual to discuss progress. Reinforce positive changes.

6) My Work-Unit Leader Recognizes Me for a Job Well Done

Heartfelt and authentic recognition and appreciation are important leader behaviors that offer intrinsic reward and gratification to colleagues. The expression of gratitude should be customized to the individual or team involved so that the means of recognition fits their personality. For some, a handwritten note is best. For others, a public story is preferable.

Leader Action Plan

✓ Create a culture of recognition within your team. Provide ongoing feedback and recognize the value of individual work within the group. Ensure that others on the team and senior leaders are informed about achievements and contributions of team members.

✓ Track progress in light of individual goals and the work group's goals. Communicate progress and the value it has to the group. Set aside time during individual and group meetings to recognize staff.

✓ When giving verbal praise and recognition, be specific, focus on concrete accomplishments, and provide feedback/recognition in a timely manner.

✓ Genuinely thank health care professionals on your team for their efforts and results. Help them understand how their work is contributing to a greater good and shaping their career progression trajectory.

Appendix 15.1. (*Continued*)

✓ Recognize members of your team individually as well as in public settings when appropriate and the person agrees (e.g., group meetings, larger organizational meetings, newsletters, emails to peers).

7) My Work-Unit Leader Keeps Me Informed About Changes Taking Place at Our Organization

Clear and consistent communication to health care professionals is critical for organizational success. Health care professionals not only make sense of their daily work through communication from leadership, but they also rely on direction and information from leadership regarding matters affecting them in their personal and professional lives. Inconsistent, unclear, or no communication creates stress and makes health care professionals feel less valued (or even disrespected) by management. In this case, health care professionals may disengage from their work, feel resentful toward the organization, and even engage in counterproductive behaviors. Effective leaders take time and expend effort in communicating important information. This does not mean that leaders should communicate everything or demoralize their team by repeatedly communicating financial and other operational performance measures that do not align with the altruistic motives of health care professionals. Although this information must be periodically communicated, leaders must know their employees. They should use judgment on how often to communicate such messages.

Leader Action Plan

✓ Share information about the organization's general situation, about different departments, and about the work group, even when information might be negative.

✓ Share department/division messages or communications regularly in various settings and formats (e.g., one-on-one meetings, staff meetings, weekly huddles, newsletters, email updates). These communications should include information about work-related and organizational issues, such as changes in policies and procedures, that could impact employees.

✓ Ensure that information from senior leadership cascades to all health care professionals.

✓ Set aside time during regular meetings to discuss organizational matters and the way in which these matters impact health care professionals. Discuss both positive and possible negative implications.

✓ Provide opportunities for health care professionals to raise concerns and questions and address all of them in a timely manner (personally or by other members of the management team).

✓ Serve as a role model to others in embracing change and reinforce positive impacts you see occurring at work.

✓ Use judgment in what information is communicated to the team and how often information is communicated. Align messaging to the altruistic motivations of health care professionals.

Appendix 15.1. (*Continued*)

---

8) *My Work-Unit Leader Encourages Me to Develop My Talents and Skills*

One of the key roles of an effective leader is staff development. Fostering the development of health care professionals is conducive to ensuring a high level of knowledge, skills, and abilities within the work group and has been linked to higher levels of team-based performance. Additionally, development of health care professionals is positively linked to loyalty and commitment to the group as well as to personal satisfaction.

Leader Action Plan

✓ Identify appropriate and meaningful goals and coach employees to identify formal and informal learning opportunities to meet those goals.

✓ Schedule one-on-one meetings to discuss personal development plans.

✓ Identify strengths and weaknesses.

✓ Coach and support health care professionals to identify specific short-term and long-term learning opportunities.

✓ Share information about career opportunities within the company.

✓ Track progress and development.

✓ Recognize efforts and accomplishments related to employees' learning and professional development.

✓ Encourage a realistic self-assessment in which employees identify strengths as well as limitations in skills and abilities.

✓ Identify formal and informal (on the job) learning opportunities. Learning opportunities should target competencies for the current job and future roles.

✓ Match health care professionals with mentors or coaches. Discuss leadership opportunities, if appropriate.

✓ Encourage health care professionals to take on *stretch* assignments (expanded job roles and responsibilities) or be exposed to assignments across the organization (expand skills and benefits from multiple areas of the organization), or both.

16

AGENCY ACTION: REMOVING PEBBLES

TODAY: DISTRESS

Cynthia is a dedicated nurse practitioner. She works hard, but lately her enthusiasm for work has waned. She is frustrated by communication issues on her team and a broken workflow process where what she needs to serve patients is not reliably available. She goes home frustrated most days. Cynthia is considering reducing her work effort to four days a week. She cannot see any other way to cope.

• • •

Muhammad Ali said, "It isn't the mountains ahead to climb that wear you out; it's the pebble in your shoe." We refer to frustrations and inefficiencies in our practices as "pebbles." Removing Pebbles is the second of the four Agency Actions. This action is principally focused on mitigating the drivers of burnout in order to decrease negativity. Removing Pebbles is an evidence-based and validated intervention (Linzer et al, 2015; Swensen et al, 2016).

PARTNERING TO REMOVE PEBBLES

The identification and removal of sources of frustration and inefficiency requires a partnership of leaders and health care professionals. This participative management process treats health care professionals as trusted and respected colleagues. It results in a more friendly work environment and a cohesive team that is able to more readily navigate the occupational challenges that arise.

The process of identifying and removing pebbles starts with an unrushed conversation with the health care professionals of a given work unit. This unrushed conversation should focus on asking the right questions and truly listening to the responses. It is about identifying what contributes to or detracts from professional fulfillment and esprit de corps for health care professionals. Only by understanding what really matters to them will you be able to recognize, categorize, and then remove obstacles to esprit de corps.

Common Pebbles

The local challenges that often surface in these discussions frequently involve disorganization (e.g., inefficiency of practice, clerical burden, challenges related to the electronic environment, professionals performing tasks that should be performed by other staff, dysfunctional processes, challenges with work-life integration caused by issues with scheduling, lack of flexibility). Organizational characteristics of processes that diminish meaning or that impede caring for patients (e.g., policies viewed as eroding quality of care or negatively impacting professional-patient relationships) are also common concerns.

Most pebbles are unique to local work-unit work flows and dynamics, so if you have seen *one* unit, you have seen just *one* unit. What you learn about pebbles in that unit cannot be applied to the next unit. Unfortunately, most employers fail to recognize this and also are unaware of what matters most to their employees. So start talking about removing pebbles by asking, "What matters to you?"

ASK-LISTEN-EMPOWER (AND REPEAT)

The participative management model Ask-Listen-Empower (and Repeat) is used to eliminate worker-identified sources of frustration and inefficiency, and its foundation is based on organization-sponsored practice improvement initiatives conceived, developed, and implemented by local (unit) staff members (Figure 16.1).

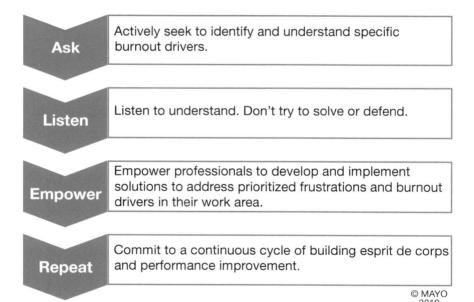

Ask — Actively seek to identify and understand specific burnout drivers.

Listen — Listen to understand. Don't try to solve or defend.

Empower — Empower professionals to develop and implement solutions to address prioritized frustrations and burnout drivers in their work area.

Repeat — Commit to a continuous cycle of building esprit de corps and performance improvement.

© MAYO
2019

Figure 16.1. Ask-Listen-Empower (and Repeat). (Data from Swensen S et al. Physician-organization collaboration reduces physician burnout and promotes engagement: The Mayo Clinic experience. J Healthc Manag. 2016 Mar-Apr;61[2]:105-27.)

Partnership in improving the practice environment transforms professionals' roles from followers to leaders and engages them in improving care for their patients and sustaining the organization. Ask-Listen-Empower (and Repeat) is a validated means of participative management, is a superb way to lead, and should be embedded into leadership behaviors and culture (Swensen et al, 2016).

The Ask-Listen-Empower (and Repeat) model is the tool best suited to help health care professionals improve local work systems and relationships. This model draws on principles from the fields of organizational psychology and social science. We have used it in many organizations to successfully improve work flow, address problems with team dynamics, establish fair and just accountability, and reduce burnout. Ask-Listen-Empower (and Repeat) is intended to:

- Nurture the psychological needs of choice, camaraderie, and excellence.
- Foster healthy professional-organization relationships.
- Identify drivers of burnout.
- Alleviate burnout by improving team dynamics, processes, and systems of care.
- Facilitate teamwork.
- Support development of clinician leadership.
- Increase health care professionals' engagement in the shared organization mission.

The technique is simple and requires primarily the time and attention of leaders.

Ask

- Convene focus groups of frontline health care professionals from a given work area and inquire about unique local opportunities to improve the care of patients and mitigate the drivers of burnout in the work unit.
- In a psychologically safe setting, ask health care professionals about their frustrations and what could be better in their work lives.
- Questions that can be used to help start the conversation include:
  o What frustrates you in this work area (i.e., what are the pebbles in your shoes)?
  o What are the inefficiencies in your day-to-day work?
  o What else is not going well?
  o Which of the following drivers of burnout is the greatest issue for you and why: excessive workload and job demands; inefficiency and inadequate resources; lack of control and flexibility; problems with organizational culture and values; isolation, loneliness, and lack of social support at work; and difficulties with work-life integration?
  o Which of these is the biggest challenge in your unit?
    ▪ What does that challenge look like in your unit?
    ▪ Which are the biggest contributing factors that are under local control?
  o If you could work on one thing under your control to make your life better in three months, what would it be?
  o What saps meaning from your work?

Listen

- Listen to understand health care professionals' concerns.
- Do not be defensive or try to solve problems, just record and acknowledge.
- After a number of opportunities have been identified by the group, ask the group to coalesce around a single, meaningful, and actionable local challenge as a place to start and make an improvement. Get consensus.

Empower

- After the results from the session have been synthesized, empower professionals to develop and implement solutions to address their prioritized issue in their work areas.
- Once a place to start has been identified, appoint a local clinician to lead this effort and to work in partnership with local leaders on the prioritized initiative.
- Assemble a team (task force) of individuals interested in helping develop a better way in this area.
- Allow the team to find a solution or refine a process that could be piloted.
- Conduct a pilot of this new approach.
- Evaluate outcomes. Did the intervention achieve what was hoped? Are refinements needed?
- Communicate results (successes and failures) to all staff members in the unit.
- Recognize accomplishments and celebrate, as indicated.

Repeat

- Commit to a continuous cycle of performance improvement and to enhancing esprit de corps.
- Revisit findings from focus groups (or reconvene) to identify the next round of improvement work related to burnout drivers.

Case Study: A Mayo Clinic Model for Success

When a division chief at Mayo Clinic began her leadership tenure, the doctors, nurses, and other team members in her division were struggling. Their burnout rates were among the highest in the institution. There was no esprit de corps. Within three years, she and her leadership team had taken the division from the worst to the best decile for professional burnout.

The division chief's approach is a model for success. Her first move in improving the esprit de corps of her colleagues was to understand the challenges. So she convened a multidisciplinary half-day retreat where the leadership team listened to all of the professionals: nurses, doctors, advanced practice providers (APPs), administrative assistants, and appointment coordinators. Problems and frustrations of all groups were described.

The physicians in the division agreed to prioritize the needs of members of the point-of-care team first. They believed that by relieving the clerical burden on these team members (e.g., nurses, medical assistants, appointment coordinators, administrative assistants), the care team could use the time saved to unburden the physicians of some tasks that did not require their level of expertise.

The leadership team responded by empowering the staff to act. They asked, "What are the pebbles in your shoes?" and "How can we make work life in our division better for you and for our patients?" The leaders listened to the responses. Then, they empowered the teams to start making improvements. For example, nurses in the clinic received many unnecessary patient phone calls every day that often reflected lack of communication in the hospital. The calls took nurses away from their teams and their current patients, which could have been avoided. The team analyzed the calls and confirmed their suspicions that patients and families weren't always regularly receiving information about follow-up and post-hospital care. To fix this, the team first created a call center, staffed by existing personnel. Second, they designed materials and a checklist so that nurses and care team members in the hospital would know what to communicate to patients at discharge and verify that they had done so.

The work life of the whole team improved because their days flowed more smoothly with fewer interruptions. And all the leaders had to do was start the dialogue:

"What brings you meaning in work?"
"What saps that meaning?"
"What is the pebble in your shoe?"
They asked.
They listened.
They empowered.
They removed the pebbles.

Respect for People

Fundamentally, removing pebbles is about trusting and respecting health care professionals to improve their work processes, their well-being, and the well-being of patients. It engages frontline workers in daily improvement and problem solving, while demonstrating that frontline leaders have confidence in the team's abilities to be true partners—the only way to achieve lasting benefits. The Ask-Listen-Empower (and Repeat) technique begins with the assumption that systems and behaviors are the problem, not people. Although many organizations use this approach to improve quality and productivity, we have found that few (almost none) do it with the specific and primary purpose of improving the work life of the care team. The case study that follows illustrates the successful implementation of the Ask-Listen-Empower (and Repeat) approach.

Case Study: Improving Workflow

Removing pebbles often involves improving work flow that threatens work-life integration, fairness and equity, safety, communication, and healthy team dynamics. Sometimes it is about increasing the efficiency of practice. HealthPartners, an urgent care clinic in Minneapolis, Minnesota, made a concerted effort to improve the efficiency of the practice environment for their health care professionals. Their efforts shortened the clinical work day for health care professionals by one hour (every day!) through practice redesign improvement efforts.

- They did not accomplish this by working harder.
- They did not achieve this by cutting corners.
- They did not realize this by spending less time with patients.
- They did this by asking busy clinicians about their frustrations and then together removing them, one broken process at a time.

The answers involved adding printers in every examination room, putting in larger monitors to make using the electronic health record easier, making changes to the physical space, and reengineering the way teams worked together, interacted, and communicated. This allowed the value-added clinical work to be achieved with less time and energy expenditure. Had they made assumptions about what needed to be changed, this might not have been a success story. The key to their success was in asking the people at the point of care what changes would improve the work environment and in doing what was in their control (i.e., their sphere of influence; see Chapter 9 "Assessment") to make the change happen.

SIX LEVELS OF OPPORTUNITY

Opportunities to reduce frustration (remove pebbles) and improve esprit de corps can be found at the individual, leader, team, work-unit, organizational, and executive levels. Frustrations should be categorized according to which of these groups is best suited to correct the problems or communicate the problems to others (Figure 16.2). Examples of opportunities the six groups might be assigned follow:

1) Individual: Improve performance by developing individual skills and efficiency in documentation, including use of the electronic health record.
2) Leader: Practice the five leader behaviors. Communicating transparently and expressing an interest in the ideas of team members will create a culture conducive to identification and removal of frustrations.
3) Team: Pilot the Ask-Listen-Empower (and Repeat) model for removing pebbles.
4) Work unit: Empower teams to improve work flows, scheduling, and team interactions.
5) Organization: Sponsor task forces to determine how, for example, to reduce clerical work associated with electronic health records. Measure and hold leaders accountable for the five leader behaviors. Revise policies to increase flexibility.
6) Executive: Work with, for example, the Centers for Medicare & Medicaid Services, vendors of electronic health records, and accrediting agencies to reduce regulations and public reporting measures that do not add value.

In our experience, most opportunities identified by staff to remove frustrations and inefficiencies in each of these categories do not require a large budget. The

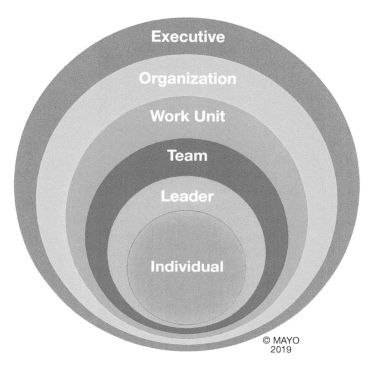

Figure 16.2. Action Groups for Removing Pebbles by Sphere of Control.

primary resources they require are the support of leadership, team time, and attention. Examples of these types of frustrations include:

- Workflow inefficiencies
- Process defects
- Suboptimal team dynamics
- Hand off imperfections
- Ordering, follow-up communication process, and call schedules
- Patient scheduling and triage
- Team-based collaborations
- Communication deficiencies
- Overly complicated, irrelevant, or duplicated guidelines
- Equity gaps in enforcement of policies or assignments
- Missed opportunities for transparency
- Care processes and tasks allocated to the wrong team members
- Lack of flexibility in scheduling
- Inefficiency and inequality in call schedules, hospital assignments, or cross-coverage (i.e., nights, weekends, and coverage for vacation)
- Rigid, local policies that don't match the care need (e.g., all support staff stay until the last patient leaves)
- Inconsiderate behavior by some care team members that adversely impacts other care team members (e.g., routinely overbooking patients at 5:00 PM)

Workflow Interventions

We developed and used the Ask-Listen-Empower (and Repeat) approach to decrease burnout at Mayo Clinic, deploying it at scale beginning in 2013. Using this approach to remove pebbles, teams at Mayo Clinic reduced burnout and dissatisfaction among health care professionals over a several-year period. They fixed broken communication systems and inefficient workflows. In 217 clinical units (about 11,000 staff), morale improved 17%, burnout decreased 21%, and teamwork increased 12% (Figure 16.3) (Swensen et al, 2016; Swensen and Shanafelt, 2017).

Work-life integration, time pressure, workplace chaos, work control, and clinician (i.e., physicians, nurse practitioners, and APPs) outcomes for burnout and satisfaction were also studied in a cluster randomized trial in 34 primary care clinics in New York City and the Midwest. The clinics that focused interventions on workflow improvements or targeted quality improvement projects saw significantly reduced rates of burnout. The clinics that chose to address improvements in communication saw increased rates of clinician satisfaction (Linzer et al, 2015).

What is fundamental to the success of such interventions is engaging health care professionals as partners in the improvement work. It does not work as well (or create the best team dynamics) if someone else repairs the local environment for them. Team-based quality improvement work is an important part of reducing burnout and cultivating professional fulfillment. Point-of-care leaders with their teams can improve efficiency of practice while simultaneously promoting esprit de corps (Box 16.1).

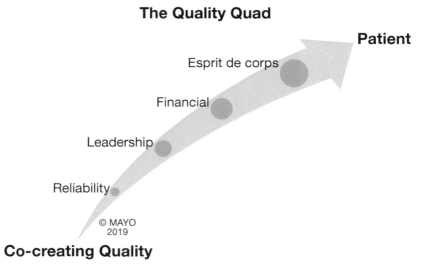

Figure 16.3. Co-creating Quality and Esprit de Corps With the Quality Quad. There are four dividends that accrue from teams that co-create quality: 1) reliability (i.e., processes are more dependable with less waste and variation); 2) leadership (i.e., Ask-Listen-Empower [and Repeat] is an effective action-learning, leadership-development technique); 3) financial (i.e., systems are more profitable with less waste and variation as well as fewer defects: "Quality is Free" [Philip B. Crosby]); and 4) esprit de corps (i.e., team-based co-creation of quality engenders camaraderie, flexibility and control, trust and respect, and meaning and purpose). All four of these dividends benefit the patient.

Box 16.1. Nurse-to-Nurse Bedside Hand Offs

Question: How often does communication across various transitions of care fail?
   Answer: At least 40% of the time.

   Patient hand offs between nurses at shift change are an important process in clinical nursing practice. Hand offs allow nurses to exchange patient information to ensure continuity of care and patient safety. A simple change in the location of the hand off discussion at Mayo Clinic a decade ago (to the bedside rather than in the work room) improved the transmission and receipt of information between nurses and removed a large staff frustration. Moving the discussion from the work room to the bedside allowed the incoming nurse to meet the patient and ask questions of the outgoing nurse, and it allowed patients to be more actively involved in their care and related decisions. The result was more consistent and compassionate communication during shift changes and improved patient care. It cost nothing!

   A minor change driven by the health care professionals on the unit improved efficiency, quality, and both patient and nurse satisfaction.

Case Study: Institute for Healthcare Improvement

One of the founding fathers of improvement work, W. Edwards Deming, Ph.D., believed that management's overall aim should be to create a system in which everyone takes joy in their work. For Deming, joy is a product of quality improvement work and high-quality systems. Frustrations are removed.

Joy in Work is an integral part of the Institute for Healthcare Improvement (IHI). In 2015, IHI (personal communication, Jessica Perlo, M.P.H., director) recognized the increasing burnout crisis and decided to use the iterative, applied science of improvement with their own staff to learn how to support other organizations in decreasing professional burnout. At that time, IHI was already a joyful place to work, as evidenced by an 87% excellent rating by staff (national averages are about 49%). However, chief executive officer and president, Derek Feeley, believed IHI could do better: "To move the needle on burnout for our partner organizations, we need to walk the talk and test what we're learning here in our office." Within a year, they aimed to have 95% of staff agree that IHI was an excellent place to work. As part of the process, IHI also set out to reduce the gap between white staff and nonwhite staff in response to this question (there was a 23% disparity).

   IHI began by asking their staff what mattered to them. Senior leaders hosted coffee meetings, had one-to-one conversations with anyone interested, and formed teams to focus on testing alternative approaches and studying the results. The teams tested a host of improvement initiatives, from training on "undoing racism" to more flexible work hours.

   To get real-time feedback and measure daily progress, IHI did something simple. During the time when they were implementing improvements, they asked staff to report if their day had been good or bad (good day = improvements occurring) by dropping color-coded marbles into a jar at the end of each day. By counting the marbles, IHI knew if staff were having days filled with progress or setbacks and frustration. This allowed them to see whether the changes they were testing were resulting in improvement. On bad days, supervisors had conversations about what had gone wrong and discussed ways to improve.

At one year, 92% of staff agreed that IHI was an excellent place to work, and the gap between white and nonwhite staff was nearly eliminated. However, the work is ongoing: IHI leadership decided not to stop their improvement efforts until their organization is one where 100% of staff thrive and achieve their full potential and until they can translate their experiences to improve joy in work for their entire health care workforce.

Case Study: East London National Health Service Foundation Trust (Personal Communication, Amar Shah, M.D., Consultant Forensic Psychiatrist and Chief Quality Officer)

East London National Health Service (NHS) Foundation Trust (ELFT) delivers mental health, community health, primary care, and some specialist services to 1.5 million patients in a densely populated and culturally diverse part of London. The organization has roughly 6,000 employees working in more than 100 locations.

For the past decade, ELFT has prioritized staff experience as one of three strategic objectives. In support of this, the organization developed a clear strategy focused on the following elements designed to remove frustrations among staff:

- Dyad relationships: Clinician leaders are supported by managers.
- Patient involvement: Each directorate in the organization has a structure for ensuring that the patient voice is included in planning, delivering, assuring, and improving services. This work has been extended to include patient involvement on all interview panels, training, and quality-assurance work.
- Accessibility: The ELFT executive team has tried to ensure that it is accessible and in touch with health care professionals at the team level through regular open forums and weekly executive WalkRounds.
- Effective teamwork: ELFT has encouraged all teams to find regular times for reflection. Almost all teams have a regular full or half day away approximately every three months.

In 2014, ELFT introduced quality improvement as a key mechanism to support its staff and patients, as well as to contribute to improving the quality of care provided. Multidisciplinary teams were encouraged to identify a complex quality issue that mattered to staff and patients. Teams were then supported to apply a systematic quality improvement method to test ideas and see what worked. This approach brought teams together around a shared purpose, thus enhancing effective teamwork. All teams were strongly encouraged to involve patients. As ELFT's quality improvement work grew, staff experience improved. Staff were less frustrated. In national NHS staff survey data for 2014 and 2016, ELFT had the highest scores for staff feeling able to contribute towards improvements at work and the highest overall staff engagement score.

ELFT then expanded their work by adopting the *IHI Framework for Improving Joy in Work* as a key strategic improvement priority. Leadership used a systematic method for quality improvement, with support from both improvement advisors and organizational development experts. With the goal "to improve staff satisfaction and well-being so that staff is better able to meet the needs of their patients," teams identified ideas for change and areas that frustrated them and pilot tested them using full transparency within the work unit.

ELFT developed a mobile app used for the global outcome measure (i.e., the proportion of staff reporting that they had a "good day"). With the mobile app, staff could easily submit change ideas via their phones, see progress against change ideas, and track their own and their team's experience at work.

The result was success. The proportion of health care professionals who reported "I had a good day" each day increased from 55% at baseline to 75%. ELFT scaled up their joy-in-work initiative to another group of 21 teams in 2018, and 17 teams completed the program in 2019, with an overall increase of 8% of staff reporting a good day at work.

THE DMAIC STRATEGY

Another strategy used by organizations to remove waste and inefficiencies in their systems is DMAIC, which is the acronym for *define* the problem, *measure* process performance, *analyze* the process, *improve* process performance, and *control* the improved process (George et al, 2004). DMAIC, a component of the Six Sigma toolkit, is a data-driven strategy that can be used to guide quality improvement projects related to waste and inefficiencies (removing pebbles) (Swensen et al, 2009). A full understanding of Six Sigma is not necessary to use DMAIC as a guide and checklist to improve systems and processes. DMAIC can be successfully used by teams without years of training or experience. This structured methodology is fully compatible with the Ask-Listen-Empower (and Repeat) process and should be employed when the work environment issue lends itself to a more robust, deliberate approach. There are five steps to the DMAIC process with various methods that can be used to accomplish the strategy, which have are described elsewhere (Smith, 2003; George et al, 2004; IHI, 2019) (Figure 16.4).

1) Define the problem.
   - What is the process targeted for improvement?
   - What are the project goals?
   - What will success look like?
2) Measure process performance.
   - Quantify the problem.
   - Define and establish metrics.
3) Analyze the process.
   - What are the root causes of variation?
   - What causes poor performance and defects?
   - Don't jump to solutions before looking at potential issues.
4) Improve process performance.
   - Understand and eliminate the identified root causes.
   - Brainstorm solutions, pilot process changes, and implement solutions.
   - Confirm there is measurable improvement.

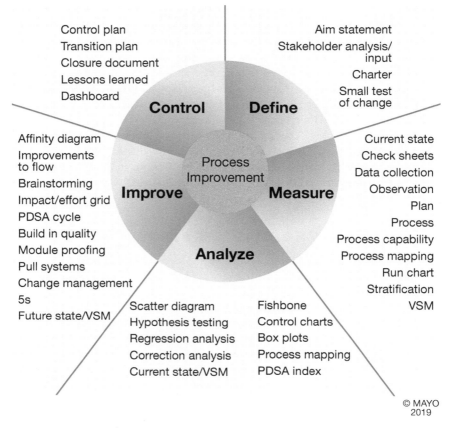

Figure 16.4. DMAIC (Define, Measure, Analyze, Improve, Control). Within the individual phases of a DMAIC project, various quality-management tools are used, including tools from the Six Sigma toolkit (Smith, 2003; George et al, 2004; IHI, 2019). PDSA indicates plan, do, study, act; 5s, sort, set in order, shine, standardize, and sustain; VSM, value-stream map.

5) Control the improved process.
  • Maintain the solution.
  • Continue measuring the success of the updated process.

If there appears to be an obvious solution, some of the DMAIC steps can be eliminated. For instance, if the team identifies a clear solution for a problem and all potential unintended outcomes have been identified or mitigated, then proceed.

Case Study: Virginia Mason Medical Center

Innovation is a pillar of Virginia Mason Medical Center's strategy. As a result, its leaders understand the necessity of co-creation between leadership and staff. Virginia Mason uses the *lean* methodology (i.e., continuous improvement and respect for people while eliminating waste in all areas of the organization) as the platform for innovation to build on current processes and measure success. The organization invests in training clinicians on idea-generating techniques to harvest robust information and ideas. Clinicians participate in rapid-cycle improvement workshops. At these workshops, frontline clinicians learn and work together to redesign care processes in a "see/feel experience of self-discovery." This process of team-based quality improvement is therapeutic. Virginia Mason also sponsors innovation grants to encourage improvement.

Virginia Mason leadership partners with teams that use value stream mapping, the lean-management tool, to identify processes and systems that are not adding value to the organization. This flowchart tool is especially helpful in finding and eliminating waste in systems because it requires users to map an item according to its added value. When clinicians used this tool, they had to look at an entire process or system and then work across boundaries within the organization to eliminate any system or part of a system that wasn't adding value. Besides eliminating waste and increasing quality, this type of thinking engendered trust and interconnectedness among the health care professionals involved.

CONCLUSION

Removing Pebbles, the second of four Agency Actions, involves engaging and empowering frontline health care professionals to identify and solve local sources of frustration. Participative management with collaborative action planning is an authentic gesture of confidence by leadership in the point-of-care team's abilities to be true partners in improving daily operations to better serve the needs of patients and the care team. Various ways exist to implement true partnering, including Ask-Listen-Empower (and Repeat) and DMAIC, both of which engender trust and respect for the entire team. Trust and respect of health care professionals are core principles for removing pebbles (Box 16.2).

In addition to removing sources of frustration, the dividends of using a team-based approach based on Ask-Listen-Empower (and Repeat) for process improvement are many and include:

- An important message from leadership
  o We are listening.
  o We trust and respect you.
- Self-discovery among team members
  o We know what the problems are.
  o We can develop solutions together.
- Camaraderie
  o We are in this together.
- Meaning and purpose in work
  o We are improving the practice environment to allow us to better serve our patients.
  o We can make a difference.

TOMORROW: FULFILLMENT

Cynthia's work-unit leader asked her and members of her team what frustrated them. It turns out that her peers had similar sources of irritation. Most of the issues could be dealt with by redesigning several of the unit's workflows. As the team reengineered the work flows together, morale improved, and they had more time to spend with patients. Team members finished their workday by 45 to 60 minutes earlier almost every day. Cynthia and her team felt like they were in control of their destiny. Cynthia decided to keep working full time and continue to improve the work environment. This was a much better solution for Cynthia and for the organization.

Box 16.2. The Playbook

- Meet with small groups of individuals from your work group.
- Identify pebbles (sources of frustration) using the Ask-Listen-Empower (and Repeat) framework.
- Chose one "pebble" that is within your work unit's sphere of control that can be addressed with several months of attention.
- Develop an approach to "remove the pebble" by work flow or system redesign.
- Implement or pilot test the new approach.
- Evaluate impact; celebrate success; learn from failure and try again.
- Repeat.

SUGGESTED READING

Barry MJ, Edgman-Levitan S. Shared decision making: pinnacle of patient-centered care. N Engl J Med. 2012 Mar 1;366(9):780–1.

Crosby PB. Quality if free: the art of making quality certain. New York (NY): New American Library; 1979.

Dilling JA, Swensen SJ, Hoover MR, Dankbar GC, Donahoe-Anshus AL, Murad MH, et al. Accelerating the use of best practices: the Mayo Clinic model of diffusion. Jt Comm J Qual Patient Saf. 2013 Apr;39(4):167–76.

George ML, Rowlands D, Price M, Maxey J. The lean six sigma pocket toolbook. New York (NY): McGraw-Hill; 2004.

Institute for Healthcare Improvement. Quality improvement essentials toolkit [Internet]. 2019 [cited 2019 Jul 3]. Available from: http://www.ihi.org/resources/Pages/Tools/Quality-Improvement-Essentials-Toolkit.aspx.

Linzer M, Poplau S, Grossman E, Varkey A, Yale S, Williams E, et al. A cluster randomized trial of interventions to improve work conditions and clinician burnout in primary care: results from the Healthy Work Place (HWP) Study. J Gen Intern Med. 2015 Aug;30(8):1105–11.

Oakley E, Krug D. Enlightened leadership: getting to the heart of change. New York (NY): Fireside; 1994.

Smith B. Lean and six sigma: a one-two punch. Qual Prog. 2003 Apr;36(4):37–41.

Swensen S, Kabcenell A, Shanafelt T. Physician-organization collaboration reduces physician burnout and promotes engagement: the Mayo Clinic experience. J Healthc Manag. 2016 Mar-Apr;61(2):105–27.

Swensen SJ, Dilling JA, Harper CM Jr, Noseworthy JH. The Mayo Clinic value creation system. Am J Med Qual. 2012 Jan-Feb;27(1):58–65.

Swensen SJ, Dilling JA, McCarty PM, Bolton JW, Harper CM Jr. The business case for health-care quality improvement. J Patient Saf. 2013 Mar;9(1):44–52.

Swensen SJ, Dilling JA, Milliner DS, Zimmerman RS, Maples WJ, Lindsay ME, et al. Quality: the Mayo Clinic approach. Am J Med Qual. 2009 Sep-Oct;24(5):428–40.

Swensen SJ, Shanafelt T. An organizational framework to reduce professional burnout and bring back joy in practice. Jt Comm J Qual Patient Saf. 2017 Jun;43(6):308–13.

17

AGENCY ACTION: INTRODUCING CONTROL AND FLEXIBILITY

TODAY: DISTRESS

Jennifer has had enough of being a private practice physician. She despises the pressure of a production compensation model that conflicts with her desire to spend as much time with each patient as they need. She does not like seeing other doctors as competitors. She does appreciate the control she has over much of her professional life, although her group is small and she takes a lot of call. At this stage in her career, Jennifer has decided to work for the large medical center in town as an employed physician with a salary. Her biggest fear is the prospect of losing the one attribute that she likes most about private practice: her control and flexibility.

◆ ◆ ◆

In this chapter, we describe ways to nurture control and flexibility by actions that strengthen teams and are patient centered.

FLEXIBILITY AND STANDARD WORK

As described in Chapter 12 ("Agency Ideal Work Element: Partnership"), research shows that control and flexibility are good for health care professionals and for organizational effectiveness. Organizations should provide flexibility in regard to how staff work, how much they work, when they work, and where they work. Thought must be given to what is practical for the professionals, their specialties, their teams, and the organization.

There is a healthy tension between standard work, which is controlled, and flexible work. Standardization of processes that improve quality and safety is good for patients. Flexible work in other areas is good for employees' mental and physical health. Executed properly, standard and flexible work can be complementary.

Standard Work

It is important for health care professionals to recognize the benefits of standard work. A few of the numerous benefits of properly determined and appropriately maintained standard work for health care professionals include:

- Standard work makes the workflow more efficient.
- More efficient workflow should free up time for professionals.
- Standard work reduces rework from defects of care.
- Fewer defects engender meaning and purpose in work.
- Creating and improving standard work as a team builds camaraderie and reinforces flexibility.

The best standard work will free up time for members of the care team to plan ways to improve more work and to have more time for activities that are meaningful for them.

Standard work tasks and protocols should be created and maintained by the care team at the point of care. They should not be blindly imported from another organization. You cannot assume that a protocol from another institution will work in your institution. It may, but generally all work tasks need to be adapted for optimal workflow, patient safety, and professional fulfillment. What is considered standard work will also change as experiences, workflow, research findings, and team dynamics evolve.

If the care team is responsible for standard work, they inherently have more control over their work lives. If the care team continually evaluates standard work, they get needed flexibility. Metrics and feedback can be provided to document and uphold high standards. Health care professionals continually review the latest literature to improve care; they should also continually assess their workflows.

Another reason to champion standard work is innovation. The two depend on each other. Innovation builds from a standard work platform using hypothesis-driven inquiries that a flexible environment then allows to be tested. In addition, a change to improve practice can only be understood and evaluated if there is a standard work baseline for comparison. The capacity to innovate is an attribute of professionally satisfying control and flexibility.

However, guidelines, pathways, and processes (and even artificial intelligence) cannot replace the clinical judgment and shared decision making of health care professionals in collaboration with their patients. Leaders must continue to bring standardization for processes that enhance quality, increase practice efficiency, create value for patients, and free up time for professionals; but, they must also simultaneously respect the clinical judgment of professionals and permit control and flexibility rather than require pedantic adherence to processes that could undermine quality care. They must remember that medicine cannot always be standardized, given the complexity of medical care and the unique values, aspirations, and comorbid conditions of each patient.

For example, it makes sense to have standard protocols for prophylaxis of deep venous thrombosis that have proven effective for a large proportion of patients and will save lives. Although the approach to prophylaxis can be standardized for most patients, the treatment of thromboses is typically more nuanced. Patients have different genomes, and some have chronic conditions and unique disabilities that may be risks for life-threatening hemorrhage. So flexibility is needed for professional staff to opt out of standard protocols. In fact, professional staff should be encouraged to opt out for patient-centered reasons, but they should also be tasked to help make protocols better by communicating their rationale and ideas to their peers and to organizational leaders.

ORGANIZATIONAL DESIGN

Earlier, we cited W. Edwards Deming's principle, "Every system is perfectly designed to get the results it gets." Health care organizations must design their operations so that their professionals feel they have some control and are not just being told what needs to be done. Without a cooperative relationship, the organization will "get" what it designed: inferior results. In our experience across multiple organizations, professionals will thrive when they are treated as respected team members who are asked to co-design the work environment rather than as just workers whose thoughts and ideas don't matter.

How can systems be designed that create control and flexibility for health care professionals? Some principles and practices that promote such an environment will be discussed in Chapter 23 ("Coherence Action: Selecting and Developing Leaders") and include:

- Health care professionals as leaders. Health care leaders should still have clinical roles in the organization.
- Egalitarian leader selection process. Leaders should be selected through a transparent approach that involves meaningful input from the people they will lead.
- Organizational democracy. Involve frontline health care professionals in co-creation of work settings and decision making.
- Rotational leadership. Set terms for leaders so that their focus is on servant leadership and stewardship rather than on building their own empires. There is a reason this principle is the cornerstone of democracies around the world. It is good for organizations, too.

Outcomes vs. Processes

In a collaborative environment, leaders and organizations create increased flexibility for health care professionals when they focus more on outcomes than on specific processes.

The most successful organizational leaders understand that giving some control to the people closest to patients cultivates an environment conducive to the best patient care at the lowest cost. Local control and individual flexibility are virtues of great leadership, as long as the strategies and tasks promote patient-centeredness and good outcomes. Organizations should specify "why" and "what," and let their professionals develop and own the "how." We like the mantra, "Wide guard rails, thin rule book . . . and lose the middle manager mentality."

As Bill Gates said, "Leaders need to provide strategy and direction and to give employees the tools that enable them to gather information and insight from around the world. Leaders shouldn't try to make every decision."

Case Study: Manager vs. Leader

In one clinical department at Mayo Clinic, the recent transition to a new chair resulted in a dramatic improvement in burnout and satisfaction ratings. The salient difference between the old and new department chairs was that the first acted as a *manager* who focused on process, and the second acted as a *leader* who focused on outcomes.

The *manager chair* said, "The reason we must do this is because senior leaders have told us to." The physicians had no control or flexibility. In contrast, the *leader chair* said, "We are doing this because it is the right thing to do for the outcomes we need to deliver to be good stewards of our role in Mayo Clinic's integrated group practice. Let's talk about the reasons why it is important and figure out the best way to do it." He provided opportunities for voice, input, and feedback and gave physicians more control over their work lives. Under the new leadership, departmental productivity (both clinically and academically) rose. In parallel, physician satisfaction and engagement improved, and the prevalence of burnout dramatically declined!

The leader chair knew the force-multiplying power of the mantra: "Wide guard rails, thin rule book . . . and lose the middle manager mentality."

DECISION MAKING

How decisions are made at all levels of the organization substantially determines the degree of control and flexibility in the workplace. To engage health care professionals, decision making must be characterized by mutual trust and commitment, transparency, and sincerity. Any autocratic pronouncement will disengage health care professionals, whereas consensus decision making through committees or work groups will engage them.

This does not mean that every decision should be consensus driven. There are certainly times when leaders need to make tough decisions on their own, or urgency precludes having time to engage the team. In those instances, the trust engendered from a baseline of team co-creation will serve the group well.

There is a continuum of decision making—from purely democratic (majority wins), to consensus, to advise and decide, and finally to authoritarian—and each type of decision making has its place. But the more leaders can connect with health care professionals to co-create policy and direction, the better the team result.

Organizational Democracy

Organizational democracy is a boundaryless approach that is designed to take full advantage of the health care team. The approach is associated with higher levels of innovation, clinician involvement, commitment, and satisfaction. Organizational democracy combines participative management for leaders and professionals and patient-centered decisions. Although we are not advocating conversion to organizational democracy for health care management, we believe lessons and elements from that approach may be beneficial for eradicating professional burnout and promoting esprit de corps. For example, the collective and often consensus decision making manifested in the Leader Behavior Index and the use of committees and task forces are relevant examples.

Committees and Task Forces

Rather than telling clinicians what to do (control), where appropriate, ask them first (flexibility). Strategic use of committees and task forces are approaches that can engage professionals in co-creation via participative management. Committees and task forces are a structured and visible means to understand the perspective and ideas of professionals doing the real work of caring for patients, and decisions result from the rich perspective of the entire team.

One of the most important functions of leaders is to have those working for them feel valued. Approximately half of American employees do not feel valued at work. Not feeling valued puts health care professionals at higher risk of burnout, lower engagement, and less discretionary effort. Shared decision making in committees is one way to show employees that they are valued.

Committees may, however, slow organizational decision making. One of the few criticisms Aristotle and Plato had in their treatise on democracy (*demokratia*) related to the slowness of decision making (Swensen et al, 2016). In general, the slower speed of committee decision making is outweighed by the merit of the quality of the decisions, the value of collaboration, the power of engagement, the inherent change in management, and the interwoven leadership development. Ensuring that committees and task forces are of optimal size helps mitigate this drawback. Economists and social scientists have developed elaborate formulas to express the trade-offs of efficiency, effectiveness, accuracy, consensus, expense, speed, and engagement of committees. The optimal group size for decision making is approximately 7 (±2) members. And the best decisions are made when the groups have discipline, thought, ethnic diversity, and gender diversity.

Once decisions are made, leaders should remove barriers to executing a committee's plan (e.g., create time, resources, compensation) and commit administrative backing (e.g., hire data clerks, improvement experts, project managers). Do whatever is within the organization's power to show that the professionals' opinions and decisions are valued. If something cannot be done, explain why and ask for feedback to mitigate the potential issues of control.

Case Study: Ascension Medical Group (Personal Communication, Joseph Cacchione, M.D., Executive Vice President; Baligh Yehia, M.D., Chief Medical Officer)

Ascension Medical Group is one of the leading nonprofit health systems in the United States. The organization includes approximately 156,000 associates and 34,000 providers delivering care at 2,600 sites of care and over 150 hospitals in 21 states.

Ascension has recognized that its clinical practices and health care professionals have different needs. Although their organization has over 34,000 care providers, they have resisted the temptation of rigid standardization. Instead, they have pursued a portfolio approach to care, helping each market identify practice models that best match the needs and preference of their local population (using consumer and geo-mapping insights). The seven archetype practices are virtual care, direct primary care, traditional primary or specialty care, enhanced primary or specialty care, integrative medicine, comprehensive care clinics, and home-based primary care.

The leaders at Ascension subsequently developed and optimized the practice plan, care team, and staffing model for each of these practice types. This approach represents astute and dynamic leadership on behalf of a large practice organization—to simultaneously blend choice and flexibility with consistency and structural optimization. It also opened the door for clinicians to grow with the organization, allowing them to pursue different practice types as their professional and personal pursuits changed.

Although still an evolving process, the model is a paragon of partnership and collaboration between leaders and clinicians working in concert to tailor the organizational approach to the unique needs of each practice/group.

A CULTURE OF COACHING

A culture of coaching can help health care professionals gain control and flexibility and promote esprit de corps. Coaching starts with a genuine interest in the well-being of the person being coached and is based on the principle of helping recipients discover for themselves the best direction and answers. This tactic allows for personal control of decisions. The path taken may not be any different than if someone had autocratically said what to do, but the outcome is typically far better. The process basically involves inquiry and dialogue between the coach and recipient. Once recipients have made a decision, coaches should help guide them toward committing to actions to achieve their goals.

At Mayo Clinic, all newly transitioned leaders are offered executive coaching. Coaching is done in the spirit of supporting good leaders and setting them up for success. Except for senior leaders, most executive coaches are internal staff (Mayo Clinic has trained more than 2,000 physicians and administrators to be coaches).

Key characteristics of a culture of coaching include:

- Respectful communications
- Openness to inquiry and questions
- Focus on strengths
- Learning environment
- Mutual, collaborative problem solving

The coach should always have some sample questions and prompts ready to start a dialogue (Box 17.1). Of course, coaches must remember to listen reflectively, which gives the recipient control of the conversation.

Mayo Clinic not only provides coaching for new leaders, but it also trains new leaders in the skill of coaching so that they can use the skills in their roles as leaders. This organizational coaching culture increases the focus on helping teammates, improves sharing and utilization of knowledge, and leads to more participative and transparent decision making. The coaching framework inherently demonstrates several key leader behaviors (i.e., inquire, develop, and include) and drives superior leadership, team, and organizational performance and relationships. Research also indicates that a coaching culture improves individual productivity and satisfaction with work (Swensen et al, 2016).

JOB CRAFTING

Job crafting is another method that leverages control and flexibility for better well-being. As we described in Chapter 14 ("Agency Ideal Work Element: Control and Flexibility"), physicians who spent at least 20% of their time focused on the aspect of work they find most personally meaningful have burnout rates that are about half that of those who spent less than 20% of their time doing what is most meaningful to them (Shanafelt et al, 2009).

Job crafting is a perfect means to reap this dividend. Through a conversation with the leader to whom you report or on your own, explore how you can craft your job to spend 20% of your time doing what is particularly meaningful to you. You can do this by changing relationships (e.g., choosing to work with people you admire or with people who are more positive), by working across boundaries (e.g., choosing to teach or mentor

---

Box 17.1. Sample Coaching Questions and Prompts

✓ What have you tried?
✓ What do you think would make a difference?
✓ What would have to change to make that happen?
✓ What are the road blocks?
✓ How will you overcome that?
✓ Who could be a strategic partner to help you achieve this?
✓ What would progress look like?
✓ What's the key next step?
✓ Who will be impacted—positively or negatively—by these potential changes?
✓ Who has expertise in this area and would be willing to offer you feedback?
✓ Tell me more about that . . .
✓ Let me make sure I understand what you are saying . . .
✓ I'm curious about . . .
✓ Tell me more . . .
✓ Could you describe this further?
✓ What is the biggest challenge for you?
✓ What areas do you want to strengthen, improve, or develop?
✓ What do you want me to hold you accountable for as you pursue this?
✓ What are the two most important things you would like to accomplish right now?
✓ What would you do today if time was not an issue?
✓ What is your dream?
✓ Where would you like to be in your career in three to five years?
✓ When do you feel you are at your personal best?
✓ When do you feel most triggered, reactive, not at your personal best?

---

a colleague), or simply by altering your cognitive perception of your work (e.g., a custodian who sees his job as reducing infections, not just sanitizing rooms) (Berg et al, 2010).

Job crafting means taking more control of your work life, and the research is clear: Job crafting reduces burnout.

CONTROL OF WORK-LIFE INTEGRATION

As described in Chapter 14 ("Agency Ideal Work Element: Control and Flexibility"), work-life integration is a major contributor to burnout, and actions that allow for control and flexibility are the best way to solve any interference between work and personal values. Resolving work-home conflicts in favor of work is undesirable and leads to burnout. Resolving work-home conflicts in favor of personal responsibilities can also contribute to burnout (Dyrbye et al, 2011a; Dyrbye et al, 2011b). The only scenario that does not lead to burnout is a mutually acceptable solution. Health care professionals should not have to sacrifice either their personal lives or their careers. They need enough flexibility to be successful at both.

Family-friendly programs and policies are imperative for health care professionals to be satisfied and successful. Such programs include part-time work options, job-sharing options, extended hours, extended family leave, flexible scheduling, weekend surgery, and greater and lesser intensity days during the week. If appropriate and possible, consider offering work-from-home alternatives, onsite childcare, sick-child care, resources for eldercare, and concierge services for physicians.

Even when these types of benefits are offered, they are often underutilized for four common reasons:

1) Lack of awareness and limited information on eligibility or benefits
2) Workplace norms and culture that stigmatize use (and may result in punishment [e.g., lack of promotion])
3) Uninformed or unsupportive chairs
4) Concerns of shifting burden to colleagues

Mounting a general awareness campaign is often not enough to change this situation and encourage health care professionals to take advantage of the benefits. The following additional strategies can be used to promote change (Fassiotto et al, 2018; Shauman et al, 2018):

1) Structure programs to drive broad use (e.g., normalize participation in programs).
2) Tailor programs to each career track.
3) Make information readily available (e.g., distribute through multiple sources— the organization's intranet, department websites, links from personal health pages).
4) Publicize the programs through emails, stories on the intranet, postings on departmental web pages or bulletin boards, and staff meetings.
5) Make programs and materials easy to access (e.g., online forms, a physical office for the program).
6) Train chairs and underscore the value/importance of supporting the programs.
7) Build in redundancy in the work team to allow coverage and ensure that everyone knows that redundancy exists.
8) Make sure that leaders address gender and culture issues that may impede equitable use of benefits.

Case Study: Stanford University School of Medicine

Leaders at the Stanford University School of Medicine examined work-life flexibility of their faculty. Two major sources of conflict for faculty were identified:

1) Work-life conflict, caused by clashing demands of career and home
2) Work-work conflict, caused by competing organizational priorities and associated with the research, education, and clinical missions

A pilot program was developed to mitigate work-life and work-work conflict using human-centered design principles. The program was based on two strategies:

1) Integrated career-life planning that entailed coaching to create a customized plan to address both career and life goals

2) A time-banking system that rewarded behaviors that promoted team success with benefits that mitigated work-life and work-work conflicts (e.g., concierge services for staff, laundry or food preparation, delivery services)

The program was a tremendous success and increased the perception of flexibility, wellness, and professional development (Fassiotto et al, 2018). It also resulted in better professional performance and results. As one example, the academic faculty participating in the program received more grant funding awards than nonparticipants.

CONCLUSION

Creating the Ideal Work Element of control and flexibility is an important part of the Agency Action Set. Designing organizational systems and approaches that provide individual flexibility and personal input meet the human need for control over work life. They also facilitate work-life integration. When properly balanced with the best interests of the patient, the organization, and other team members, substantive benefits occur for the physical and emotional well-being of health care professionals (Box 17.2).

TOMORROW: FULFILLMENT

Jennifer's first day at work was amazing! The physician leader of the department and her administrative partner welcomed her and shared the philosophy of the group: Wide guardrails with a thin rule book! They explained their group needed to work as a team to deliver the best quality patient care. At their weekly lunch meetings, they would decide together how to improve their work life to make the best care the easiest to provide. Jennifer was amazed. She had all the flexibility and control she needed to be professionally satisfied. And she was able to co-create with colleagues the refined workflows and standardization that allowed her to be the best doctor that she could be. Jennifer is now recruiting her friends from private practice to join her.

Box 17.2. The Playbook

- Allow the local unit to define and improve the standard work.
- Review and update your organization's policies to promote flexibility and work-life integration.
- Be democratic instead of autocratic.
- Think: "Wide guardrails, thin rule book . . . and lose the middle manager mentality!"
- Use principles and guidelines instead of rules and policies whenever possible.
- Ask teams to meet outcomes, not leader-determined processes, when appropriate for the best care.
- Job craft: Help yourself or a colleague spend more time on what is most meaningful.

SUGGESTED READING

Berg JM, Grant AM, Johnson V. When callings are calling: crafting work and leisure in pursuit of unanswered occupational callings. *Org Sci.* 2010 Sep/Oct;21(5):973–4.

Burgard SA, Lin KY. Bad jobs, bad health? How work and working conditions contribute to health disparities. *Am Behav Sci.* 2013 Aug;57(8):1105–27.

Dyrbye LN, Freischlag J, Kaups KL, Oreskovich MR, Satele DV, Hanks JB, et al. Work-home conflicts have a substantial impact on career decisions that affect the adequacy of the surgical workforce. *Arch Surg.* 2012 Oct;147(10):933–9.

Dyrbye LN, Shanafelt TD, Balch CM, Satele D, Sloan J, Freischlag J. Relationship between work-home conflicts and burnout among American surgeons: a comparison by sex. *Arch Surg.* 2011a Feb;146(2):211–7.

Dyrbye LN, Sotile W, Boone S, West CP, Tan L, Satele D, et al. A survey of U.S. physicians and their partners regarding the impact of work-home conflict. *J Gen Intern Med.* 2014 Jan;29(1):155–61.

Dyrbye LN, West CP, Satele D, Sloan JA, Shanafelt TD. Work/home conflict and burnout among academic internal medicine physicians. *Arch Intern Med.* 2011b Jul 11;171(13):1207–9.

Fassiotto M, Simard C, Sandborg C, Valantine H, Raymond J. An integrated career coaching and time-banking system promoting flexibility, wellness, and success: a pilot program at Stanford University School of Medicine. *Acad Med.* 2018 Jun;93(6):881–7.

Greenhaus JH, Beutell NJ. Sources of conflict between work and family roles. *Acad Manag Rev.* 1985;10(1):76–88.

Lee B-J, Park S-G, Min K-B, Min J-Y, Hwang S-H, Leem J-H, et al. The relationship between working condition factors and well-being. *Ann Occup Environ Med.* 2014;26:34.

Linzer M, Visser MR, Oort FJ, Smets EM, McMurray JE, de Haes HC, et al. Predicting and preventing physician burnout: results from the United States and the Netherlands. *Am J Med.* 2001 Aug;111(2):170–5.

Shanafelt TD, West CP, Sloan JA, Novotny PJ, Poland GA, Menaker R, et al. Career fit and burnout among academic faculty. *Arch Intern Med.* 2009 May 25;169(10):990–5.

Shauman K, Howell LP, Paterniti DA, Beckett LA, Villablanca AC. Barriers to career flexibility in academic medicine: a qualitative analysis of reasons for the underutilization of family-friendly policies, and implications for institutional change and department chair leadership. *Acad Med.* 2018 Feb;93(2):246–55.

Swensen S, Gorringe G, Caviness J, Peters D. Leadership by design: intentional organization development by physician leaders. *J Manag Dev.* 2016;35(4):549–70.

Yandrick RM. High demand, low-control jobs reduce productivity and increase workplace disability costs. *Behav Healthc Tomorrow.* 1997 Jun;6(3):40–4.

18

AGENCY ACTION: CREATING A VALUES ALIGNMENT COMPACT

TODAY: DISTRESS

Phillip is an affiliated physician with the flagship hospital in his metropolitan area. He used to like taking care of his patients at this hospital until "the administration" started setting expectations for his behavior and performance. Although he knew the hospital viewed him primarily as just a "revenue center," he liked his autonomy. Those days are gone, and it is upsetting to him. The hospital administrators have decided to create a Values Alignment Compact, and Phillip is skeptical. He is looking into requesting privileges at the other area hospital so that he "can do his own thing again."

◆ ◆ ◆

Creating a Values Alignment Compact is the final Agency Action. For optimal performance, health care professionals and their organizations must have values that align (i.e., providing healing and high-quality care to the patients and community they serve). Health care professionals typically approach their work with a sense of calling, most often centered on healing, relieving suffering, and demonstrating compassion for fellow human beings experiencing illness. Health care professionals are also loyal to their community (i.e., their neighbors, family members, and co-workers). They must believe that their organization is also committed to these goals and values. If leaders can help health care professionals recognize how their personal and the organizational values intersect, they will create engagement.

Values alignment forms a powerful bond between individuals and an organization—one that cultivates meaning and purpose in work. Values alignment is central to well-being, mitigates burnout, and promotes esprit de corps. This alignment of values must be authentic. A polished mission statement is meaningless if the organization's actions and behaviors are incongruent. Health care professionals will see through the charade. If leaders primarily communicate about subjects such as payer mix and net operating income, health care professionals will recognize the organization's true values, which will create a chasm between the work professionals aspire to do and the motivation of those to whom they report. Such values misalignment creates cognitive dissonance and moral distress.

PROFESSIONAL VALUES ALIGNMENT COMPACT

In health care, a professional Values Alignment Compact is a structured conversation between medical center leaders and clinicians that results in a mutual understanding (and a document) articulating shared goals. The Values Alignment Compact also clarifies roles: what clinicians expect from their organization and what their organization expects in return. The process of developing a compact is a dialogue that nurtures the culture of "interdependency" of leadership (administration) and health care professionals (Silversin and Kornacki, 2000; Kornacki and Silversin, 2012). Once developed, the compact can be used to help assess the current state and serve as a guide for future decision making. Joyce K. Lammert, M.D., of the Virginia Mason Medical Center, stated it this way, "What matters is living by the compact and sticking to it over time. That's how the culture is changed."

Different disciplines in health care have both shared and distinct values, and to achieve optimal accordance, Values Alignment Compacts must address both aspects. This can be achieved by developing separate compacts for the different groups of health care professionals (e.g., nursing, physicians, administrators) or by having subsections within an overall compact for different disciplines. All Values Alignment Compacts:

1) Should be explicit, written, and developed through multiple iterations by both parties (e.g., committees, task forces).
2) Should articulate the expectations that health care professionals have of the organization and that the organization has of the professionals.
3) Must be aligned with the stated mission and vision of the organization. This should be unambiguously affirmed.
4) Must be embraced and the principles of the compact modeled by all leaders and health care professionals.
5) Must be co-created by health care professionals and leaders.

The Mayo Clinic Compact

Mayo Clinic has had well-crafted mission, vision, and organizational value statements for decades. In 2011, we realized that these statements were not the same as and could not substitute for a Values Alignment Compact between Mayo Clinic and its people.

The Compact (Box 18.1) Mayo Clinic made with its voting staff was co-created by clinicians, scientists, and administrators over a two-year period of discussion and reflection. The process was led by one of us (T.D.S.) and engaged approximately 2,000 staff (e.g., through focus groups, surveys, department dialogues, task forces), over 95% of whom endorsed the principles and concepts it espoused (Shanafelt and Noseworthy, 2017). The feedback included constructive ideas for how Mayo Clinic could better realize its stated aspirations.

The Compact was built on the Mayo Clinic principle that administrators and physicians are dyad partners. It articulates what Mayo Clinic stands for, its core values, how administrators and physicians will work together, and how change will be approached. Producing and maintaining a Values Alignment Compact ensures culture and values alignment.

Case Study: Working in Partnership

Robert R. Waller, M.D., served as Mayo Clinic president and chief executive officer (CEO) between 1986 and 1999. During his tenure, he successfully moved the responsibility for *continuous improvement*, one of the tenets of the Mayo Clinic Compact, from the Quality Academy and 300 systems engineers to one of a shared responsibility across 40,000 staff from all disciplines and in all job classifications.

Box 18.1. The Mayo Clinic Compact

Mayo Clinic, and its physicians and scientists, have a shared commitment to achieve Mayo Clinic's mission, which is built upon:

A Patient-Centered, Integrated Practice

- We will treat all patients with respect and compassion.
- We will communicate with patients using language they understand.
- We will consider the whole person and not just the diagnosis.
- We will integrate community-based care with the supporting expertise of tertiary referral centers to provide optimal care to patients.
- We will integrate the expertise of multiple disciplines to meet the patient's health care needs.

A Commitment to Excellence in Patient Care, Research, and Education

- Patient care, research, and education are all essential for Mayo Clinic to succeed.
  - ○ Patient care: Delivery of the highest quality patient care is the primary goal of Mayo Clinic.
  - ○ Research: Delivery of the highest quality care depends on innovation and scientific discovery that improve our current knowledge.
  - ○ Education: Delivery of the highest quality care requires that we train the next generation of physicians and scientists.
- Delivery of the highest quality care requires that our physicians stay current with new discoveries that allow us to rapidly translate advances into our practice.
- The success of our education and research programs is part of our competitive edge and allows us to recruit and retain the best physicians and scientists.

An Inclusive Culture of Professionalism, Collegiality, and Mutual Support

- We will provide support to our colleagues as they strive to provide the highest quality patient care.
- We will invest in the professional development of our colleagues by sharing knowledge and providing constructive feedback.
- We will address disagreements about patient care promptly, directly, and privately.

A Framework of Trust and Accountability

- We will cultivate an environment of mutual trust where leaders trust staff and staff trust leaders.
- We will trust the professional integrity of our physicians and scientists.
- Our physicians and scientists are accountable to adhere to the highest standards of professional behavior commensurate with this trust.

(continued)

Appendix 15.1. (*Continued*)

A Commitment to Continuously Improve the Value and Efficiency of Care Delivered

- We will strive to optimize the efficiency and productivity of our physicians by having them do what only physicians can do.
- We will strive to relieve physicians and scientists of administrative tasks to allow them to stay focused on practice, education, and research activities.

An Expectation That All Physicians and Scientists Are Leaders and Role Models

- The behavior and professionalism of our physicians and scientists define our culture and are examples that other employees will follow.
- Regardless of formal title, all physicians and scientists are leaders whose words and actions should model professionalism to other members of the care delivery team and organization.

A Belief That We Are Stronger as a Team Than as Individuals

- We believe the resources, environment, and collective expertise of Mayo Clinic maximize the abilities of our individual physicians and scientists to provide optimal patient care.
- We believe that the collective expertise of our physicians and scientists should be used to develop consistent approaches for patients seeking care at any Mayo Clinic site.
- All members of our care delivery team are critical to delivering optimal patient care and should be valued.
- We will communicate respectfully and clearly with all members of the multidisciplinary health care team.
- Although a collaborative approach requires sacrificing some autonomy, we strive to consider the input of physicians and scientists as we develop and refine the consensus-driven approach.
- We believe in the value of rotating physician leadership and administrative partnerships.

Opportunity for Professional Development and Career Fulfillment

- We are dedicated to creating an environment of opportunity and professional development that allows physicians and scientists to continually improve.
- Although professional development and career fulfillment cannot be guaranteed, opportunities to pursue these goals will be provided.

Open Dialogue and Information Sharing

- Bidirectional communication between Mayo Clinic's leaders and physicians and scientists is essential to the success of the organization.
- This communication should be delivered in a direct, timely, and respectful manner.

Appendix 15.1. (*Continued*)

A Commitment to Staff Members' Health and Personal Well-being

- We value the well-being of our staff.
- We believe personal well-being contributes to sound clinical judgment and is therefore important for our physicians to provide optimal clinical care.
- Medicine is a demanding profession, and we must be dedicated to care for ourselves and each other.
- We are committed to providing timely assistance to physicians and scientists who experience distress because of personal or professional challenges.

A Commitment to Adapt to Change Together in a Manner Consistent With Our Values

- The medical delivery system is influenced by many factors outside our control and is constantly changing.
- We will be innovative and adapt to these changes in a manner that is consistent with our principles and allows us to achieve the Mayo Clinic mission.
- Successful innovation requires our staff to work in partnership with leaders.

The Mayo Clinic Compact has helped define, articulate, and elucidate the culture for the entire Mayo Clinic workforce.

One day, Waller came back to his office after a late meeting. A group of custodians was on dinner break, and he joined them for a chat. After a few minutes, one of the custodians excused himself, saying he had to go to a continuous improvement meeting (evidently, that was more important than dinner with the CEO!).

Waller later said, "That was it! I knew then that we would be all right. The culture of continuous improvement was embedded deep in the organization. We had partners everywhere."

This anecdote is a perfect example of values alignment between individuals and their organization. This group of custodians was trusted and treated with respect. Because they were treated as partners, they behaved like partners. They understood that they had two jobs: to do their work and to improve their work. This was their Values Alignment Compact. The leaders were sending the following message to the continuous improvement teams: "Your work matters and we trust you." Through partnerships, Waller was aligning values at all levels of the organization.

CONCLUSION

Creating a Values Alignment Compact, the final Agency Action, is critical for creating esprit de corps and reducing burnout. Values misalignment creates cognitive dissonance, which leads to moral distress, and is a major cause of burnout. Compacts created through an organizational dialogue are an effective tactic to align values and nurture a patient-centered culture. Mayo Clinic has long been recognized as one of the best organizations in the United States for which to work. This recognition is the result of decades of relentless focus on caring for the caregivers (Berry and Seltman, 2008). It is part of the compact Mayo Clinic leadership has with its people.

TOMORROW: FULFILLMENT

In his discussions with the clinical leaders about the Values Alignment Compact (he no longer calls them "the administration"), Phillip came to understand that patient care could be much better if they all worked together on the common ground of aligned values. The organization pledged to support his well-being and to focus on quality patient care in all standardization conversations. He was able to discuss his concerns about being considered a revenue center as part of the values alignment conversation. Phillip now understands that choosing to work in the flagship hospital and embracing the expectations of medical staff will make him a better doctor, and he appreciates the mutual understanding that resulted from the conversation around the Compact. He feels respected as a professional who has ideas that can help not just his team and department thrive, but the whole organization.

Box 18.2. The Playbook

- Consider creating a professional Values Alignment Compact.
- Start with a conversation between senior leadership and professional staff leaders.
- Discuss these questions in a series of conversations:
  - What matters to you most as a health care professional?
  - What is the purpose of our organization?
  - How do your values as a health care professional and the mission and purpose of our organization align?
  - What are our core values? What do we stand for?
  - What qualities describe how we should work together?
  - What should health care professionals expect to receive from the organization? What should the organization expect from its people?
  - How will we approach change?
- After initial discussions, allow all parties involved to co-create a draft compact. Seek broad feedback and input to refine and improve the document. Have the right bodies endorse/approve the compact. These conversations and the process of developing the compact are often as important as the written compact document.

SUGGESTED READING

Berry LL, Seltman KD. Management lessons from Mayo Clinic: inside one of the world's most admired service organizations. New York (NY): McGraw-Hill; 2008.

Kornacki MJ, Silversin J. Leading physicians through change: how to achieve and sustain results. Tampa (FL): American College of Physician Executives; 2012.

Shanafelt TD, Noseworthy JH. Executive leadership and physician well-being: nine organizational strategies to promote engagement and reduce burnout. Mayo Clin Proc. 2017 Jan;92(1):129–46.

Silversin J, Kornacki MJ. Creating a physician compact that drives group success. Med Group Manage J. 2000 May-Jun;47(3):54–8, 60, 62.

Virginia Mason Institute. Improving your organization's relationship with your physicians [Internet]. 2012 [cited 2018 Dec 5]. Available from: https://www.virginiamasoninstitute.org/2012/05/part-1-would-you-like-to-improve-your-organizations-relationship-with-your-physicians/.

19

COHERENCE ACTION SET: INTRODUCTION

People who are truly strong lift others up.
People who are truly powerful bring others together.
—Michelle Obama

Coherence is an organizational state in which all the parts fit together comfortably to form a united whole. The elements needed for Coherence (i.e., organizational culture, leaders, policy, and process) limit Agency, the capacity of individuals or teams to act independently, which we described in previous chapters. The ultimate work situation encompasses a healthy, dynamic equilibrium between individual and team agency with organizational coherence. Establishing the most fruitful balance of Coherence and Agency is a fundamental challenge for leaders in nurturing esprit de corps.

The Coherence Action Set is designed to mitigate or eliminate known specific drivers of professional burnout and to develop supportive leaders and systems that foster the interrelated Ideal Work Elements.

Primary burnout drivers addressed by Coherence Actions:

1) Excessive workload and job demands
2) Inefficiency and inadequate resources
3) Difficulties with work-life integration

Ideal Work Elements cultivated by Coherence Actions:

1) Professional development and mentorship (Chapter 20)
2) Fairness and equity (Chapter 21)
3) Safety (Chapter 22)

Coherence Actions:

1) Selecting and developing leaders (Chapter 23)
2) Improving practice efficiency (Chapter 24)
3) Establishing fair and just accountability (Chapter 25)
4) Forming safe havens (Chapter 26)

In this section, we will present the three germane Ideal Work Elements followed directly by the four aligned Coherence Actions.

20

COHERENCE IDEAL WORK ELEMENT: PROFESSIONAL DEVELOPMENT AND MENTORSHIP

> Leadership is about making others better as a result of your presence and making sure that impact lasts in your absence.
> —Sheryl Sanberg

The first Ideal Work Element in the Coherence Action Set is professional development and mentorship. For organizations, professional development and mentorship are about investing in individuals, unlocking and developing their talent, and harnessing that talent to help the organization achieve its mission. Once this occurs, people will be better connected to the meaning and purpose of their work and equipped to achieve their ambitions more effectively. When individuals experience professional fulfillment and esprit de corps, extraordinary care and organizational performance will follow.

Professional development and mentorship are fundamentally about creating human and social capital. Human capital is the reservoir of competencies, knowledge, and personality attributes necessary to perform important work and create value that results from a combination of talent, education, and experience. Social capital is the extent to which human capital is knitted together to harness the power of synergistic interconnectedness, mutual respect, and trust to accomplish a common purpose.

STRONG-LINK SPORTS AND WEAK-LINK SPORTS

In a strong-link sport like basketball, a dominant player (e.g., LeBron James, Diana Taurasi) can take over games and create a winning team almost single handedly. In contrast, in a weak-link sport like soccer, the aggregate strength of the team is more important than having a superstar. In fact, having a superstar (e.g., Alex Morgan, Cristiano Ronaldo) does not guarantee that you will have a winning team, because in these types of sports (i.e., larger teams and more interaction), the outcome is more dependent on the collective play. A single weak link (e.g., a poor defensive player guarding the left side of the soccer field) can be exploited by the opponent and result in a goal. In this low-scoring sport, that goal may be sufficient to win the game. Indeed, the weakest link is as or more important to the outcome than the strongest link (e.g., the opposing team exploits the weak link) (Gladwell, 2017).

Health Care as a Weak-Link Sport

Health care is like a weak-link sport. The ultimate patient outcome is less dependent on the skill of a single, talented superstar than on the collective talent and excellence of a team of care providers. Even the greatest superstars in health care (e.g., unusually talented surgeons) are dependent on their teammates (i.e., the anesthesiologist, surgical scrub team, pathologist, and postoperative care nurses). Accordingly, to build a strong team, the skills and expertise of the entire team must be developed for the best patient outcomes, beginning with orientations and onboarding for new hires and then continuing education and maintaining certifications for existing employees.

Leadership development is essential to professional development, and we will discuss this in detail in Chapter 23 ("Coherence Action: Selecting and Developing Leaders"). Identifying those moving along the leadership trajectory and helping them develop leadership skills will create a healthy leader pipeline with culturally aligned, ready-now, diverse candidates in the key succession pools. The best approach to leadership development (and the one used at Mayo Clinic) should be multidisciplinary, with physicians, nurses, and administrators in programs together. The best organizational approach to leadership development should be consistent and engage leaders from all sites and locations across the organization. Each leader position has a succession pool of candidates that is rated for readiness, leader behaviors, and ethnic and gender diversity. The clinicians in each pool are selectively given leader experiences, coaching, mentoring, and coursework to help them develop and advance as value-aligned, team-oriented, and patient-centered servant leaders.

MENTORSHIP AND COACHING

Mentor was a figure described in Greek mythology as an older, caring man who was trusted by Odysseus to look after his son, Telemachus, and help him develop into a thoughtful young man while Odysseus was away at war. Today's mentors must also be caring people who voluntarily give their time and attention to teach, support, encourage, and develop less-experienced individuals. We believe that mentorship and coaching should be employed as part of a comprehensive professional and leadership development culture. However, effectively developing others through mentoring and coaching requires a variety of skills for which health care professionals, including clinical leaders, often receive the minimal training.

Coaching is complementary to but different from mentorship. Mentoring involves advising, recommending, and shepherding (e.g., "I think you should reorganize your leadership team like this . . . "). Coaching is characterized by inquiry and problem solving (e.g., "What do you think would be the best structure for your leadership team? Why? How would that make a difference? Is there another approach that might work better?"). Coaching helps individuals discover their own best approaches (see Chapter 17, "Agency Action: Introducing Control and Flexibility" for additional information on a culture of coaching) rather than giving advice or instruction.

The best professional development cultures blend mentorship and coaching. A blended mentoring-coaching culture supports individual, team, and organizational development and performance. The key characteristics of a mentoring-coaching culture include respectful communication, a spirit of inquiry (i.e., asking questions), a focus on strengths and learning, and mutual, collaborative problem solving. Mentors and coaches do not have to be anyone in the employee's reporting structure, and individuals can serve in both roles. Research indicates that mentoring and coaching improve overall productivity, employee satisfaction, and customer satisfaction. Together, mentoring and coaching result in improved relationships, good feelings, teamwork, and quality (McGovern et al, 2001; Phillips and Phillips, 2005) (Box 20.1).

Individuals are ultimately responsible for their professional development. However, most employees achieve much more with mentors and coaches than by themselves. It is important that health care professionals believe that their leaders care about them and have an interest in their careers. Mentoring and coaching are examples of how leaders can show that they care. Appendix 15.1 (Chapter 15, "Agency Action: Measuring Leader Behaviors") gives specific actions for how leaders can provide useful feedback and coaching and how leaders can encourage professionals to develop their talents and skills.

Box 20.1. Facilitating Professional Development

One Saturday morning after a junior surgeon completed his patient hospital rounds, he was surprised to be paged by his department chair who asked him what type of coffee he wanted.

The chair had come to the hospital to help this junior colleague assemble material for his academic appointment proposal for promotion to associate professor. When the chair delivered the coffee and they sat down to work together on the promotion letter, the junior surgeon cried . . . from joy. He said he had never dreamed a department chair would come in on the weekend to help him and, on top of it, buy him a cup of coffee.

The chair did much more by this action than just help the junior surgeon with his promotion proposal. He showed the junior surgeon how to be an amazing mentor.

CONCLUSION

Professional development and mentorship, an important Ideal Work Element, are facilitated by Coherence Actions that help unite the workforce. Health care professionals need to know that those leading them are interested in helping them develop. Organizational activities that promote and grow mentorship, coaching, and skills to facilitate professional development should be part of every health care organization's professional and leadership development culture. If your organization hasn't begun offering these activities, get started now.

> The best time to plant a tree was 20 years ago.
> The second best time is now.
> —Chinese proverb

SUGGESTED READING

Gladwell M. My little hundred million [Internet]. 2017 [cited 2019 Jul 3]. Available from: https://blog.simonsays.ai/my-little-hundred-million-with-malcolm-gladwell-s1-e6-revisionist-history-podcast-transcript-e1942c633432.

Gladwell M. Outliers: the story of success. New York (NY): Little, Brown and Company; 2011.

Harter JK, Schmidt FL, Hayes TL. Business-unit-level relationship between employee satisfaction, employee engagement, and business outcomes: a meta-analysis. J Appl Psychol. 2002 Apr;87(2):268–79.

IBM. Capitalizing on complexity: insights from the global chief executive office study [Internet]. 2010 [cited 2019 Mar 29]. Available from: https://www.ibm.com/downloads/cas/1VZV5X8J.

Johansen B. Get there early: sensing the future to compete in the present. San Francisco (CA): Berrett-Koehler Publishers; 2007.

McGovern J, Lindemann M, Vergara M, Murphy S, Barker L, Warrenfeltz R. Maximizing the impact of executive coaching: behavioral change, organizational outcomes, and return on investment. Manchester Rev. 2001;6(1):3–11.

O'Leonard K, Loew L. Leadership development factbook 2012. San Francisco (CA): Bersin and Associates; 2012.

Petrie N. Future trends in leadership development [Internet]. 2011 [cited 2019 Mar 29]. Available from: http://www.isacs.org/uploads/file/article%20CCL%20white%20paper%20Petrie%20vertical%20development.pdf.

Phillips C, Phillips JJ. Measuring ROI in executive coaching. Int J Coach Organ. 2005; 3(1):53–62.

Swensen S, Gorringe G, Caviness J, Peters D. Leadership by design: intentional organization development of physician leaders. J Manag Dev. 2016;35(4):549–70.

Yip J, Ernst C, Campbell M. Boundary spanning leadership: mission critical perspectives from the executive suite [Internet]. 2015 [cited 2019 Mar 29]. Available from: https://www.ccl.org/wp-content/uploads/2015/04/BoundarySpanningLeadership.pdf.

21

COHERENCE IDEAL WORK ELEMENT:
FAIRNESS AND EQUITY

I think perfect objectivity is an unrealistic goal; fairness, however, is not.
—Michael Pollan

The second Ideal Work Element in the Coherence Action Set is fairness and equity.

INNATE SENSE OF FAIRNESS

A famous experiment at Emory University involved capuchin monkeys, a species known for their intelligence (de Waal and Davis, 2003). The monkeys were consistently given cucumbers as a reward for successfully completing tasks. The monkeys could see each other and the consistent reward process. It seemed fair to them.

Then something changed.

In full view of a comrade, one of the monkeys was given sweet grapes, a more desirable reward, for completing the same task. The second monkey became very upset. The system was no longer equitable. In protest of the injustice, the monkey who felt cheated threw its cucumber at the trainer!

The monkeys rejected unfair treatment.

FAIRNESS

Human beings also reject unfair treatment. We have an innate sense of fairness and a desire to be treated equitably. Health care organizations and providers have a collective responsibility to do everything possible, within the scope of their influence, to treat everyone fairly. If this aspiration is successful, health care teams will function better and patients' experiences will be better. When leaders treat professionals with fairness, they engage staff in ways that enable trust, vulnerability, authenticity, and community.

To build confidence among health care professionals that the organization is treating them with fairness, leaders should be transparent in all matters that are appropriate. In our discussion of intrinsic motivation (Chapter 29, "Camaraderie Ideal Work Element: Intrinsic Motivation and Rewards"), we emphasize that money and benefits are not among the top motivators of discretionary effort. However, money and benefits are *dis-satisfiers* when professionals feel like they are being treated unfairly.

The best organizations are transparent with quality, financial, and salary data. They allow everyone to know the criteria used to make management decisions. This transparency applies to pay scales, privileges, work and call schedules, academic promotions, and other factors. Like others, health care professionals often fill in the blanks when information is not shared openly. They also tend to assume the worst (e.g., that others may be getting a better deal). Once information is available for all to see, comparisons are less likely to be "the thief of joy" (Theodore Roosevelt). Thus, transparency prevents misinformation and leads to a mutual growth in trust and understanding. Transparency reassures employees that the organization has a moral compass and will treat its people fairly (Box 21.1).

FAIR AND JUST ACCOUNTABILITY

Another facet of evenhandedness is the practice of fair and just accountability. It is also an important attribute of a supportive work environment and needs to exist in the health care workplace to mitigate burnout and promote esprit de corps. In such a culture, human limitations are acknowledged and a framework employed of compassionate improvement, not shame and blame. The foundation of fair and just accountability is, for example, appropriately dealing with individuals involved in adverse patient events who made expected human factors errors within imperfect systems. Properly instituted, fair and just accountability also promotes psychological safety and routine reporting of all adverse events and near misses. The action of implementing fair and just accountability will be presented in Chapter 25 ("Coherence Action: Establishing Fair and Just Accountability").

CONCLUSION

Fairness and equity are important elements of the ideal work environment. Health care professionals need transparency in all matters that make sense including the way pay, privileges, and work schedules are determined. This Ideal Work Element also requires fair and just accountability to provide support when clinicians experience a traumatic patient adverse care event (regardless of whether the cause was a systems failure or anticipated human error). Behaviors and actions that grow fairness and equity should be embedded into the functional infrastructure of leadership and organization and will be described in Chapter 23 ("Coherence Action: Selecting and Developing Leaders"), Chapter 25 ("Coherence Action: Establishing Fair and Just Accountability"), and Chapter 26 ("Coherence Action: Forming Safe Havens").

Box 21.1. Salary Transparency at Mayo Clinic

At Mayo Clinic, all physician salaries are set with a methodology that is transparent to all. Salaries are based on two factors: specialty and length of service (independent of academic rank, relative value unit generation, gender, and age). Incremental salary steps occur in years one to five; after year five, salaries within the specialty and annual adjustments are the same for everyone. National benchmarks for each discipline determine salaries, not productivity/throughput. With a pure salary system, there is no financial conflict of interest with the needs of patients. Surgeons are not paid more or less because they do or do not recommend an operation or expensive test or treatment. Specialists are not paid more if they order more tests or expensive therapies. There is no guessing about which team member is making more, no comparisons made among staff, no concern about gender inequity, no need to argue for pay or raises, and no need to explain the importance of contributions made.

Everyone is treated in a consistent and equitable manner.

SUGGESTED READING

de Waal FB, Davis JM. Capuchin cognitive ecology: cooperation based on projected returns. Neuropsychologia. 2003;41(2):221–8.

Hall LW, Scott SD. The second victim of adverse health care events. Nurs Clin North Am. 2012 Sep;47(3):383–93.

Marx D. Patient safety and the "just culture": a primer for health care executives. New York (NY): Columbia University; 2001.

Swensen SJ, Dilling JA, Milliner DS, Zimmerman RS, Maples WJ, Lindsay ME, et al. Quality: the Mayo Clinic approach. Am J Med Qual. 2009 Sep-Oct;24(5):428–40.

Thomas KW. Intrinsic motivation at work: what really drives employee engagement. San Francisco (CA): Berrett-Koehler Publishers; 2009.

22

COHERENCE IDEAL WORK ELEMENT: SAFETY

You do your best work when you feel safe.
—Julianna Margulies

The third Ideal Work Element in the Coherence Action Set is safety. Health care professionals need to feel both physically and psychologically safe at work. Although there is still much room to improve, most organizations tend to do better attending to physical safety than they do to psychological safety, so let's begin with the weakest link.

PSYCHOLOGICAL SAFETY

Psychological safety for health care professionals forms part of the bedrock of esprit de corps. Psychological safety includes a work environment where professionals are comfortable speaking up and sharing their perspectives without feeling insecure or embarrassed or fearing retribution. A psychologically safe environment is also one where disruptive and abusive behavior is absolutely unacceptable. Dismissive behavior and incivility, which are insidious and prevalent, cannot be tolerated. These behaviors are the acids that corrode esprit de corps.

Health care professionals need to feel there is safe haven when adverse events occur because of system failures or expected human factors errors. They must work in an environment where support exists for emotional distress triggered by medical errors or poor patient outcomes, which are inevitable. In a psychologically safe environment, health care professionals know that they won't be punished when they make a mistake or speak their mind.

In a two-year survey conducted by Google on team performance, the highest performing teams were found to have one trait in common (Schneider, 2017). The trait was not charismatic leaders, extraordinary IQs, free meals and dry cleaning, or dollar value of resources. The trait was psychological safety: a mutual respect and a team culture that made it comfortable for all to contribute. Everyone was respected regardless of personality, gender, creed, or color.

Unfortunately, many health care organizations are far from providing a psychologically safe environment. In survey data from 382,834 hospital respondents across 630 hospitals, 68% of employees indicated that they were "afraid to ask questions when something does not seem right" (AHRQ, 2018). If all staff were comfortable asking questions and shared their insights or perspectives, they could prevent harm or even save a patient's life. If their perceptions are incorrect, the dialogue nonetheless serves as a learning experience that facilitates professional development and deeper expertise, which enhances the collective effectiveness and well-being of the care team and may benefit future patients.

Organizations need to ensure that psychological safety is part of the work culture if they hope to eliminate moral distress and burnout among their employees and provide superlative patient care (Box 22.1).

Box 22.1 Moral Distress and Psychological Safety

A patient in the intensive care unit (ICU) is struggling to hang onto life. The doctors, with deep knowledge of her medical condition, know that there is a reasonable (20%) chance of recovery and believe they should provide aggressive care for the next 72 hours to see if she will respond. They have not, however, discussed this with other team members. The ICU nurses incorrectly assume the care is futile. They are with the family all day, and the patient's husband and children are uncertain, anxious, and wondering if continuing care is the right thing to do. Seeing the aggressive treatment continue has caused the nurses moral distress. They are unable to sincerely reassure the family or re-enforce a consistent care team message because no one has shown the respect and wisdom of involving them in developing the plan.

If the physicians had shared the medical information with the nurses about the likelihood of recovery and the plan to pursue aggressive care for only 72 hours, this moral distress would likely not have occurred. The nurses could have explained their concerns and the family's anxiety to the physicians on the team. The team could have set up a care conference with the family and all care team members to collaboratively develop a unified plan. The physician and nurses could have sent a consistent message to the family.

In this example, creating psychological safety is primarily the physician's responsibility because of the high power-distance index (i.e., the measure of the distribution of power between persons in different roles). The physician should have set the tone for open two-way communication among members of the care team and shown respect and value for the expertise of the nurses by involving them in the discussion of the treatment plan. The failure of the team to communicate perpetuated the family's anxiety, created moral distress for the nurses, and robbed the physicians of valuable insights from the nursing team that may have improved medical decision making.

Safe Haven

To help maintain the emotional well-being of health care professionals, organizations must also deal with preventable harm in a just manner—one that addresses factors contributing to defective care rather than assumes that an individual is to blame. The primary goal of a supportive team culture is creation of a safe haven that mitigates the emotional trauma of clinicians involved with patient deaths and adverse events. The components and actions involved in such a culture will be described in Chapter 26 ("Coherence Action: Forming Safe Havens").

Organizations that establish multidisciplinary improvement teams to address root causes of harm events gain substantial dividends from the time and resources invested. The first dividend is a safer system (usually with a lower cost structure). The teamwork cultivated through the process of identifying and eradicating the system variables and processes that cause harm events increases camaraderie, which is a second dividend.

PHYSICAL SAFETY

What industry has the highest rates of occupational injury in the United States?

Manufacturing? Mining? Professional sports?

Nope.

Health care!

Evidence from the U.S. Bureau of Labor Statistics shows that hospitals are one of the most hazardous places to work (OSHA, 2013). Hospitals have a higher rate of "days away" among workers than construction, manufacturing, or private industry. In addition, health care professionals suffer occupational injuries at nearly three times the rate of employees in the professional and business sectors and approximately double the rate of private industry overall (OSHA, 2013).

This was not the case just two decades ago. These statistics indicate that, even as safety in other sectors has improved, the health care industry is falling short in caring for and protecting its professionals. What protective measures do health care professionals receive for the occupational risks they are exposed to, including burnout and exposure to human suffering?

Physical safety means that clinicians can work on highly functional teams within well-designed systems without fear of injuring themselves. This includes avoiding such problems as needle sticks, back injuries, and occupational overuse injuries. Organizations have an obligation to address these physical safety issues for health care professionals. Addressing safety sends a strong message to staff that leadership cares, which contributes to esprit de corps in three fundamental ways:

1) It communicates to health care professionals that their well-being is a priority for the organization.
2) It connects leaders and clinicians in pursuit of a common goal.
3) It teaches the discipline of addressing systems issues, which is also needed to eradicate most burnout drivers.

Violence and Mistreatment in the Workplace

Workplace violence is another important aspect of physical safety for all professionals. Threats and violence from patients or their family members are increasing. This mistreatment can take the form of verbal abuse, racial or gender discrimination, sexual harassment, or physical threats. Patients with behavioral disorders and those using illicit drugs are more likely to be violent against members of the caregiver team. However, mistreatment and abuse is happening across health care broadly and is not limited to such patients or clinical work areas.

Hospital leaders should know of potential risks and provide appropriate staffing, physical space, and security to simultaneously meet the needs of all patients and ensure the safety of the caregivers. Leaders should take a holistic approach to support and protect their people as they deal with these challenges.

Organization best practices should include primary prevention (de-escalation training), tracking and early detection (part of morning huddles and hand offs), appropriate responses (address the behavior and support the individual who experienced the mistreatment), and secondary prevention (instituting measures that preclude recurrence). This integrated approach is best accomplished through collaboration of security officers, nursing leaders, medical team leaders, behavioral health teams, the patient experience office, human resources, and the legal team.

Case Study: Alcoa and Safety

The transformative story of Alcoa (Aluminum Company of America) under the leadership of Paul O'Neill makes a good case study for increasing physical safety in the health care industry. From his first day at the company, O'Neill focused relentlessly on worker safety to renovate the entire business and its culture. He told employees and shareholders that profits were not as important as worker safety. Thus, Alcoa became one of the safest workplace cultures in the world (Duhigg, 2014).

In the end, O'Neill proved what he knew at the onset: making employee well-being and safety the top priorities increased employee engagement, lowered costs, increased profits, and led to greater quality and productivity. When Paul O'Neill retired 14 years later to become the U.S. Department of the Treasury secretary, Alcoa's annual net income and the value of the stock were five times larger than before he arrived. Doing the right thing can, indeed, be good for both the organization and its people.

PSYCHOLOGICAL AND PHYSICAL SAFETY INTERTWINED

In some instances, the psychological and physical well-being of health care professionals is intertwined. When stress levels of health care professionals are higher, for example, patients and professionals themselves don't fare as well. For patients, there are higher rates of physical injury, medical and medication errors, falls, and decubitus ulcers. For clinicians, there are higher rates of on-the-job accidents, motor vehicle accidents, and burnout. Burnout is associated with diffuse aches, insomnia, memory and concentration difficulties, profound fatigue, anxiety, irritability, and absenteeism. Given these facts, it is imperative that organizational leaders address factors that increase levels of psychological and physical safety in the workplace.

Case Study: Social Pollution

Jeffrey Pfeffer, professor at the Stanford Graduate School of Business, coined the term "social pollution of the workplace," defined as workplace stress, long hours, no health insurance, layoffs, job insecurity, toxic cultures, no job control, micromanagement, and high job demands. According to Pfeffer, the social pollution employees experience in the workplace is the fifth leading cause of death in America (Pfeffer, 2018)! He estimates that 120,000 deaths each year and 5% to 8% of annual U.S. health care costs may be attributable to how companies treat their workforce. For these statistics to change for the better, Pfeffer believes that companies should focus on eliminating the management practices that lead to "social pollution" of the workplace rather than expecting the workers to find their own solutions.

CONCLUSION

Physical and psychological safety are important elements of the ideal work environment for health care professionals. Health care organizations should regularly assess both types of safety in their clinical work environments and mitigate factors that erode these qualities. Improving physical and psychological safety is central to creating Coherence and must be embedded into the leadership and organization infrastructure.

SUGGESTED READING

Agency for Healthcare Research and Quality (AHRQ). Hospital survey on patient safety culture: 2018 user database report [Internet]. 2018 [cited 2019 Oct 31]. Available from: https://www.ahrq.gov/sites/default/files/wysiwyg/sops/quality-patient-safety/patients afetyculture/2018hospitalsopsreport.pdf.

Duhigg C. The power of habit: why we do what we do in life and business. New York (NY): Random House; 2014.

Occupational Safety and Health Administration (OSHA), U.S. Department of Labor. Caring for our caregivers: facts about hospital worker safety [Internet]. 2013 [cited 2019 Apr 2]. Available from: https://www.osha.gov/dsg/hospitals/documents/1.2_Factbook_508.pdf.

Occupational Safety and Health Administration (OSHA), U.S. Department of Labor. Worker safety in your hospital [Internet]. 2013 [cited 2019 Apr 2]. Available from: https://www.osha.gov/dsg/hospitals/documents/1.1_Data_highlights_508.pdf.

Pfeffer J. Dying for a paycheck: how modern management harms employee health and company performance and what we can do about it. New York (NY): Harper Collins; 2018.

Savic I. Structural changes of the brain in relation to occupational stress. Cereb Cortex. 2015 Jun;25(6):1554–64.

Schneider M. Google spent 2 years studying 180 teams: the most successful ones shared these 5 traits [Interent]. 2017 [cited 2019 Apr 2]. Available from: https://www.inc.com/michael-schneider/google-thought-they-knew-how-to-create-the-perfect.html.

23

COHERENCE ACTION: SELECTING
AND DEVELOPING LEADERS

TODAY: DISTRESS

Cordelia is an oncologist. She feels like her supervisor, a hospital administrator with little clinical knowledge, behaves like a "boss" rather than a leader or mentor. Her supervisor is not interested in her ideas or her career. She does not feel valued. She and her colleagues don't understand what is going on with the organization broadly or how the efforts of their group fit into the plan. They are told how many patients they are expected to see and what needs to be done without explanation or dialogue. Cordelia does not have a say about her work life. She feels trapped in the organization and has resigned herself to just show up and try to do her best for her patients.

◆ ◆ ◆

Selecting and Developing Leaders is the first of four actions designed to create Coherence and cultivate the three Ideal Work Elements just presented. In this chapter, we will discuss the importance of selecting and developing leaders with high emotional intelligence and behaviors that cultivate esprit de corps.

Canada Geese

Canada geese are amazing migratory birds that are a wonderful example for humans regarding collective leadership. The geese fly in a V-shaped formation. When geese fly in formation, they conserve a substantial amount of energy because of aerodynamic efficiencies. They can fly at a speed of 40 miles per hour but can accelerate to 60 miles per hour. During migration, they fly more than 1,000 miles per day at an altitude of approximately 3,000 feet. But they cannot do this alone. The team is much stronger than the sum of the strength of the individual members.

The geese rotate in and out of the lead position as they tire, sharing responsibility and fairly distributing the extra burden and work of leading. No single bird knows the entire route. But collectively they can find destinations hundreds of miles away. Canada geese are also better able to communicate with each other while in V formation. They use body language and at least 10 different sounds for communication. The geese need the whole team to accomplish their migratory mission. It takes a flock.

The best human leaders, teams, and organizations share many of these qualities. The culture of Canada geese offers a wonderful example for humans in collective rotational leadership, an approach to leadership that will be described in this chapter.

LEADING IN A VUCA WORLD

The basic tenets of leadership haven't changed much over the last decades. Effective leaders share a fundamental set of core traits. They act with integrity, lead with vision, inspire followers to achieve results, communicate clearly, and build relationships based on trust and respect.

Although the core components of leadership have not changed, the world in which they lead has undergone substantial change. Today, ours is a *VUCA* world (Bennett and Lemoine, 2014):

V, volatile (change is rapid and widespread)
U, uncertain (the future cannot be predicted with accuracy)
C, complex (issues are multifaceted with compound causes and solutions)
A, ambiguous (best approach and effects are unclear)

In a VUCA world, leaders must have more adaptive thinking capabilities than before. In fact, the growing complexity of the current working environment was cited as the top concern of over 1,500 chief executive officers (CEOs) (Bennett and Lemoine, 2014). Most of the CEOs, including those of health care organizations, indicated that their organizations were not equipped to cope with this complexity.

Leadership Development Business Case

Organizations with leadership development programs defined by evidence and best practices consistently outperform those with poor or nonexistent strategies (Jones and Olken, 2005; Goodall, 2011). They are equipped to cope with the changes in a VUCA world. Organizations with effective leadership development and selection programs outperform organizations without such programs in numerous ways:

- Overall employee turnover is 18% lower.
- Turnover of high-performing employees is 62% lower.
- Ratings of leaders are two to three times higher.
- Productivity and financial performance are more consistent.
- Downsizing during the last recession was one-half the rate of their peers with such programs.

Organizations with best-practice leadership development programs are not just developing leaders. They are creating human and social capital as well as high-performing, sustainable organizations (Swensen et al, 2016a) by engaging teams as well as building trust and the interconnectedness of staff. Some timeless best practices for developing leaders to meet the challenges of a complex and rapidly evolving environment are described in Box 23.1.

LEADER SELECTION

To thrive in a VUCA world, organizations must choose their leaders carefully. Because leaders have such a central role in organizational culture, professional

---

Box 23.1 Timeless Best-Practice Strategies for Leadership Development

- Ensure the commitment and engagement of executive leadership in the vision, strategies, and tactics to be used for leadership selection and development with intent to cultivate esprit de corps.
- Align leadership development and selection strategies with organizational culture.
- Connect the business strategy to a portfolio of experiential, action-learning–based key leadership talent programs (i.e., doing real, prioritized work as opposed to case studies or simulations).
- Attend to diversity and inclusion among leaders and team members to provide a broader array of ideas, perspectives, and insights necessary for optimal leadership development and decision making.
- Build a culture of coaching with internal coaching expertise, facilitated leadership roundtables, and coaching skills development at all levels to drive leadership development (see Chapter 20, "Coherence Ideal Work Element: Professional Development and Mentorship").
- Accelerate the development of the entire leadership pipeline to leaders at all levels (i.e., collective leadership).

---

fulfillment, and esprit de corps, leader selection is critical. Traditionally, physician leaders were selected because of seniority, national reputation, research expertise, or skill as a physician. They were not selected because they had the skills, demeanor, and aptitude to lead people. This situation is changing, but slowly.

Selection of clinician leaders is an opportunity to engage staff. The leader selection process should include the health care professionals who will report to the new leader, and the process must be transparent and meaningful to ensure the best results for clinician engagement. If practicing clinicians are consulted in or co-lead the process of leadership selection, they feel more like partners and less like employees. Conversely, if leaders are selected strictly by administrators (without consulting clinical staff), social capital among clinicians softens and engagement decreases. Worse, without buy-in of the staff who will be led, the newly appointed leader is set up to struggle needlessly, flounder, or fail. Of course, ultimately it will be the health care professionals who decide whether a person in a leadership role truly will be their leader.

This principle was well stated by Reverend Theodore M. Hesburgh, C.S.C., president emeritus of the University of Notre Dame, Congregation of Holy Cross. Before the press conference where he was going to announce Lou Holtz (who is now in the College Football Hall of Fame) as the new head coach of the football team, he told Mr. Holtz, "I'm going to announce that you are the new football coach at Notre Dame. I cannot announce to the world that you are the leader of the Notre Dame football team. I can give you a title, but the players will determine if you are a leader."

At Mayo Clinic, physician leaders are selected for a robust and meaningful partnership by the staff they will have the privilege of serving. Before the planned transition of an existing physician leader, each member of the department is interviewed by a physician who works in another department. The interview includes the question, "Who would make a good leader of your group?" The confidential results are pooled and the top three to four candidates identified by the department are then interviewed in a formal search committee process led by physicians from a department other than the one in leadership transition. Whoever is appointed as chair is set up for success because that person already has the trust and respect of the colleagues they will be serving in the entire integrated practice.

LEADERSHIP DEVELOPMENT

An integral part of an esprit de corps strategy is a constructive organization-clinician relationship bolstered by effective and aligned leadership development. Investment in leadership development for health care is a decade or more behind that of other business sectors, even though it is possible to effectively grow leader talent while advancing strategy and delivering a measurable return on investment. The effectiveness of frontline clinician leadership is one of the most critical ingredients for organizational success. The performance of clinician leaders affects not only the productivity of each work unit but also the well-being of those they have the privilege of leading and with whom they co-produce ideal work-life results.

Leadership Pipeline

For the long-term durability of an organization, a focus on a leadership pipeline is critical (Figure 23.1). The best and most resilient organizations manage a succession pool for every important leader position. Mayo Clinic, for example, has a well-developed leader pipeline for all key positions across the organizations (i.e., for physician leaders this involves 242 physician-leader roles). The talent in each succession pool should be measured for competency, readiness, ethnic diversity, and gender diversity.

The competency assessment should include how well the person demonstrates the five leader behaviors in their current position using the Leader Behavior Index (Chapter 15, "Agency Action: Measuring Leader Behaviors"). This is a key predictor of future success. These leader behaviors can be taught, and they should be used for leader selection. Feedback should be provided to frontline leaders on an ongoing basis (i.e., not just once a year). The constructive and supportive opportunities for leadership improvement should be shared by the frontline leader's supervisor. Organizations should then provide resources (e.g., improvement science mentoring, executive coaching, meeting facilitation skills, time-management workshops) to help leadership teams continue to develop through participation on quality improvement teams and through executive coaching and other programs specifically designed to enhance a clinician leader's capacity to demonstrate the five leader behaviors.

At Mayo Clinic, individuals identified as future leaders are also offered assignments, coaching, and development opportunities that further strengthen their skills and prepare them for their next leadership role. Leaders move through the pipeline if the organization asks them to take on a leadership role and they choose to accept this responsibility in their careers. Every newly transitioned Mayo Clinic physician leader is offered and encouraged to work with an executive coach. This is an investment in leaders and the esprit de corps of their staff that keeps the pipeline fresh and vital.

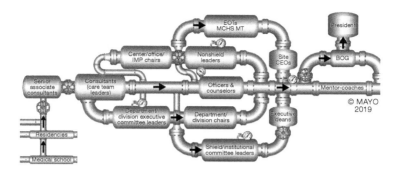

Figure 23.1. The Leadership Pipeline at Mayo Clinic. The physician leadership pipeline concept represents the developmental flow of junior to senior leaders in designated leadership positions. At each position along the pipeline, a succession pool of leaders is assessed for readiness to move to the next level, for leader behaviors, and for ethnic and gender diversity. The pipeline starts at the senior associate consultant status (newly hired staff). During a three-year period, these staff members undergo dozens of hours of communication, quality improvement, and professionalism training. They also undergo emotional intelligence and 360-degree assessments. They have opportunities to be involved with a variety of leadership activities. At each juncture in the pipeline—from new hires to the president—leaders are assessed, developed, mentored, and coached with the goal of preparing them for their next leadership position. The intent is to have a qualified, ready-now diverse group of leaders who have the capacity to engage colleagues, cultivate professional fulfillment for those they lead, grow social capital, and engender esprit de corps. BOG indicates board of governors; CEO, chief executive officer; EOT, executive operations team; IMP, integrated multispecialty program; MCHS, Mayo Clinic Health System; MT, management team.

Five Leader Behaviors

Leaders who wish to demonstrate a caring attitude that engenders esprit de corps and reduces burnout must develop the five leader behaviors described in detail in Chapter 15 ("Agency Action: Measuring Leader Behaviors"): include, inform, inquire, develop, and recognize. These leadership traits are within reach of every leader. They are not rocket science. They are common sense—just not common practice.

Although these are far from all the skills leaders require, they are the aspects of leadership most critical to cultivating engagement and professional fulfillment among those they lead. If all an institution did was select and develop leaders for these five behaviors, health care professionals would know their leaders care about them, they would be empowered to improve and co-create the work environment, burnout rates would plummet, and patient outcomes would improve.

If you care about someone, you should know what matters to them, and in health care, that means understanding professional ambitions of those you supervise. We have asked hundreds of frontline leaders of health care professionals (e.g., division chairs, section heads, nurse managers, clinic leaders) if they know the specific aspect of work that motivates and provides meaning to each of the health care professionals they lead. To a person, they have honestly replied they do not. We have challenged them to reflect about whether they can effectively lead people and maximize their potential, engagement, and discretionary effort without knowing what motivates them. We challenge them to reflect on how to engage those they lead individually in a conversation—by asking them what inspires and motivates them . . . what brings them joy in work.

Leaders can use the information about what matters to each colleague to explore together how that interest might be developed and applied for the good of the individual, the work unit, the organization, and patients and their families.

Emotional Intelligence

Emotional intelligence is the ability to be aware of, understand, and manage emotions and to master interpersonal relationships judiciously and empathetically. It is fundamental to both personal and professional success and can be learned and improved. When leaders have higher emotional intelligence, team members have lower levels of anxiety, stress, and burnout. Leader emotional intelligence promotes team satisfaction, engagement, productivity, well-being, effectiveness and, ultimately, better patient care and esprit de corps.

Emotional intelligence should be a criterion for leadership. Programs to assess and enhance emotional intelligence for all newly hired health care professionals are feasible and effective. At Mayo Clinic, all physicians undergo a standardized, nationally benchmarked emotional intelligence assessment at the end of the first of their first three years on staff before a permanent commitment is made for their employment. These assessments are an opportunity for physicians to self-reflect and become better team members and patient caregivers. Although the assessments are not pass-fail, the physicians understand that they must be respectful and sensitive to the emotions, needs, and psychological comfort of patients and care team members to fit in the patient-centered culture of Mayo Clinic. Coaching and course offerings in emotional intelligence and empathy are available to all staff.

In addition, all physicians undergo a 360-degree evaluation at the end of the second of the three-year onboarding period. This is basically a qualitative emotional intelligence assessment. Each physician receives anonymous and confidential feedback from co-worker team members (i.e., nurses, managers, social workers, trainees, administrators, and other doctors). The message is that extraordinary care is a team sport, and the intent is to optimize interpersonal dynamics in order to cultivate esprit de corps.

Humble Inquiry

Thriving leaders regularly demonstrate a genuine interest in the ideas of the entire professional health care team in both informal, standard work settings and in more formal settings, such as an annual review. One way to show this interest is through *humble inquiry*, a term coined by Edgar Schein, an international authority on organizational culture and leadership. Humble inquiry refers to an attitude of interest, curiosity, and vulnerability. Humble inquiry reflects a desire to build a collaborative relationship and is predicated on the belief that leaders are dependent on those they lead and need to learn from their experiences and insights to be effective.

Humble inquiry is a mindset and skill derived from intentionality, self-confidence, and humility (i.e., traits that are required to ask for honest feedback). Humble inquiry is part of participative management and entails leaders asking colleagues for their ideas on how to improve leadership and work life. Whenever possible, humble inquiry should also encompass empowering clinicians to develop and put their ideas into action in collaboration with other team members. Beneficial outcomes for the work unit that result from these activities provide opportunities for achievement and recognition. Engaging clinicians in the co-creation of a better work environment is a flattering form of recognition that acknowledges that they are trusted. It leverages their intrinsic motivation and reduces burnout.

Developing Clinical Leaders Through Ask-Listen-Empower (and Repeat)

Participative management with collaborative action planning is a natural fit with leadership development, action learning, and esprit de corps. The Ask-Listen-Empower (and Repeat) improvement process, discussed in detail in Chapter 16 ("Agency Action: Removing Pebbles"), is an important technique for leader development. This process is an effective way for leaders to demonstrate humble inquiry, harness people's passions, empower them, and help them develop. It also provides an opportunity for clinicians considering leadership to try out and improve their people and process skills, all while doing real work that makes life better for colleagues and for patients.

We recommend using this active learning process along with coaching, mentoring, assignments, assessment, evaluation, feedback, and thoughtful planning of goals as central components of organizational leadership development.

NURTURING SOCIAL CAPITAL

Nurturing social capital is a fundamental responsibility of leaders. Therefore, leadership development must involve cultivating these skills. Leadership development programs themselves should also generate trust and interconnectedness of the participants. This can be achieved with multidisciplinary, team-based activities that involve professionals from different geographic regions and disciplines.

The trust and interconnectedness of health care professionals can also be expanded by leadership development focused on two simple approaches: the five leader behaviors and the Ask-Listen-Empower (and Repeat) process. Social capital is good for the organization (i.e., better diffusion, learning, and productivity), good for the individual (i.e., greater resilience and camaraderie and less burnout), and good for patients (i.e., safer and more reliable care). Formidable social capital is a primary source of sustainable competitive advantage for any organization. Leaders should be the primary force multiplier for the development of social capital.

Physicians, nurses, advanced practice providers, and other health care professionals tend to be highly engaged with their work. That engagement, however, does not necessarily mean they are committed to their organization (e.g., "I can be a nurse anywhere."). Addressing this discrepancy results in greater volunteerism and teamwork, more involvement in process improvement, lower burnout rates, less turnover, and better patient outcomes and can be done by improving clinician-organization partnerships.

Leadership Dyads and Triads

No clinical leader can prosper without partnership. Leader dyads and triads are models in health care where physician leaders, as well as other clinical leaders, partner with administrators to form a dyad or with administrators and nursing leaders to form a triad. These models allow clinicians to maintain a meaningful clinical presence while serving in a leadership role.

A practicing clinician (e.g., physician, nurse, social worker, pharmacist, technologist) is in a superior position to connect with people in the work area compared with individuals without clinical expertise and an active practice. Practicing clinician leaders understand the real current work of hospitals and clinics. With the support of an administrative partner, they are also more readily able to continue to work alongside their colleagues and engage them as partners instead of as employees.

Leadership dyads and triads render clinical leaders more effective and help them retain credibility with those whom they lead. Mayo Clinic has used the dyad model for over a century.

EXPANDING LEADER COMPETENCIES

The most valuable competencies future leaders will need are evolving and reflect the need to adapt in a VUCA world (Figure 23.2). In health care, the necessary skills, abilities, and attributes leaders must have now include adaptability, self-awareness, engaging employees, collaboration, and systems thinking across the traditional boundaries of organizations.

Nearly 90% of senior executives believe it is "extremely important" for them to work effectively across all types of boundaries, including horizontal boundaries of function and expertise, as well as geographic, demographic, and stakeholder boundaries. However, only 7% of these executives believe they are currently "very effective" at doing so. This underscores the need for leaders to move out of their comfort zones, form alliances both internally and externally, and become more comfortable in dealing with diverse people and opinions.

COLLECTIVE LEADERSHIP DEVELOPMENT

At some point during their career, most people have experienced the joy and observed the dividends of exceptionally well-prepared leaders. Most have also suffered the agony of missed opportunity and witnessed the attendant emotional and financial costs when struggling or failing leaders have fallen short. They have first-hand experience with the prima facie case for investment in leadership development. Prepared leaders deliver results. Building the leadership capabilities of an organization is a clear differentiator. It happens in the context of the whole system and is unique to each organization's culture, strategies, processes, and people.

As important as it is to develop individual leaders, it is perhaps even more important to develop the collective leadership of an organization. This requires a strategy

Today	Tomorrow
Burnout as a problem for clinicians to address	Esprit de corps as a leading indicator of organizational effectiveness
Quality as a necessary expense	Quality as a business strategy
Leader as a position and a title	Leadership as behaviors and attributes
Reluctant leaders	Passionate and purpose-driven leaders
Cognitive skills: deductive reasoning, analytical problem solving	Creative problem solving with values-driven thinking
Knowledge base and experiences for independent leadership	Ability to ask the right questions, give and receive feedback, handle ambiguity
Influence through authority, decree, memorandum, announcements, and job title	Influence through communication, trust, confidence, authenticity, and humility-servant leadership
In-depth local health care knowledge and connections	Empathetic understanding of cultural abilities
Ability to lead face-to-face teams	Ability to lead virtual and face-to-face teams
Deep general management, functional competencies, and commensurate knowledge	Deep functional expertise plus broader thinking to deal with complexity
Managing: doing things right	Leading: doing the right things
Responsible for managing change	Learn and adapt: flexibility
Heroic individual efforts	Collaborative team efforts
Status quo	Creativity and innovation
Individual achievement	Team achievement
People told what to do	Humble inquiry to find solutions
Direct reports	Engaged colleagues and team members
Smartest person in room with all the answers	Ability to ask the right questions and invite participation
Individual leadership development	Collective leadership development
Human resources and manager responsible for development	Leaders responsible for their own development
Fixed burnout mindset	An esprit de corps mindset based on aspiration

© MAYO
2019

Figure 23.2. Changes in Leadership Qualities: Today and Tomorrow.
(Adapted from and informed by data from Petrie N. Future trends in leadership development: a white paper [Internet]. 2011 [cited 2019 Apr 8]. Available from: http://integralleadershipreview. com/ 7264-nick-petries-future-trends-in-leadership- development-a-white-paper/.)

to develop all leaders, formal and informal, at all levels so that all people in the organization can be committed to the same mission and moving in the same direction. Given the increasingly complex health care industry in the VUCA world, the challenges and demands are too great for a small number of senior leaders to handle on their own. The traditional focus on individual leader as hero is shifting to collective, boundaryless, and connected capacity for leadership across the organization.

CONCLUSION

People don't leave organizations. They leave ineffective leaders. When an organization and its leaders are trusted, there is a direct correlation with improved overall performance of the organization and the health care professionals they have the privilege of serving. Participative management is a social approach to leadership that engages colleagues, individually and on teams, to face challenges and then to work together to advance mission-aligned goals.

When medical institutions organize their systems and structure to promote a mindset of collective stewardship and hire and develop clinicians who exhibit civility, have community-building skills, and are socially and emotionally intelligent, they enable boundarylessness and are set up to succeed. This leadership approach is a cultural match for health care professionals as it acknowledges their expertise and desire to improve the work environment to better meet the needs of patients. Selecting and developing leaders with team-driven, psychologically safe, consensus-building skills is an evidence-based and validated action in the Coherence Action Set that will combat professional burnout and promote esprit de corps (Box 23.2).

TOMORROW: FULFILLMENT

The parent company of Cordelia's health care organization realized that the staff morale was poor throughout the organization, and it was especially bad in Cordelia's department. They instituted a dyad leadership model and replaced her supervisor with a clinician leader and an administrative partner. Cordelia's new leader does not behave like a boss at all. She understands Cordelia's concerns, is interested in her ideas, and shares all the work-unit data with the team so that they can figure out the best way forward together. She has emotional intelligence. Last week she actually scheduled a time for them to meet to discuss what brings her joy in work. Cordelia has regained her passion and excitement about work because she feels respected and is treated as a colleague. Others in her unit feel the same way, and esprit de corps is increasing in the department.

Box 23.2 The Playbook

- Consider adopting a leadership dyad or triad model that allows practicing clinicians to lead in partnership with administrators and nursing leaders as appropriate.
- Consider term limits and role rotations for all organization and clinical leaders.
- Consider engaging clinicians in the selection of all leaders who impact clinical matters.
- Make certain all senior leaders understand and role model the five key leader behaviors that promote professional fulfillment.
- Begin leader development of the five behaviors through assessment, feedback, training, sharing best practices, skill building activities, and coaching.
- Consider annual staff surveys for frontline clinicians to assess how well leaders demonstrate the five behaviors.

SUGGESTED READING

Bennett N, Lemoine GJ. What VUCA really means for you. Harv Bus Rev. Jan/Feb 2014. Available from: https://hbr.org/2014/01/what-vuca-really-means-for-you.

Goodall AH. Physician-leaders and hospital performance: is there an association? Soc Sci Med. 2011 Aug;73(4):535–9.

Jones BF, Olken BA. Do leaders matter? National leadership and growth since World War II. Q J Econ. 2005;120(3):835–64.

O'Boyle EHJ, Humphrey RH, Pollack JM, Hawver TH, Story PA. The relation between emotional intelligence and job performance: a meta-analysis. J Organ Behav. 2011; 32(5):788–818.

Petrie N. Future trends in leadership development: a white paper [Internet]. 2011 [cited 2019 Apr 8]. Available from: http://integralleadershipreview.com/7264-nick-petries-future-trends-in-leadership-development-a-white-paper/.

Schein EH. Humble inquiry: the gentle art of asking instead of telling. San Francisco (CA): Berrett-Koehler Publishers, Inc; 2013.

Swensen S, Gorringe G, Caviness JN, Peters D. Leadership by design: intentional organization development by physician leaders. J Manag Dev. 2016a;35(4):549–70.

Swensen S, Kabcenell A, Shanafelt T. Physician-organization collaboration reduces physician burnout and promotes engagement: the Mayo Clinic experience. J Healthc Manag. 2016b Mar-Apr;61(2):105–27.

24

COHERENCE ACTION: IMPROVING PRACTICE EFFICIENCY

TODAY: DISTRESS

Samir is a primary care physician who used to love going to work. He had time to connect with his patients and had lunch with his care team several times per week. Those days are gone. The electronic environment has changed his life for the worse. The new requirements for documentation seem endless and without purpose. The administrative and clerical work have become overwhelming, and there is no longer time to connect with patients or colleagues or even consider reading a good book. His day used to end at 6:00 PM, with family dinner starting at 6:30 PM. Now, he usually arrives home 15 minutes late for dinner and always has a few more hours of charting and documenting to do after the kids are in bed. Every night he wonders, "How much longer can I keep doing this?"

• • •

Improving Practice Efficiency is the second of four Coherence Actions. In this chapter, we will provide a roadmap to successfully implement this action and show how it combats professional burnout and fosters esprit de corps.

IMPACT OF IMPROVING PRACTICE EFFICIENCY

Case Study: Virginia Mason Institute (Personal Communication, Sarah Patterson, M.H.A., F.A.C.M.P.E., Executive Director)

The best way to start this chapter is with this story from Sarah Patterson. Sarah has been a health care leader at Virginia Mason Institute for over 30 years. She believes burnout among health care professionals is often caused by the failure of leaders to evolve—to advance their mindsets, management methods, and systems fast enough to keep up with the increasingly challenging complexities in health care.

Virginia Mason has long prided itself on being an exceptional place to work. Founded nearly 100 years ago as a physician group practice, Virginia Mason has maintained a culture that values teamwork and quality. They have a foundational belief that practicing in a group setting allows physicians to work collaboratively to provide the best possible care for patients. Under the leadership of chairman and chief executive officer Gary Kaplan, M.D., Virginia Mason staff have spent the past 20 years working to adopt a management system based on the core principles of continuous improvement, eliminating waste and defects, and demonstrating respect for people by giving staff the opportunity and expectation of driving improvement efforts. Given the absence of health care exemplars when they began their journey, Virginia Mason looked to industry and manufacturing companies for ways to best accomplish their goals.

Sarah notes, "When we began to change our mindsets as leaders, our teachers from industry encouraged us to see what was happening on the front lines. They asked us just to observe: no talking, no asking people questions, just observe. Gradually, we were able to see the chaos and waste endemic in our organization. I saw nurses in the hospital leaving patient rooms multiple times to find supplies and standing in line to get patient medications from the dispensing units. I watched physician assistants frequently interrupted by pages from nurses and residents. I saw physicians in clinic hurriedly reviewing patient records to see what preventive tests needed to be ordered while the patients waited in front of them. I observed doctors apologizing to patients for how long they had waited to get an appointment and then watched patients wait again to be taken to a room."

Sarah recalls her industry teachers asking questions such as, "What are you doing about the rework (waste) that these nurses, doctors, and medical assistants have to manage? It is very disrespectful to your team members to do so many wasteful things because the processes are poorly designed. Addressing that is your job as the leader." This fundamentally changed Sarah's view of what her role as an administrative leader was and where she should focus her time. Today, Virginia Mason's system has substantially reduced waste and is a patient-centered organization. Staff and patients are measurably better off.

Creating Efficiency

Creating an efficient practice environment is about genuinely respecting health care professionals and working with them to improve their workplace. Improving practice efficiency goes far beyond reducing clerical work or optimizing the electronic environment—it involves optimizing workflows and eliminating waste in all forms. The best approach is to:

1) Observe the clinical work being done.
2) Assess administrative work to determine whether it adds value from a patient perspective and, if not, stop it.
3) Identify the administrative work that does add value but requires the greatest time and burden for health care professionals.
4) Reduce the time and energy expenditure for this work by providing necessary resources and staffing and by streamlining and optimizing workflow, processes, efficiency, variation, and defects.
5) Repeat the process.

In too many organizations, patients and providers suffer from the absence of a sustainable management system and the lack of urgency to implement continuous, meaningful process improvements to enhance efficiency of practice (Figure 24.1). Processes that are often inefficient include triage, scheduling systems, room usage and assignment, computerized order entry, referrals, insurance preapproval, documentation, medication refills, and message documentation in patient portals. For practices that involve

Efficiency of Practice =

$$\frac{\text{Value-Added Clinical Work Produced}}{\text{Time + Energy Expended}}$$
to Accomplish It

© MAYO
2019

Figure 24.1. Efficiency of Practice.

invasive and noninvasive procedures, inefficiencies can also be found in scheduling and availability of the operating and other procedure rooms, turnaround times, staffing, and teamwork (including consistency of procedure-room teams). Systematically improving the efficiency of each of these processes and workflows can reduce burnout of professionals by removing the frustration of inefficiency and wastefulness.

Practice inefficiency is a target-rich environment for identifying and removing frustrations of health care professionals and creating value for patients (see Chapter 16, "Agency Action: Removing Pebbles"). Patient-centered, value-added processes should be evaluated in relation to the time and energy expended to accomplish them and the ratio improved, if practical. If a coronary artery bypass operation is performed via a streamlined process with no defects and no wasted energy in a short period of time, but the procedure was *not* clinically indicated, then the efficiency of practice is zero! If a nurse spends three and a half hours on multiple phone calls to secure insurance payment for an expensive medication for inflammatory bowel disease that is lifesaving and evidence based, then the value is high, but the efficiency (value divided by the time and energy expended to accomplish it) is low. Low-efficiency activities are opportunities to create value for patients and time for professionals. They are also rich opportunities to reduce burnout.

Case Study: Finish Work Before Going Home (a Novel Idea)

Atrius Health prioritized reducing burnout among its health care professionals as being essential to its future. Perhaps the most ambitious workflow improvement project underway at Atrius Health is redesign of their internal medicine practice model. The goal of this initiative is for all clinicians to finish the day's work *during the day* to free up evening and weekend time for themselves.

The goals of the redesign process are to 1) have all health care professionals working at the top of their licensure (e.g., better teaming), 2) remove unnecessary or redundant work from physician inboxes (e.g., eliminate carbon copies of notes), 3) automate the workflow process for specific tasks (e.g., medication refills), 4) track care gaps and adopt standard work, and 5) facilitate optimal workflow at all practice locations.

Much time and effort must be spent to redesign workflow and commit to developing and sustaining an environment of well-being and support. Historically, Atrius Health viewed struggling health care professionals as weak. Now, they work relentlessly to improve systems efficiency to benefit all their professionals and prioritize projects. They have successfully found that fundamental organizational change occurs when leadership commits to marshaling and focusing resources in a sustained manner to combat drivers of burnout and promote esprit de corps.

ELECTRONIC TECHNOLOGY

Before we explore the dark spaces of the current electronic world, we should emphasize that much of the electronic environment improves satisfaction and productivity. Many of you remember the days of the paper chart (which often didn't arrive with the patient). Today's access to results of laboratory tests and imaging results in the examination room at the time of the patient visit profoundly improves efficiency. Having digital, fingertip access to PubMed (the free online search engine that accesses the U.S. National Library of Medicine at the National Institutes of Health MEDLINE database of biomedical literature) and UpToDate, a robust clinical decision-making support tool, is a good thing. Mobile devices, used appropriately, can improve work-life integration by providing mobility, flexibility, efficiency, and productivity benefits that help both clinicians and patients.

Clinicians actually anticipate the day when practice efficiency will be further improved by more automated decision support, artificial intelligence, electronically assisted team-based care, patient engagement with telemedicine, and excellent voice-recognition dictation and transcription services. Until that day, however, improving the efficiency of the electronic environment starts with recognizing and avoiding five common mistakes.

Five Mistakes

Leaders make five common mistakes in assessing how to mitigate the human toil of the electronic environment:

1) Confusing efficiency with productivity. Many administrators assume that higher patient volumes or relative value unit generation per provider is a measure of a more efficient clinic. However, these are actually measures of a more productive clinic. Efficiency results from how much effort it takes to deliver that productivity.
2) Assuming all clerical burden is due to the electronic environment and neglecting to identify clerical burden associated with the workflow processes (e.g., scheduling, check in, rooming, ordering, patient education, documentation, triage of inbox messaging, billing).
3) Assuming that the electronic environment is a ubiquitous and necessary evil that cannot be reckoned with. Leaders who make this assumption assume a victim mindset and miss the opportunity to address actionable characteristics related to function and use of the electronic health record (EHR) as well as to workflows, which would improve the well-being of health care professionals.
4) Focusing narrowly on the EHR and failing to recognize the toll associated with the electronic environment as a whole (e.g., email, mobile devices, audible notifications and alarms, interruptions).

5) Concluding that EHR tools themselves are the only culprit for the inefficiencies associated with the EHR. In fact, a large portion of the increased burden is from regulatory, payer, and public reporting requirements as well as in how the organization's compliance department interprets these requirements (typically in the most conservative way possible).

An Untamed Electronic Environment

For every hour physicians spend face to face with patients, they spend nearly two more hours updating EHRs and doing clerical work. EHR tasks often get shifted from work time to personal time. Time-stamp studies of the EHR suggest that the average physician spends nearly 30 hours per month interacting with the EHR on nights and weekends to complete charting and to review results and inbox messaging (DiAngi et al, 2017). Emergency department physicians in a community hospital setting spend substantially more time entering data into the EHR than on any other activity, including direct patient care. During a busy 10-hour shift in the emergency department, total mouse clicks equaled about 4,000 (Hill et al, 2013).

The error too many leaders make is to assume incorrectly that there is no recourse. There are many ways to mitigate the administrative and clerical burden, including those described in the *Patients Before Paperwork* initiative of the American College of Physicians.

Hidden Effects of the EHR

In addition to the associated clicks and clerical burden, the EHR has also fundamentally altered the way clinicians work. Even in the examination room, studies indicate that nearly 40% of the encounter is spent with physicians interfacing with the EHR rather than interacting, examining, and engaging in dialogue with patients, which has been the bedrock of the profession for centuries (Sinsky et al, 2016). The increased time charting also often results in spending less time interacting with colleagues and other team members, which can result in a sense of isolation. All of this increases the risk of professional distress.

To overcome this deleterious effect, leaders must make intentional efforts to restore health care professionals' connections with patients and colleagues. Organizational approaches to cultivate collegiality and connection with colleagues in today's practice environment are considered in Chapter 30 ("Camaraderie Action: Cultivating Community and Commensality"). Restoring connection with patients can be achieved by minimizing interruptions and distractions in the examination room. This includes providing assistance with documentation and order-entry tasks so that physicians can focus their time and attention on the patient and medical decision making.

Case Study: Radiology

The precise way in which the EHR has changed the nature of work varies by discipline. Radiology is an illustrative example.

Before EHRs, radiologists "held court" every morning to review images and discuss patient cases with clinicians caring for the patients. This was a community event: The radiologist taught, and the team provided clinical context. Follow-up discussion of cases from the previous day and the outcomes of workups were reviewed.

After images went digital, all of this changed. Radiologists were initially happy about digitized images, as they had a bit more time in their work day. Soon however, they realized their work had changed forever. They were more isolated. They were less connected with colleagues. The direct exchange of expertise and application to patients happened less often. In today's world, the radiologist reading an image may not even be in the same state (or continent) as the treating physician!

Today, the most common means for a diagnostic radiologist to review thousands of computed tomography and magnetic resonance images per day is to sit (no physical movement) in a dark room (no sunlight) with no social interactions (isolation) and no input about whether this imaging examination was appropriate or not (cognitive dissonance). When a consultation is performed, it occurs via a computer workstation and phone, not in person (no oxytocin). This explains in part why radiologists are in the five specialty disciplines at highest risk for burnout.

So what can be done about it? Radiologists certainly cannot and should not go backwards. Radiology practices and physicians should intentionally consider the following actions:

- Schedule regular, short walking breaks that include sunlight.
- Deliberately plan lunch or breaks with colleagues.
- Attend clinical conferences in person and show up five minutes early to connect with peers.
- Create a work environment with options for an interpretation workstation that can be moved from a sitting to standing position throughout the day.
- Create work rooms that allow radiologists to be in physical proximity with colleagues to foster community.
- Build treadmill workstation combinations so that radiologists can interpret examinations while walking slowly (this is healthy for the radiologist and the patient because it increases interpretation accuracy) (Fidler et al, 2008).

The Compliance Department

Organization compliance departments often serve as a magnifier of EHR-related factors. The compliance department often interprets regulations, including those related to the Health Insurance Portability and Accountability Act (HIPAA), in the most conservative way possible to minimize the organization risk. Such conservative interpretations, however, often create further inefficiency for clinicians. A simple example is implementing a short automatic log-out interval in the EHR with the intent of minimizing the risk that someone will access a workstation with patient information. These short log outs, however, often result in physicians having to log back into the EHR multiple times in a single, 20-minute patient encounter. If the hospital has not implemented efficient log-in processes (e.g., tap-and-go), these interruptions can consume 2 to 3 minutes (i.e., 10%-15%) of the encounter and fragment the office visit. The source of the inefficiency is not the EHR but overly strict interpretation of regulations by the compliance department.

Similarly, the compliance office of many organizations suggests that only physicians enter electronic orders (American Medical Association [AMA]), even though the Centers for Medicare & Medicaid Services (CMS) eliminated this requirement for eligible hospitals and critical access hospitals in 2017 (AMA). The CMS also did not include computerized physician-order entry as an objective within the advancing care information performance category; thus, physician-order entry is not required for reporting by clinicians who are eligible for MIPS (merit-based incentive payment system for Medicare reimbursement). Although objective measures for the computerized physician-order entry remain required for the Medicaid EHR incentive program to successfully attest to meaningful use, that program states that "any licensed health care provider or a medical staff person who is a credentialed medical assistant or is credentialed to and performs the duties equivalent to a credentialed medical assistant can enter orders in the medical record per state, local, and professional guidelines" (CMS, 2018).

Having the compliance department of many health care organizations re-evaluate their automatic log-out interval and update their internal policies regarding computerized order entry are simple and no-cost interventions that have the potential to profoundly decrease administrative burden related to the electronic environment.

IMPROVING INEFFICIENCIES OF THE EHR

Even though EHR-related clerical work and inefficiencies are ubiquitous issues, organizational actions can be taken to mitigate EHR impact on human performance. EHR-related work should be guided by the principle of creating value for patients and minimizing impact on professionals. Best practice is to appoint a practicing physician and nurse who will have the sole responsibility of streamlining and reducing clerical work in the EHR. The clinicians in that role should be members of the appropriate decision-making bodies.

Selecting Metrics

The first step to improving practice efficiency is to select the metrics by which efficiency will be assessed. The optimal measures may vary by setting (e.g., clinic vs. hospital inpatient vs. operating room), occupation, and specialty. Examples from the EHR to include are time physicians spend documenting and interfacing with the inbox, click counts (i.e., per day or necessary to complete common tasks), work after work, proportion of different team-member interactions with the EHR, and operating room turnaround time. Once the metric is identified, it can be applied to assess the baseline state. This assessment often reveals heterogeneity across like units, which can allow leaders to initially focus their attention on the areas where things are working less optimally. These metrics can also serve as a framework to facilitate root cause analysis of the factors contributing to inefficiency as well as a metric to evaluate the effectiveness of improvement work or the impact of ecological events (e.g., move to a new facility, implementation of a new EHR system), or both.

Identifying Inefficiencies

The clinicians who are responsible for streamlining and reducing clerical work in the EHR should focus relentlessly on the following questions:

1) Must this process be performed?
   - Is it a patient safety issue?
   - Is it a regulatory requirement? Are the regulations being correctly interpreted? If not, eliminate the process now!
2) If the process must be performed, make it as efficient as possible.
   - Can we reduce the number of clicks required to accomplish this task?
3) Finally, could the work be executed by someone other than a physician, advanced practice provider, or nurse? This is the opportunity to engage all professionals at the top of their licensure and optimally integrate the full care team in patient care. Having each member of the care team practice at the top of their licensure and capabilities distributes the clerical work that is truly necessary to do.
   - Who is the best team member to complete this task?
   - Which degree should the person hold: an M.D., D.O., R.N., N.P., P.A., or M.A.? Or, could the person be a medical assistant or appropriately trained scribe?

Scribes

In every business sector that has undergone computerization, productivity gains have been reflected in a reduction in workforce. This situation has not yet occurred in health care. Health care organizations have actually had to increase their workforces to adapt to current EHR technology. Only in health care have we found a way to use a fifth century approach (scribes) to address the problems created by our twenty-first century technology.

Nonetheless, scribes have been shown in many practice settings to make sense on multiple levels. Primary care and emergency medicine practices have made a business case for hiring scribes to assist with clerical work for busy professionals. Studies actually suggest scribes increase patient satisfaction, increase provider satisfaction, and improve efficiency all while being cost neutral or net positive (Taylor et al, 2019). There are now many ambulatory practices where primary care physicians never touch a computer for clinical work during their work days.

The practice of enlisting scribes makes financial sense when the expense is offset by productivity gains. The typical rule of thumb in the outpatient setting is that a physician needs to see two additional patients per day to cover the cost of adding a scribe to the payroll. Virtual scribes (e.g., via a listening device or Google glass) typically are cost neutral at one to one-and-a-half extra visits each day and may offer greater flexibility and simplify hiring/staffing. In many primary care settings, physicians with scribes indicate they are working far fewer hours and enjoying medicine again even though they are seeing two incremental patients each day. Many practices have found that having trained medical assistants perform documentation assistance allows the person scribing to take on other duties (e.g., order entry) that result in enhanced team-based care.

At Mayo Clinic, the philosophy is that incremental human resources can be added to a work unit only after the work environment has been formally assessed for optimal efficiency. The mantra is "no new resources to an unexamined process." This has served patients and professionals well for decades. This philosophy has made it possible for a nonprofit organization to be a good steward of its responsibility to the public. An additional mantra can extend the stewardship: "No additional work should be added to an unexamined or unimproved practice." Basically, this means that we should not ask professionals to work harder in a system that we have not first optimized so that it can accommodate the additional work. These two principles of practice efficiency honor the pledge to improve provider well-being at every patient-centered opportunity. Thus, Mayo Clinic uses scribes in work units that have examined and optimized their processes, determined that scribes are the right incremental resource, and developed a strategy to implement scribes seamlessly into the workflow process.

Case Study: University of Colorado Department of Family Medicine

Redesigning clinical care models so that some of the work is performed by partners on the care team and then determining the necessary staffing level for those partners is a tactic to reduce professional burnout. This is exactly what family medicine care teams at the University of Colorado have done. They call the process APEX, which stands for Ambulatory Process Excellence.

The teams started by identifying structured processes involved in patient encounters (i.e., data collection, medication reconciliation, patient education, and visit documentation). The care team decided that, described and properly structured, these important tasks could be efficiently and effectively completed by a trained medical assistant. The new care model developed by APEX necessitated hiring incremental medical assistants and deploying new training and communication systems. The ratio of medical assistants to physicians increased from 1:1 to 2.5:1, but the additional assistants were paid for by the increase in patient visits per day. This advance allowed physicians and nurses to spend more time with patients, where they could create the most value.

Six months after APEX was instituted, burnout rates dropped from 53% to 13%! APEX also resulted in improvement in the rates at which patients received appropriate preventive health measures (e.g., mammography, colonoscopy, vaccinations) as well as in shorter patient wait-room times.

Creative thinking can make a difference for patients and for professional burnout.

Case Study: Intermountain Healthcare Team Approach

Intermountain Healthcare has established a team of professionals called a Super User Support Program to help clinicians with electronic environment interactions. The support staff reviews EHR use at all Intermountain Healthcare hospitals and clinics to identify the physicians who use the most mouse clicks to chart a given condition or spend the most time charting on nights and weekends. They then provide additional support to those physicians. They offer to individually coach and provide EHR skills training with the goal to improve the physician's work life. It works! Consistently, there is a real reduction in EHR time and a reduction in frustration for the doctors who participate. The Super User Support Program focuses on four factors:

1) Efficiency of navigation. How many mouse clicks does it take to chart requirements for a patient with otitis media? The range is 35 to 65 mouse clicks. After coaching, everyone is at 35 clicks. This assessment can be scaled and diffused for the most common conditions within each specialty, and the time savings add up.
2) Workflow. The best practice is to chart and complete order entry immediately after each patient is seen rather than work in batches later in the day. Optimizing workflow in this manner is more efficient for the care team and better for quality control.
3) Elimination of multitasking. Professionals need to understand that efficiency gains from multitasking are a myth. Multitasking actually reduces quality and productivity. Physicians should receive coaching on how to sequence tasks during the clinic visit and daily workflow so that their focus can be on a single task to the greatest extent possible.
4) Elimination of interruptions. Here again, observation is a powerful tool and can help identify how pages, phone calls, and other tasks lead to interruptions and how to reduce them (e.g., holding nonurgent messages, calls, and pages and creating set times each day to address them).

"Honey, Did You Get Fired?"

One Intermountain Healthcare team member tells the story of a physician's wife who noticed a big change in her husband's availability for dinner and the time he had for family activities on nights and weekends (he was part of the Super User Support Program). She asked him, "Honey, did you get fired?" Because he was now home more, she assumed something bad had happened at work! Nope, he was just supported by an organization that cared and made improving his efficiency an organizational priority.

Improvements in efficiency reduce workload, work hours, and cognitive dissonance. They recover time for patients and co-workers, increase meaning and purpose in work, and facilitate work-life integration. Done well, EHR pajama time decreases and the Saturday date night with the EHR comes off the calendar.

CONCLUSION

Improving practice efficiency cultivates coherence and the work elements necessary to support esprit de corps. The EHR is not the sole cause of practice inefficiency. Other sources of administrative burden, low-value work, and inefficiency must be comprehensively identified and relentlessly reduced. This includes identifying efficiency metrics, applying them to assess the current state, identifying opportunity areas, and then having a laser-like focus on improving those areas. Often, this involves eliminating some tasks, reassigning others to the most appropriate member of the care team, and then streamlining the tasks. Staff may need to be increased in some categories to provide an adequate team to handle the reallocated work. The electronic environment and other sources of inefficiency must be tamed if we want to demonstrate respect for people. Many organizations have already made a measurable difference for clinicians. Yours can, too (Box 24.1)!

TOMORROW: FULFILLMENT

Samir is now regularly home for dinner with his family, and he has taken up reading again. His practice implemented a care redesign effort to optimize workflow and also added scribes. Even though he sees a couple extra patients each day, he is able to give patients his undivided attention during their visit and still finishes his work day an hour earlier than before. Even more amazing, he almost never has to log in from home to finish his charting. He loves being a physician again.

Box 24.1 The Playbook

- Identify a group of clinician super users and technology professionals dedicated to improving efficiency of the electronic health record (EHR).
  - Support their time.
  - Identify clinicians who are struggling with the electronic environment by survey or surveillance.
  - Approach clinicians identified in a spirit of support and partner with them to improve their electronic work.
- Use EHR time-stamp data to identify specialties and clinics with the greatest work-after-work documentation time. Create a task force to evaluate how this time could be reduced through changes in workflow, care-team redesign, or documentation assistance. Have the courage to develop criteria and an approach for a pilot study of scribes or medical assistants to assist with documentation. Evaluate the impact, adapt, and, if appropriate, scale across the unit.
- Support one to three large, systems-level, practice-efficiency improvement projects per year (these complement the unit-based removing pebbles work). Most of these projects should identify common themes that transcend frontline work units and are issues that were escalated from unit-based, removing pebbles focus groups (see Chapter 16, "Agency Action: Removing Pebbles").
- Identify basic technology investments that can save clinicians time (e.g., tap-and-go log on, printers in each room, wider screens) and prioritize investment in these resources.
- Have executive leaders engage the Compliance Department and request that they partner with super users to identify ways in which regulations have been interpreted in a manner that is burdensome to physicians. Potential targets:
  - Automatic log out time
  - Internal policies regarding who can enter electronic orders (to be reviewed and signed by the appropriate provider)

SUGGESTED READING

American Medical Association. Computerized provider order entry (CPOE) myth [Internet]. 2019 [cited 2019 Jul 8]. Available from: https://www.ama-assn.org/practice-management/medicare/computerized-provider-order-entry-cpoe-myth.

Arndt BG, Beasley JW, Watkinson MD, Temte JL, Tuan WJ, Sinsky CA, et al. Tethered to the EHR: primary care physician workload assessment using EHR event log data and time-motion observations. Ann Fam Med. 2017 Sep;15(5):419–26.

Centers for Medicare & Medicaid Services. Medicaid eligible professionals: promoting interoperability program modified. Stage 2 objectives and measures [Internet]. 2018 [cited 2018 Jul 8]. Available from: https://www.cms.gov/Regulations-and-Guidance/Legislation/EHRIncentivePrograms/Downloads/TableofContents_EP_Medicaid_ModifiedStage2_2018.pdf.

DiAngi YT, Lee TC, Sinsky CA, Bohman BD, Sharp CD. Novel metrics for improving professional fulfillment. Ann Intern Med. 2017 Nov 21;167(10):740–1.

Fidler JL, MacCarty RL, Swensen SJ, Huprich JE, Thompson WG, Hoskin TL, et al. Feasibility of using a walking workstation during CT image interpretation. J Am Coll Radiol. 2008 Nov;5(11):1130–6.

Gidwani R, Nguyen C, Kofoed A, Carragee C, Rydel T, Nelligan I, et al. Impact of scribes on physician satisfaction, patient satisfaction, and charting efficiency: a randomized controlled trial. Ann Fam Med. 2017 Sep;15(5):427–33.

Hill RG Jr, Sears LM, Melanson SW. 4000 clicks: a productivity analysis of electronic medical records in a community hospital ED. Am J Emerg Med. 2013 Nov;31(11):1591–4.

Shanafelt TD, Dyrbye LN, Sinsky C, Hasan O, Satele D, Sloan J, et al. Relationship between clerical burden and characteristics of the electronic environment with physician burnout and professional satisfaction. Mayo Clin Proc. 2016 Jul;91(7):836–48.

Sinsky C, Colligan L, Li L, Prgomet M, Reynolds S, Goeders L, et al. Allocation of physician time in ambulatory practice: a time and motion study in 4 specialties. Ann Intern Med. 2016 Dec 6;165(11):753–60.

Taylor KA, McQuilkin D, Hughes RG. Medical scribe impact on patient and provider experience. Mil Med. 2019 Feb 27 (Epub ahead of print).

25

COHERENCE ACTION: ESTABLISHING FAIR AND JUST ACCOUNTABILITY

TODAY: DISTRESS

Samantha is a competent, conscientious, hard-working nurse in the intensive care unit. She always follows guidelines and protocols. She never comes to work impaired. She goes the extra mile for her patients and for her team. She has always been a model health care professional.

Then one day about a year ago, she was involved in a calcium chloride overdose of an infant. The infant died, and Samantha was devastated.

By all standards and from all perspectives, the death was related to medication ordering and labeling. It was the result of a systems issue that failed to protect a patient from the fallibilities of clinicians who are human beings. Any competent nurse in the system where Samantha was employed could have been involved with this event. She happened to be working when the factors contributing to the event aligned. In a culture with fair and just accountability, the family and professionals affected would be consoled, and the germane processes and systems that allowed the event to occur fixed.

Instead, Samantha was isolated and treated as if she were to blame for this patient's death. She was neither consoled nor offered professional support for her grieving. A malpractice lawsuit followed. Samantha was not supported.

She considered her options. She considered changing hospitals. She considered leaving nursing.

Instead, she began to think suicide. It seemed to be the only option.

◆ ◆ ◆

Establishing Fair and Just Accountability is the third of four Coherence Actions. In this chapter, we describe how to instill fair and just principles into the work culture. What does this have to do with professional burnout? Everything. Without fair and just accountability, health care organizations cannot foster esprit de corps.

SYSTEMS AND PROCESS DEFICIENCIES

Systems and process deficiencies have been shown to cause the vast majority of adverse events and serious safety events (Swensen et al, 2010). To feel comfortable reporting near misses and adverse events, health care professionals need to be in a nonhostile work environment where they trust the integrity of the leadership and reporting system. They must believe that the system is designed to lead to improved systems of care. Fair and just accountability nurtures such an environment.

Many health care professionals are detail oriented, compulsive, and perfectionistic. They take their responsibilities and the trust patients place in them very seriously. When they make a mistake, they frequently ruminate about the event and self-criticize. Research has shown that health care professionals are at increased risk for burnout as well as suicide after they make or think they have made a medical error (Shanafelt 2011; Hall and Scott, 2012). Therefore, procedures and practices that support fair and just accountability, including consoling health care professionals after human error, are important for reducing the likelihood that an adverse event will result in negative consequences for the involved health care professional (i.e., secondary distress).

Case Study: Insufficient Checks and Balances

Not too many years ago, a group of health care professionals were involved in the preventable death of a young child (ISMP, 2009). The child received an overdose of a normally lifesaving medication used to treat a blood disorder. The health care professionals involved were competent, conscientious, hard-working people. They followed the existing safety and procedure protocols. No one cut corners. No one was impaired. Unfortunately, the protocols were flawed and had not been reviewed in years. There were insufficient checks and balances to protect this patient from the frailties of normal humans.

The lead professional was convicted, fined, stripped of his license, and incarcerated. Although this case may sound extreme, we regularly hear of similar stories of patient deaths and medical errors. In some cases, fault is difficult to determine. In this case, however, the child died because the system was broken. Yet rather than look to the health care system to take responsibility for this adverse outcome, the legal system held an individual solely responsible and disrupted his life in a culture of shame and blame.

To make meaningful improvements in the quality and reliability of health care and the well-being of clinicians, issues in the system must be addressed and health care professionals assisted in situations like the one described.

Consoling Health Care Professionals

The principles of fair and just accountability center on consoling health care professionals involved in adverse patient events caused by systems failures or expected human factors errors. In an organization with a culture of fair and just accountability, leaders recognize the difference between risky or reckless behavior and human factors errors and defective systems and processes (Marx, 2001).

When a health care professional experiences a traumatic adverse patient care event, the professional should be treated fairly. If the professional involved in an adverse event followed procedures and was competent (yet made an anticipated human factors error) or the cause was a systems failure, then the person should be consoled and the flawed systems and process deficiencies addressed. The individual in these situations should not be blamed for adverse effects. This is a central tenant of fair and just accountability (Figure 25.1). If risky or reckless behavior was involved, then there should be different consequences, including coaching and corrective action.

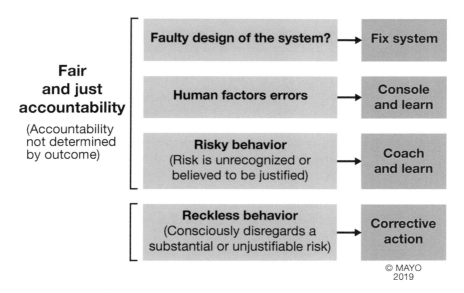

Figure 25.1. Fair and Just Accountability.
(Data from Leonard MW, Frankel A. The path to safe and reliable healthcare. Patient Educ Couns. 2010;80(3):288-92 and Marx D. Patient safety and the "just culture": a primer for health care executives. Report of the medical event reporting system-transfusion medicine prepared by David Marx, JD, for Columbia University under a grant provided by the National Heart, Lung, and Blood Institute. 2001. Available from https://www.chpso.org/sites/main/files/file-attachments/marx_primer.pdf.)

Organizations that want to reduce burnout and promote esprit de corps must establish fair and just accountability as a top organizational priority. These qualities impact individuals involved in an adverse event and their co-workers, who observe how the involved health care professional is treated. If the principles of fair and just accountability are followed, health care professionals should feel comfortable reporting all near misses and adverse events. Such reporting allows the organization to learn from the events to improve quality and safety for patients.

HOSTILE WORK ENVIRONMENTS

Without fair and just accountability, the work environment can become hostile—a situation that is unsafe for patients and toxic to members of the care delivery team. A hostile work environment results in:

- Teams without psychological safety
- Social isolation
- Moral distress
- Compassion fatigue
- Cognitive dissonance
- Inequity
- Malpractice suits

Inappropriate behavior in operating rooms and other clinical care areas is still too common (e.g., verbal threats, invasion of personal space with intent to intimidate, physical assault). In a large survey of surgical personnel in seven countries, including the United States and Canada, 44.5% of respondents had been exposed to at least one abusive event in an operating room in the preceding year (Villafranca et al, 2017).

However, abusive team members are only the most obvious problem. Most psychologically unsafe environments are caused not by overtly hostile, bullying, or abusive behavior. They are more often the result of subtle condescension, sarcasm, humiliation, shame, and other dismissive behaviors. Unit and senior leadership have a moral imperative to identify such hostile work environments and to address them through appropriate actions including, where necessary, dismissal of staff members who refuse to change their behavior. Such behaviors create a vicious cycle that hurts patients and clinicians (Figure 25.2). Staff surveys can include questions about mutual respect, safety climate, and esprit de corps to help identify units that are struggling with poor teamwork and psychological safety.

Handling Disruptive Behavior

Disruptive or disrespectful behavior is serious and a critical matter for leaders to address immediately and with deliberate action. Evidence indicates that burnout increases the likelihood of individuals behaving disrespectfully and that disruptive behavior can be a cause of burnout in others.

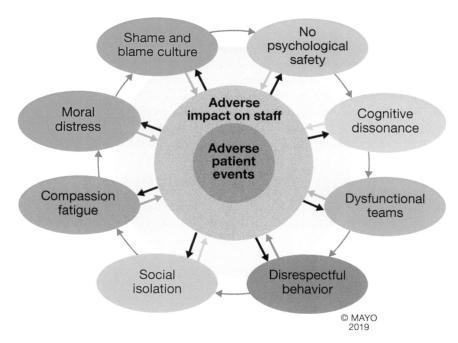

Figure 25.2. The Vicious Cycle of Adverse Events in a World Without Fair and Just Accountability.

The first step in handling disruptive behavior is to ensure that a fair and just process exists for those accused of unprofessional behavior. That process should recognize that there are typically two sides to a story and should allow for collecting as complete and accurate information as possible. There should be a consistent and principled approach to dealing with individuals who have patterns of unprofessional behavior, with a goal of remediation. An authentic appeals process should also be included in this procedure, especially when the complaints against an individual are anonymous in nature.

In the initial stages of investigation, those responsible must make sure the disruptor does not need help (e.g., for substance abuse, burnout, depression) and strive to understand the disruptor's perspective on the alleged incident or behavior. The disruptive behavior may be a sign of someone reaching out for help. Disruptive persons should be given the help they need, even as they are counseled that this type of behavior will not be tolerated and they will be held accountable for their unacceptable actions.

The second step (assuming the behavior was indeed out of line) is to (with absolute clarity) set expectations for the person's future behavior and set the consequences if the standards are not met. The graduated performance management plan (with corrective actions) should indicate that the consequences are suspension or ultimately dismissal if the individual cannot or will not meet the behavior expectations.

Health care professionals must have confidence that the process is designed to seek truth and is consistent and appropriate in the corrective actions taken. Lack of attention to these characteristics creates a psychologically unsafe work environment and causes health care professionals to lose confidence in the integrity of their organization. Few things destroy the trust between health care professionals and their organization more quickly than watching colleagues or co-workers be treated unfairly. There is nothing that sends the message that the organization is serious about upholding the highest standards of mutual respect and professional behavior than walking one or two people who are unwilling to uphold such standards out the front door. There is also nothing that says the organization cares about perception over truth and justice than treating someone unfairly. Just like the criminal justice system, nothing destroys the faith of health care professionals in their organization faster.

Esprit de corps is dependent on leaders addressing disrespectful and disruptive behavior in a consistent, fair, and just manner.

COLLABORATIVE EFFORT (FOCUS GROUPS)

Leader attention to a just and accountable culture yields real dividends for health care professionals and for patients. At Mayo Clinic, more than 200 clinical units and more than 10,000 staff have been engaged collaboratively in focus groups to improve patient safety, fair and just accountability, workplace morale, hand offs, and teamwork. The process involves team-based collaborations to identify common pain-point issues, which are addressed by the group. The clinical units engaged in this manner have successfully improved leadership, patient safety, and teamwork measures. Specifically, the *absolute* workplace morale score improved 17%, the teamwork score improved 12%, and satisfaction with hand offs improved 11%. After seeing these outcomes, senior leadership supported the complete rollout to over 800 work-unit teams involving 61,000 staff.

THE VIRTUOUS CYCLE

A virtuous cycle of support for health care professionals has the principles of fair and just accountability as a central component. As the culture-transition work becomes a reality, there will be fewer adverse patient events, less secondary distress, and fewer malpractice suits. These better working conditions also reduce staff turnover, improve camaraderie, build teamwork, increase efficiency, and, ultimately, create esprit de corps. Professional fulfillment begets more engagement and leads to a virtuous cycle of meaning, efficiency of practice, and camaraderie. The work environment becomes even more clinician friendly, and the organization has lower turnover and better experiences, safety, and outcomes for their patients.

CONCLUSION

Instilling principles of fair and just accountability into the work culture enhances Coherence, which cultivates work elements necessary for combating professional burnout and creating esprit de corps. These actions are evidence based and validated. The emotional stakes are high for individual health care professionals dealing with the consequences of human error and system defects. The stakes are also high for organizations dealing with such events—indeed, their integrity and credibility with their staff are at stake. Health care professionals must feel that they and their co-workers are supported and being treated fairly and consistently. When a culture of fair and just accountability is suboptimal, health care professionals feel socially isolated and stressed, and patient harm events increase, as does the risk of burnout.

For optimal esprit de corps, health care leaders must also actively seek to identify and eradicate hostile work environments and disrespectful clinicians. This requires anonymous or confidential processes to report inappropriate behavior and systematic assessment of mutual respect, teamwork, and safety climate on annual surveys. However, a fair and just process, recognizing two sides for every story, must exist for those accused of unprofessional behavior. The process should include a means for appeals and incorporate discipline, including dismissal, when necessary (Box 25.1).

TOMORROW: FULFILLMENT

After the infant's death, Samantha was consoled by members of her team. She was given some time off and offered the support of a psychologist. Two senior leaders, the chief nursing officer, and the chief executive officer arranged a brief meeting with her to express their empathy and assure her that the organization was committed to her as well as to addressing the factors in the work environment that contributed to the event. She was provided resources and support for the lawsuit.

A multidisciplinary team conducted a thorough root cause analysis. They reviewed all of the systems, processes, behaviors, and technology involved in medication administration in the intensive care unit. They found seven previously unrecognized process defects. The team was astounded that professionals had been working in this high-risk setting with such systems set up for failure. System changes were rapidly deployed not only in Samantha's unit but also in similar units across the organization.

Samantha felt validated because the organization recognized that system factors contributed to the error. More importantly, the organization demonstrated that they were more focused on preventing future patient harms than on finding a scapegoat to blame for the previous event.

Samantha was still devastated. But her team and leaders supported her. She briefly thought of suicide, but her focus rapidly shifted to getting back to caring for patients and improving the system for future patients. She knew that she wanted to continue to care for patients, and her colleagues knew that they did not want to lose her. Because she worked in a culture with a high level of esprit de corps, Samantha recovered from the trauma and rejoined the team.

Box 25.1 The Playbook

- Include measures of psychological safety and teamwork climate on annual staff surveys.
- Review work-unit results to determine where there are problems with psychological safety and fair and just accountability.
  - Meet with team members to understand opportunities for improvement and address them as needed.
- Determine whether organization policies, the sentinel-event reporting system, and the root cause analysis process are consistent with the principles of fair and just accountability rather than shame and blame.
- Address deficiencies.
- Create a process that provides an avenue for confidential or anonymous reporting of unprofessional and inappropriate behavior.
- Develop a fair and just process to engage an individual accused of unprofessional behavior. That process should recognize both sides of the story. Ensure that there is a consistent and principled approach to dealing with individuals who have patterns of unprofessional behavior.

SUGGESTED READING

Hall LW, Scott SD. The second victim of adverse health care events. Nurs Clin North Am. 2012 Sep;47(3):383–93.

Institute for Safe Medication Practices (ISMP). An injustice has been done: jail time given to pharmacist who made an error [Internet]. 2009 [cited 2019 Nov 4]. Available from: https://www.ismp.org/resources/injustice-has-been-done-jail-time-given-pharmacist-who-made-error.

Marx D. Patient safety and the "just culture": a primer for health care executives [Internet]. 2001 [cited 2019 Apr 11]. Available from: https://nursing2015.files.wordpress.com/2010/02/mers.pdf.

Shanafelt TD, Balch CM, Dyrbye L, Bechamps G, Russell T, Satele D, et al. Special report: suicidal ideation among American surgeons. Arch Surg. 2011 Jan;146(1):54–62.

Swensen SJ, Dilling JA, Harper CM Jr, Noseworthy JH. The Mayo Clinic value creation system. Am J Med Qual. 2012 Jan-Feb;27(1):58–65.

Swensen SJ, Meyer GS, Nelson EC, Hunt GC Jr, Pryor DB, Weissberg JI, et al. Cottage industry to postindustrial care: the revolution in health care delivery. N Engl J Med. 2010 Feb 4;362(5):e12.

Villafranca A, Young AE, Hamlin C, Arora R, Jacobsohn E. Abusive behavior in the operating room: prevalence and predictors. Anesthesiology Annual Meeting; 2017 Oct 21-25; Boston, MA.

26

COHERENCE ACTION: FORMING SAFE HAVENS

TODAY: DISTRESS

Sam is a well-respected obstetrician who meticulously follows protocol. Last month, one of his patients, a 23-year-old woman, had a hemorrhagic stroke. She had received anticoagulation for a deep venous thrombosis that developed after childbirth. Sam and his team followed the anticoagulation protocol meticulously, but the patient's clotting factor level got too low, which caused the stroke. It is not clear if she will fully recover. Sam is struggling with this tragic adverse event. He continually reworks the case in his mind and wonders if he should have or could have done something differently. He wonders if this event would have occurred if he had adjusted the anticoagulation himself rather than used the standard protocol. He does not know whom to talk to about this. He is concerned about a lawsuit. He is having trouble sleeping and focusing at work and wonders if he has lost his edge.

◆ ◆ ◆

Forming Safe Havens is the final Coherence Action. Safe haven creates a confidential and readily accessible refuge to provide emotional support for health care professionals dealing with occupational distress due to medical errors, the consequences of which include secondary distress, compassion fatigue, depression, and risk of suicide.

In this chapter, we present a plan to create safe havens that mitigates the negative consequences of occupational distress and thus prevents the vicious cycle of self-criticism, isolation, and burnout.

CONSEQUENCES OF OCCUPATIONAL DISTRESS

Stigma and barriers make it more difficult for professionals to seek help for emotional and psychological issues related to many kinds of occupational distress. Many state/territory medical licensure applications contain questions about physician mental health (Polfliet, 2008). The presence of questions about mental health issues or problems with substance use may cause professionals to avoid or delay treatment (Schroeder et al, 2009). The barriers for women physicians are even higher. Female professionals report substantial anxiety regarding the stigma of seeking counsel and treatment. This negatively impacts both disclosure and treatment (Gold et al, 2016).

Compassion Fatigue

Health care professionals are exposed to unique stressors. Many of their patients are combating illnesses that may have limited treatment options. Other patients are living with health conditions that have substantial emotional and existential dimensions. The best health care professionals express empathy and concern for their patients and help support them and their families.

Health care professionals are also exposed to death and human suffering as well as the sometimes unrealistic demands and expectations of patients or their loved ones who, understandably, want better options for care than current medical knowledge and treatment can provide. Long hours, overnight call, and night and weekend shifts are also characteristic of the work life of many health care professionals and may deplete physical and emotional reserves. Collectively, these challenges contribute to compassion fatigue.

Compassion fatigue results from the stress of serving patients and families in distress (i.e., regular exposure to human suffering, adverse patient events, and both anticipated and unanticipated deaths). Caring for a dying patient and the emotional labor associated with discussions and shared decision making about whether a patient wishes to forgo artificial life-sustaining treatment or institute end-of-life care are primary drivers of compassion fatigue. Compassion fatigue can result in apathy, social isolation, loss of meaning and purpose in work, and burnout.

The highest rates of compassion fatigue in health care occur in the nursing profession (Sinclair et al, 2017; Zhang et al, 2018). Nurses often have a front-row seat to patient suffering and, in hospital settings, typically spend a profoundly greater amount of time with each patient and family than other members of the health care team.

Preventable Harm

Health care organizations have an obligation to disclose and support patients and families who are the victims of preventable harm (i.e., any traumatic event that affects patients, their families, and other loved ones). They also have a responsibility to support clinicians experiencing secondary emotional distress triggered by these traumatic events. To minimize deleterious emotional consequences, organizations must show that they are committed to dealing with preventable harm in a just manner—one that addresses the factors that contributed to the defective care and does not simply blame the individual who provided the care (see Chapter 25, "Coherence Action: Establishing Fair and Just Accountability").

Secondary Distress

Most occurrences of preventable harm also cause secondary distress for the health care professional involved in the adverse clinical event or medical error. Health care professionals are motivated to help others and typically have pursued a medical career to heal and relieve suffering. They take the responsibility and trust patients place in them seriously and are substantially affected by adverse events.

The risk of depression for health care professionals triples in the three months after they perceive they have made a major medical error (Shanafelt et al, 2011). Many experience symptoms consistent with posttraumatic stress disorder or burnout. Burnout increases the risk of future errors. This situation has led some (Barnes et al, 2019) to suggest that the third person harmed in this scenario is the next patient of the health care professional who was not supported and healed. Therefore, creating psychological safety and a supportive environment are fundamental for the well-being and survival of health care professionals and their patients and for breaking the destructive chain of events when preventable harm occurs.

Suicide

The likelihood of physicians committing suicide is substantially higher than that in the general population. Job-related stress, compassion fatigue, cognitive dissonance, moral distress, medical errors, and burnout contribute to suicide risk. Studies of health care professionals also suggest the risk of suicide doubles in the three months after a major medical error and increases if a malpractice suit, a very public event, is filed (Shanafelt et al, 2011).

Health care organizations are typically aware when their people are involved in an adverse event (e.g., an error, when a patient dies) or are named in malpractice suits. Unfortunately, despite this knowledge, most organizations fail to respond at those times in a manner commensurate to the risk of harm.

SAFE HAVEN STRATEGY

Creating a safe haven for health care professionals is central to their well-being. A safe haven is a refuge that allows professionals to share personal emotions experienced as a result of adverse clinical events and to receive structured emotional support, not blame, from trained peers and colleagues. These actions and resources can mitigate the negative repercussions of preventable patient harm and adverse events on health care professionals. The best safe haven strategy includes the following components:

- A supportive team culture
- A psychologically and emotionally safe work environment
- An on-call institutional support team
- Peer-support programs
- Confidential, information-protected counseling services
- Enhanced support for professionals named in malpractice suits
- Multidisciplinary teams to address root causes of patient-harm events

Supportive Team Culture

Organizations have an obligation to nurture a supportive work environment. Today's health care professionals work in teams and, when a crisis occurs, they are likely to reach out to or confide first in members of their team. Because team members know the affected individual and have a relationship that predates the traumatic event, they are more likely to be a source of support.

The primary goal of supportive team culture is to mitigate the emotional trauma of health care professionals involved in anticipated adverse effects and unanticipated or tragic deaths. Some of the attributes of a supportive team culture include psychological and emotional safety, respectful team dynamics, authenticity, ability to be vulnerable with one another, and camaraderie. Providing team members space and a regular time to discuss the emotional challenges of their work also normalizes vulnerability and creates a safe environment to share stressors as they are experienced.

Lack of emotional safety and mutual respect in the work environment drives burnout and characterizes intimidating work environments that lead to adverse events and poor patient safety. Such unsympathetic work environments are incompatible with a supportive team culture.

Psychologically and Emotionally Safe Work Environments

Empathy and compassion for co-workers is an important and critical component of supportive teams and a successful safe haven. These qualities should be nurtured by organizations to help create a psychologically safe and supportive work environment. When physicians and nurses have compassion and empathy for patients and colleagues, their risk for burnout decreases, and their professional satisfaction, quality of life, and well-being improve (Boissy et al, 2016; Thirioux et al, 2016; Salvarani et al, 2019). Empathy and compassionate care also improve patient outcomes and family experiences. System-wide efforts to cultivate these qualities can build the collective skill of the organization and reverse the decline in empathy that often occurs among health care professionals during their training and in the arc of their career.

On-Call Institutional Support Team

Even when team support for individual health care professionals experiencing distress is optimized, there are times when the whole team is under stress. This may occur when the workload is high or after the death of a patient that affected the unit in a particularly powerful way. An on-call institutional team should be available to support units when such stress occurs. Its purpose is to provide social, psychological, and emotional support for the entire stressed unit.

Case Study: Code Lavender

Chaplains and nurses at Cleveland Clinic started a program to support health care professionals involved in adverse or stressful patient care events. They call the program Code Lavender (Poncet et al, 2007; Advisory Board, 2013; Cleveland Clinic, 2016). Code Lavender was designed to increase organizational acts of kindness for health care professionals after stressful workplace events occur. It provides a holistic, rapid response to all members of a unit in emotionally stressful times.

Any individual on the unit recognizing care-team stress can call a Code Lavender for the unit. When a Code Lavender is called, a team of support staff visit the stressed unit and provide various tools to decrease stress, including light massage, recorded music, singing, self-directed art, journaling, storytelling, guided imagery, meditation, movement and breathing exercises, acupressure, and holistic coaching.

They provide the unit Code Lavender kits that include lavender essential oil, chocolate, cards with words of comfort, and resource referral information. The Code Lavender team partners with the institution's wellness center and employee assistance program to coordinate long-term support for members of the unit. The support provided by Code Lavender is a tangible demonstration to the team that the organization cares about them, knows they are exposed to unique occupational stressors, and will be there to support and assist them.

Peer-Support Programs

Peer-support programs are low-stigma, low-barrier approaches to support health care professionals dealing with adverse events, burnout, or other personal or professional challenges. Successful peer-support programs are readily accessible and may reach some health care professionals who would not directly pursue a mental health consultation. Peer support, using a coaching framework, is an established approach that can provide support for diverse challenges and be a bridge to connect those dealing with issues to mental health professionals, if needed.

For 19 years, Mayo Clinic has provided peer support for physicians, scientists, and senior administrators through their Office of Staff Services (Shanafelt et al, 2017). The support provided goes beyond peer counseling for adverse clinical events and is available for any personal or professional issue. The peer-support resources for those experiencing distress are intentionally combined in the same physical space where resources for financial planning (e.g., retirement, tax services, college savings for children) are provided to increase awareness of the resource, normalize the use of the office, reduce the stigma of peer-support programs, and lessen barriers for those seeking assistance. Approximately 75% of staff uses the financial counseling services, and 5% to 7% access peer-support resources each year.

The office has also piloted systematic, comprehensive annual check-ups for physicians covering a range of topics intended to promote personal and emotional well-being (e.g., self-care, relationships, work-life integration) as well as professional well-being (e.g., career direction, promotion process).

Case Study: The Center for Professionalism and Peer Support at Brigham and Women's Hospital (Personal Communication, Jo Shapiro, M.D., F.A.C.S., and Pamela Galowitz)

Leaders at Brigham and Women's Hospital recognized that they could only achieve their mission if the well-being of clinicians was supported. To help provide such support, they established the Center for Professionalism and Peer Support in 2008. The focus of the center is to strengthen and support a culture of trust predicated on mutual respect for individuals, teams, the institution, and patients and their families. Three core programs were developed to support clinician well-being:

1) Peer support
2) Disclosure coaching
3) Professionalism and teamwork

The peer-support program focuses on supporting colleagues in emotionally stressful situations, such as after a medical error. The team recognized that, although health care professionals commit themselves to improving patients' lives, at some point they are likely to be involved in an event that harms a patient. The team trained dozens of clinicians who were not involved in mental health to reach out to colleagues after adverse events and other acute stressors, such as being named in a malpractice lawsuit, caring for trauma victims, experiencing patient aggression, or dealing with the illness of a colleague. The program was predicated on the belief that no health care professional should go through these events alone.

The disclosure coaching program sought to help prepare health care professionals for conversations with patients and families after adverse events by providing just-in-time disclosure coaching. Such conversations with patients and families are high stakes and emotionally charged, and most clinicians have had little or no prior experience conducting them. The coaching helps physicians prepare for these conversations and for communicating with patients and families with transparency and compassion.

The professionalism and teamwork program was based on the premise that respectful, professional behavior fosters trust, while toxic work environments negatively impact both clinician well-being and patient outcomes. Behavioral expectations at Brigham and Women's Hospital are clearly stated in the code of conduct and supported by education and training. All physicians are required to participate in facilitated, simulation-based, small-group training that illustrates professionalism challenges and ways to avoid and address them. Separate workshops help clinicians develop skills to provide difficult feedback and facilitate conflict resolution.

Confidential, Information-Protected Counseling Services

An employee assistance program that provides access to counselors and therapists available at no cost can be a work-based safe haven for health care professionals. The center should be specifically designed to identify and assist health care professionals in resolving personal emotional difficulties related to work stresses associated with clinical care and not just a generic employee assistance program, such as those found at any large employer. The interactions must be strictly confidential and the information protected (i.e., not discoverable in a malpractice suit). The steps necessary to provide such protection vary for each state and must be intentionally and carefully constructed. In some states, this requires oversight for peer-support and counseling services as part of quality improvement efforts.

Enhanced Support for Professionals Named in Malpractice Suits

Supporting health care professionals named in malpractice lawsuits is a highly specialized form of peer support. This circumstance generally requires support over a period often lasting one to three years. Clinicians involved in malpractice lawsuits should be assigned a *navigator*, a colleague with specific training in how to support a named person. Navigators are often professionals who have been involved in a malpractice lawsuit themselves. Health care professionals should be paired with navigators as soon as they are notified of a lawsuit. Navigators should explain what to expect, including that it is a lengthy process; describe commonly experienced emotions; and let the professional(s) know that they will be there to support them throughout.

Health care professionals named in a lawsuit should meet with their navigator at regular intervals. The organization should provide protected time for this as part of the malpractice process, just as they provide time for depositions related to the case. Because the timing of peak emotional response or crisis varies for each health care professional, navigators should also be on call to provide support as needed.

Multidisciplinary Teams to Address Root Causes of Patient-Harm Events

Organizations should establish multidisciplinary improvement teams to review all adverse events and identify and address the root causes. The time and resources invested will yield a meaningful return in quality of care and organizational culture. The primary dividend is a safer system. The multidisciplinary process involved in identifying and eradicating root causes augments camaraderie and boundaryless-ness. The act of working together with colleagues across disciplines (e.g., physicians, nurses, pharmacists, other team members) to prevent future harm is therapeutic and is a coherence intervention in its own right.

Case Study: OASIS (Personal Communication, Heather Farley, M.D., M.H.C.D.S., F.A.C.E.P., Chief Wellness Officer; Vanessa Downing, Ph.D., Director of Content Development and Training, Center for Provider Wellbeing, Institute for Learning, Leadership, and Development, ChristianaCare Health System)

In 2015, four colleagues in the ChristianaCare Health System decided to turn their longstanding individual concerns about burnout, compassion fatigue, vicarious trauma, and waning resilience into meaningful, tangible action. The year before, two members of the group had successfully launched a peer-support program for health care professionals involved in adverse patient care events. As the foundational work for the new project began, the team immersed themselves in data and evidence about the extent to which these issues threatened the ability of health care providers to experience meaning in their work and undermined organizational goals. The idea that emotional trauma resulting from patient-care experiences warranted an empathetic, system-based response gained surprising organizational traction and signaled a growing interest for addressing the occupational risks of trauma-rich environments.

The medical intensive care unit was selected for initial intervention on the basis of results of an employee-engagement survey and a determination of unit readiness through discussions with frontline leaders. The team identified unit champions to serve on the steering committee and involved them in the design and delivery of the interventions to address the need. OASIS was chosen as the name for the project (Opportunity to Achieve Staff Inspiration and Strength). A baseline survey of staff was conducted to measure compassion fatigue, vicarious trauma, burnout, and perceived resilience.

The backbone of the intervention consisted of delivering condensed training in eight monthly, experiential lessons. The interventions lasted five to ten minutes and were delivered in a conference room located on the unit. The interventions used colloquial, concrete language and relied upon interactive games, quizzes, and informal conversations that encouraged open sharing. The content was delivered during all shifts and to all staff (e.g., nurses, technicians, clerical staff, faculty physicians, resident physicians, advanced practice providers, respiratory therapists). The content was presented to more than 330 attendees over eight months.

In addition to these skill-building sessions, the team employed strategies to enhance recognition of co-worker distress, offer peer support after adverse events, foster camaraderie and social connection, and create operational work groups to identify and remediate sources of frustration. Finally, an OASIS room was opened within the intensive care unit that consisted of dedicated space designed by the unit champions, with the intent of providing respite space where staff could recover and reset.

Data analysis after the intervention showed a substantial decrease in turnover and monthly unplanned days off. Substantial decreases in vicarious trauma, burnout, and depression were also noted from follow-up surveys.

The results were met with enthusiasm by health system leaders, and support for programmatic expansion was pledged. As of this writing, the OASIS project is rolling out in multiple patient care units across the system.

CONCLUSION

Creating safe haven for health care professionals experiencing occupational stress, which is inherent to health care delivery, helps to create the coherence necessary for esprit de corps. Safe haven and a supportive team culture should mitigate the negative effects of occupational stress and create a refuge for health care professionals involved in adverse patient care events. Even as organizations identify and reduce the root causes of events that harm patients, they must also support the health care professionals involved in such events. Doing so prevents a vicious cycle of occupational distress, burnout, compassion fatigue, preventable harm, secondary distress, depression, and suicidal ideation. Creating safe spaces for teams to routinely discuss patient care and adverse events and to enhance the ability of team members to support each other is an important way to normalize such discussions and create vulnerability.

Forming safe havens requires a multipronged approach and includes providing a supportive team culture; a psychologically and emotionally safe work environment; an on-call institutional support team; robust peer support; confidential, information-protected counseling; and support and resources during malpractice suits; as well as addressing root causes of patient-harm events. Reducing preventable patient harm, assisting health care professionals involved in adverse clinical events when events occur, and supporting distressed health care professionals—forming a safe haven—can mitigate the drivers of burnout and promote well-being (Box 26.1).

TOMORROW: FULFILLMENT

After the adverse event involving his patient who had a hemorrhagic stroke, Sam met with a colleague in the peer-support program who provided support and connected him to a staff psychologist in the hospital's confidential clinician support program. The conversations were very helpful. Sam subsequently met with the patient and her family to express his concern and compassion. They expressed gratitude for the care he provided and his kindness and were pleased that her symptoms were improving. Sam's symptoms of compassion fatigue and burnout are improving. He is now fully engaged in his practice and helping heal and relieve the suffering of other patients.

Box 26.1 The Playbook

- Nurture a supportive team culture: team members are the first source of support after traumatic occupational events.
- Provide team members with space and a regular time to discuss the emotional challenges of their work. This action normalizes vulnerability and creates a safe environment for them to share future stressors as they are experienced.
- Establish a robust and appropriately resourced peer-support program with a hotline number or web link to connect a struggling clinician.
- Consider establishing a Code Lavender response team to support work units experiencing stress.
- Provide confidential, information-protected professional counseling for health care professionals dealing with occupationally precipitated stress.
- Establish a navigator program to support health care professionals named in malpractice suits.
- Form multidisciplinary teams to evaluate and address the root causes of patient-harm events.

SUGGESTED READING

Advisory Board. When Cleveland Clinic staff are troubled, they file 'code lavender' [Internet]. 2013 [cited 2019 Apr 12]. Available from: https://www.advisory.com/Daily-Briefing/2013/12/03/When-Cleveland-Clinic-staff-are-troubled-they-file-Code-Lavender.

Barnes R, Blyth CC, de Klerk N, Lee WH, Borland ML, Richmond P, et al. Geographical disparities in emergency department presentations for acute respiratory infections and risk factors for presenting: a population-based cohort study of Western Australian children. BMJ Open. 2019 Feb 24;9(2):e025360.

Boissy A, Windover AK, Bokar D, Karafa M, Neuendorf K, Frankel RM, et al. Communication skills training for physicians improves patient satisfaction. J Gen Intern Med. 2016 Jul;31(7):755–61.

Cleveland Clinic. Code lavender: offering emotional support through holistic rapid response [Internet]. 2016 [cited 2019 Apr 12]. Available from: https://consultqd.clevelandclinic.org/code-lavender-offering-emotional-support-holistic-rapid-response/.

Gold KJ, Andrew LB, Goldman EB, Schwenk TL. "I would never want to have a mental health diagnosis on my record." A survey of female physicians on mental health diagnosis, treatment, and reporting. Gen Hosp Psychiatry. 2016 Nov-Dec;43:51–7.

Hawton K, Agerbo E, Simkin S, Platt B, Mellanby RJ. Risk of suicide in medical and related occupational groups: a national study based on Danish case population-based registers. J Affect Disord. 2011 Nov;134(1-3):320–6.

Office for National Statistics. Suicide by occupation, England: 2011 to 2015 [Internet]. 2017 [cited 2019 Apr 11]. Available from: https://www.ons.gov.uk/peoplepopulation-andcommunity/birthsdeathsandmarriages/deaths/articles/suicidebyoccupation/england2011to2015.

Polfliet SJ. A national analysis of medical licensure applications. J Am Acad Psychiatry Law. 2008;36(3):369–74.

Poncet MC, Toullic P, Papazian L, Kentish-Barnes N, Timsit JF, Pochard F, et al. Burnout syndrome in critical care nursing staff. Am J Respir Crit Care Med. 2007 Apr 1;175(7):698–704.

Salvarani V, Rampoldi G, Ardenghi S, Bani M, Blasi P, Ausili D, et al. Protecting emergency room nurses from burnout: the role of dispositional mindfulness, emotion regulation and empathy. J Nurs Manag. 2019 May;27(4):765–74.

Schernhammer ES, Colditz GA. Suicide rates among physicians: a quantitative and gender assessment (meta-analysis). Am J Psychiatry. 2004 Dec;161(12):2295–302.

Schroeder R, Brazeau CM, Zackin F, Rovi S, Dickey J, Johnson MS, et al. Do state medical board applications violate the Americans with disabilities act? Acad Med. 2009 Jun;84(6):776–81.

Shanafelt TD, Balch CM, Dyrbye L, Bechamps G, Russell T, Satele D, et al. Special report: suicidal ideation among American surgeons. Arch Surg. 2011 Jan;146(1):54–62.

Shanafelt TD, Lightner DJ, Conley CR, Petrou SP, Richardson JW, Schroeder PJ, et al. An organization model to assist individual physicians, scientists, and senior health care administrators with personal and professional needs. Mayo Clin Proc. 2017 Nov;92(11):1688–96.

Shapiro J, Galowitz P. Peer support for clinicians: a programmatic approach. Acad Med. 2016 Sep;91(9):1200–4.

Sinclair S, Raffin-Bouchal S, Venturato L, Mijovic-Kondejewski J, Smith-MacDonald L. Compassion fatigue: a meta-narrative review of the healthcare literature. Int J Nurs Stud. 2017 Apr;69:9–24.

Thirioux B, Birault F, Jaafari N. Empathy is a protective factor of burnout in physicians: new neuro-phenomenological hypotheses regarding empathy and sympathy in care relationship. Front Psychol. 2016;7:763.

Zhang YY, Han WL, Qin W, Yin HX, Zhang CF, Kong C, et al. Extent of compassion satisfaction, compassion fatigue and burnout in nursing: a meta-analysis. J Nurs Manag. 2018 Oct;26(7):810–9.

27

CAMARADERIE ACTION SET: INTRODUCTION

Alone we can do so little; together we can do so much.
—Helen Keller

Camaraderie is the loyalty, social capital, mutual respect, teamwork, and bound-arylessness that organizations need to thrive. In this section, we explore the social connectedness inherent in camaraderie and its inextricable link with the meaning and purpose, intrinsic motivation, and personal relationships that health care professionals find in work. The Action Set for Camaraderie is designed to mitigate or eliminate known, specific drivers of professional burnout and to nurture supportive leaders and systems that foster the interrelated Ideal Work Elements.

Primary burnout driver addressed by Camaraderie Actions:

1) Isolation, loneliness, and lack of social support at work

Ideal Work Elements cultivated by Camaraderie Actions:

1) Community at work and camaraderie (Chapter 28)
2) Intrinsic motivation and rewards (Chapter 29)

Camaraderie Actions:

1) Cultivating community and commensality (Chapter 30)
2) Optimizing rewards, recognition, and appreciation (Chapter 31)
3) Fostering boundarylessness (Chapter 32)

We first present the two germane Ideal Work Elements followed directly by the three aligned Camaraderie Actions.

28

CAMARADERIE IDEAL WORK ELEMENT: COMMUNITY AT WORK AND CAMARADERIE

We are only as strong as we are united, as weak as we are divided.
—J.K. Rowling

Community at work and camaraderie, the first of two Ideal Work Elements for Camaraderie, are cultivated by actions to improve social support among health care professionals. Health care professionals thrive when they are part of a supportive community of colleagues (Swensen et al, 2016). The act of coming together and supporting one another so that patients can be best served is what community at work and camaraderie are all about.

WORKING TOGETHER

During the Great Depression, Mayo Clinic experienced a 40% decrease in patient visits to fewer than 50,000 per year. Approximately one in four of the patients who were seen did not have the money to pay for their care. Yet, all patients were served regardless of their ability to pay. Of course, this turn of events left Mayo Clinic with vast excess capacity and not enough money to pay salaries and bills. Many organizations would have "decreased the head count" to meet payroll. But at Mayo Clinic the leaders instead decided to have everyone take a pay cut to a "bare bones" salary. Because everyone was treated equally, no one felt singled out. And, everyone knew they needed to pull together as a team to make it through the difficult times. The lead administrator, Harry Harwick, reflecting on this dark time, termed it "the most unifying influence in Mayo Clinic history." Everyone was in it together.

Because humans are social creatures, community at work and camaraderie can combat burnout, foster esprit de corps, and enable people to overcome seemingly insurmountable challenges. Studies suggest that burnout can be alleviated for professionals when they spend time with colleagues in a psychologically safe setting designed to provide the opportunity for shared experience and mutual support (see Chapter 26, "Coherence Action: Forming Safe Havens") (West et al, 2014; Kim et al, 2018). Colleagues provide a special community of support that others cannot because they understand the unique challenges of their work and profession. For example, a group of nurses is best equipped to understand and support a junior nurse dealing with the emotional burden of losing a young patient she has cared for. Another pharmacist may be the best source of support for a junior colleague dealing with the stress of a systems issue that generated a medication error.

Creating a culture of mutual respect and social support is fundamental to engendering community at work and camaraderie. Health care organizations have a responsibility to create such a culture and recognize that community at work is a necessary system safeguard against occupational risks, such as emotional burden, exposure to human suffering, deaths of patients, and demanding and unpredictable fluctuations in workload. Organizations that do not attend to building and maintaining community set up professionals for failure. Organizations that foster socially connected teams of people who care for and care about each other have health care professionals with:

↑ Professional satisfaction
↑ Commitment and loyalty
↑ Engagement
↑ Productivity
↓ Exhaustion
↓ Burnout

TEAMWORK

Teamwork is an important dimension of community at work and camaraderie. Team members must value each other as human beings, not simply as role-based co-workers. They must show each other respect, authenticity, appreciation, loyalty, and recognition of each other's talents. A sense of belonging, resulting from teamwork, is a critical component of professional fulfillment that helps in providing immunity to burnout. Clinics with high multidisciplinary teamwork ratings realize superior patient experience scores, higher nurse retention rates, and lower operating costs (Swensen et al, 2013).

At Mayo Clinic, the assessment of teamwork dynamics in each work unit, with relentless focus on improvement, has paid organizational dividends over the decades. The returns include exceptional and ever-improving quality, high morale, low turnover, high professionalism, and interdisciplinary collaboration. Dividends for patients include less pain and anxiety, lower blood pressure, shorter length of hospital stay, lower readmission rates, and faster surgical wound healing (Hsu et al, 2012; Doyle et al, 2013).

Organizations and patients aren't the only ones who experience better results from teamwork and camaraderie. Teamwork creates an environment where co-workers have the opportunity to be safely vulnerable and authentic and express compassion for one another. Health care professionals who provide (or observe colleagues providing) compassionate treatment also benefit. Examples of compassion for colleagues include assisting a co-worker when the workload is high, looking out for one another, encouraging a colleague under stress, consoling someone after an adverse patient outcome, and celebrating together when good things happen.

Task Sharing

Research shows that inadequate team staffing and turnover among team members increase the risk of burnout for all members of the care team (Helfrich et al, 2017; Kim et al, 2018). One element of teamwork, task sharing, can help to reduce turnover, stabilize staffing, and mitigate burnout—when it is collaborative, equitable, team based, and multidisciplinary. The well-being of everyone on the team must be considered in this process. Task sharing and delegation should be done thoughtfully with appropriate reengineering of work flows and practice efficiency as well as consideration of the overall workload and the expertise and training of care-team members. Care-team huddles are one best practice for promoting and optimizing task sharing and teamwork.

Case Study: Two Different Types of Health Care Institutions

A physician friend of ours related the story of a patient who was also a professional musician. He received care at a world-class East Coast medical center where our friend worked. He later came to Mayo Clinic for a second opinion regarding the management of his complex medical condition. Both organizations are consistently ranked among the top five medical centers in the United States. Our friend observed that his home medical center places great emphasis on optimizing and rewarding individual performance and expertise. Physicians are paid on the basis of individual productivity and higher academic rank.

At Mayo Clinic, all physicians in the same department are paid the same salary, regardless of academic rank and productivity. The emphasis is on supporting colleagues working in a highly integrated team. Each department is expected to function as an integrated part of the whole. Patients often see seven to eight different specialists and have dozens of studies, tests, and imaging in a two- to three-day window—as outpatients. A coordinating physician organizes the interdisciplinary collaboration, and all specialists talk to one other. This level of integration is unparalleled. Rewards are team based. Patients with complex medical problems can typically have a more complete and coordinated evaluation in a couple days as an outpatient at Mayo Clinic than can be accomplished in one to two weeks in the hospital at most of the elite medical centers around the world.

After returning to the first medical center, the patient summed up his experience to his physician, "You have some world class soloists and even a few quartets. Mayo Clinic has an orchestra."

CONCLUSION

The important Ideal Work Element, community at work and camaraderie, can be cultivated by the actions that will be described in Chapters 30 through 32. Community at work and camaraderie are critical characteristics of resilient, high-functioning teams. Both can be nurtured. The most successful organizations attend to these characteristics and develop programs and leader behaviors to cultivate them.

SUGGESTED READING

Barsade SG, O'Neill OA. What's love got to do with it? A longitudinal study of the culture of companionate love and employee and client outcomes in a long-term care setting. Admin Sci Q. 2014;59(4):551–98.

Cosley BJ, McCoy SK, Saslow LR, Epel ES. Is compassion for others stress buffering? Consequences of compassion and social support for physiological reactivity to stress. J Exp Soc Psychol. 2010;46(5):816–23.

Doyle C, Lennox L, Bell D. A systematic review of evidence on the links between patient experience and clinical safety and effectiveness. BMJ Open. 2013 Jan 3;3(1):e001570.

Edwards ST, Helfrich CD, Grembowski D, Hulen E, Clinton WL, Wood GB, et al. Task delegation and burnout trade-offs among primary care providers and nurses in Veterans Affairs Patient Aligned Care Teams (VA PACTs). J Am Board Fam Med. 2018 Jan-Feb;31(1):83–93.

Egbert LD, Battit GE, Welch CE, Bartlett MK. Reduction of postoperative pain by encouragement and instruction of patients: a study of doctor-patient rapport. N Engl J Med. 1964 Apr 16;270:825–7.

Emanuel L, Ferris FD, von Gunten CF, von Roenn JH. Combating compassion fatigue and burnout in cancer care [Internet]. Excerpted and adapted from: Emanuel LL, Ferris FD, von Gunten CF, Von Roenn J, eds. EPEC-O: education in palliative and end-of-life are for oncology (module 15: cancer doctors and burnout). 2011 [cited 2018 Nov 20]. Available from: https://www.medscape.com/viewarticle/742941.

Hamrick WS. Kindness and the good society: connections of the heart. Albany (NY): SUNY Press; 2002.

Helfrich CD, Simonetti JA, Clinton WL, Wood GB, Taylor L, Schectman G, et al. The association of team-specific workload and staffing with odds of burnout among VA primary care team members. J Gen Intern Med. 2017 Jul;32(7):760–6.

Hsu I, Saha S, Korthuis PT, Sharp V, Cohn J, Moore RD, et al. Providing support to patients in emotional encounters: a new perspective on missed empathic opportunities. Patient Educ Couns. 2012 Sep;88(3):436–42.

Kelley JM, Kraft-Todd G, Schapira L, Kossowsky J, Riess H. The influence of the patient-clinician relationship on healthcare outcomes: a systematic review and meta-analysis of randomized controlled trials. PLoS One. 2014;9(4):e94207.

Kim LY, Rose DE, Soban LM, Stockdale SE, Meredith LS, Edwards ST, et al. Primary care tasks associated with provider burnout: findings from a veterans health administration survey. J Gen Intern Med. 2018 Jan;33(1):50–6.

Rakel DP, Hoeft TJ, Barrett BP, Chewning BA, Craig BM, Niu M. Practitioner empathy and the duration of the common cold. Fam Med. 2009 Jul-Aug;41(7):494–501.

Shanafelt TD. Enhancing meaning in work: a prescription for preventing physician burnout and promoting patient-centered care. JAMA. 2009 Sep 23;302(12):1338–40.

Sinsky C, Colligan L, Li L, Prgomet M, Reynolds S, Goeders L, et al. Allocation of physician time in ambulatory practice: a time and motion study in 4 specialties. Ann Intern Med. 2016 Dec 6;165(11):753–60.

Swensen S, Gorringe G, Caviness J, Peters D. Leadership by design: intentional organization development of physician leaders. J Manag Dev. 2016;35(4):549–70.

Swensen SJ, Dilling JA, McCarty PM, Bolton JW, Harper CM Jr. The business case for health-care quality improvement. J Patient Saf. 2013 Mar;9(1):44–52.

West CP, Dyrbye LN, Rabatin JT, Call TG, Davidson JH, Multari A, et al. Intervention to promote physician well-being, job satisfaction, and professionalism: a randomized clinical trial. JAMA Intern Med. 2014 Apr;174(4):527–33.

Zolnierek KB, Dimatteo MR. Physician communication and patient adherence to treatment: a meta-analysis. Med Care. 2009 Aug;47(8):826–34.

29

CAMARADERIE IDEAL WORK ELEMENT: INTRINSIC MOTIVATION AND REWARDS

We make a living by what we get, but we make a life by what we give.
—Winston Churchill

The second principal Ideal Work Element cultivated by Camaraderie is intrinsic motivation and rewards. By nature, most health care professionals are motivated by altruistic values and should receive intrinsic—rather than superficial or extrinsic—rewards and recognition. An environment and culture that encourage intrinsic motivation and rewards help alleviate burnout and foster esprit de corps. Specific actions for achieving this element are detailed in Chapter 31 ("Camaraderie Action: Optimizing Rewards, Recognition, and Appreciation").

DREAMS AND PASSION

In the late 1800s, Samuel Langley led a team that was supposed to build the first airplane. His resources included the best scientists, a full-time staff, an amazing budget of $50,000 from the U.S. Department of War, and an additional $20,000 from the Smithsonian Institution. Samuel Langley had everything he needed to win the race and wanted to be first. But he didn't win. Orville and Wilbur did.

In the winds of Kitty Hawk, North Carolina, on December 17, 1903, the Wright brothers were the first to fly. The two brothers ran a small bicycle repair shop. They had no budget, no staff, no scientists—nothing except a dream and a cartload of desire.

Samuel Langley was trying to build an airplane for fame, money, and glory. It was not a calling. Orville and Wilbur had a calling. They were chasing a dream. They were inspired to make a difference. The Wright brothers were driven by intrinsic motivation and rewards and Samuel Langley by extrinsic ones.

Dreams and passion do not always yield fame or success, but they are always the key to discretionary effort and to maximizing human motivation.

INTRINSIC VS. EXTRINSIC MOTIVATION AND REWARDS

Intrinsic motivation arises from an activity itself rather than from an external reward. Doing something for its own sake or because it aligns with one's values—such as wanting to help others, contribute to a cause, or connect to a community—are deep-rooted, intrinsic needs and have profound motivational power. The rewards are internal.

In contrast, extrinsic motivation gains its leverage from the possibility of external rewards such as money, plaques, benefit packages, awards, and bonuses. These rewards are profoundly different than intrinsic motivators such as the satisfaction that comes from doing a job well or helping someone in need. The latter might be accompanied by an extrinsic reward, but it is not motivated by it. Systems focused on extrinsic rewards are often divisive and incite competition with colleagues rather than collaboration.

With few exceptions, research has consistently demonstrated that humans are best and most effectively motivated by intrinsic drivers (Pink, 2009). One recent survey of 200,000 employees working in more than 500 organizations asked, "What motivates you to excel and go the extra mile at your organization?" (Drzymalski et al, 2014). The top seven motivators were:

1) Camaraderie: 20%
2) Intrinsic desire to do a good job: 17%
3) Feeling encouraged and recognized: 13%
4) Having a real impact: 10%
5) Growing professionally: 8%
6) Meeting customer needs: 8%
7) Money and benefits: 7%

More than 90% of employees listed one of the first six rewards, which are all intrinsic motivators. Money and benefits (extrinsic motivators) ranked last, cited by only 7%.

Excellence

Clinicians and medical centers have the pursuit of excellence as a common goal. For health care professionals to reach this goal, they must find meaning and purpose in work that stems from delivering superlative, patient-centered health care (Grant, 2008; Grant and Hoffman, 2011). Physicians, nurses, advanced practice providers (APPs), and pharmacists are generally driven and accomplished individuals who have had to demonstrate aptitude, commitment, resilience, and dedication to be selected for and to complete their professional training. With few exceptions, each cares deeply about patient outcomes (i.e., safety, quality, and experience), efficiency, and wasted resources.

Although these values often align with the priorities of their organizations, most health care professionals are initially interested only tangentially in organization level processes, systems, and priorities. Therefore, leaders and administrators have the responsibility to ensure that health care professionals understand how the aspects of their work that they care about align with organizational priorities. This intentional communication model facilitates a shared sense of purpose, collaboration, and the pursuit of excellence. Medical centers can use various approaches to engage professionals in improving systems to support optimal patient care. Examples include using data to identify areas needing improvement, engaging the professionals in that area to get their ideas on the opportunities to improve, providing visible support through leadership and resources for improving work, identifying and developing clinician champions to help engage peers, and communicating the value of the group's effort and contributions (more on this in Chapter 31, "Camaraderie Action: Optimizing Rewards, Recognition, and Appreciation").

These positive approaches to improving organization systems and excellence help cultivate engagement and esprit de corps.

Money

Question: Does money buy happiness?

Answer: According to the research of two Nobel Laureates, not if you make more than $75,000 per year (Kahneman and Deaton, 2010). Once income is adequate to provide for basic needs (e.g., safe shelter, food), additional income is not substantially related to more happiness—even though most people may think it is. A survey of 4,000 millionaires showed that 87% believed that more money would make them happier. Notably, within this group, only those with very high levels of net worth (greater than $10 million) were actually happier, and they were only moderately happier (Donnelly et al, 2018). What is striking was that the slight increase in happiness among those with extremely high net worth was related to their ability to use their money to help others and to the greater control over their time that money brought them. The researchers also found that those millionaires who created their own wealth (as opposed to inheriting it) were happier, perhaps because there was an intrinsic reward from their labor.

Although some clinicians believe that making more money would reduce burnout, this does not appear to be true. Indeed, analysis of which medical specialties have both high burnout scores and low satisfaction with work-life integration identified some of the highest paid specialties (e.g., orthopedic surgery) as well as some of the lowest paid (e.g., family medicine) (Shanafelt et al, 2015). Notably, those doing well in both dimensions included some of the lowest paid specialties (e.g., pediatrics). Thus, disparity in income by specialty does not appear to be a major cause of burnout. The myth that more money means more happiness could, however, be part of the reason why physicians overwork and why pay-for-performance models of compensation add fuel to the burnout fire.

Ironically, once burnout occurs, evidence shows that making more money might contribute to satisfaction if it allows physicians to work fewer hours (called *partially quitting*) (Shanafelt et al, 2016). This scenario suggests that our clinical practice models are so broken that dedicated, intrinsically motivated clinicians often use the spoils of extrinsic rewards to work less than full time to avoid burnout (Shanafelt et al, 2016).

Case Studies: Hand Sanitizer

Two recent studies on hand sanitation further illustrate the ability of intrinsic and extrinsic rewards to motivate health care professionals (Grant and Hofmann, 2011).

In the first study, signs were attached to hand sanitizer dispensers throughout the hospital. Each sign had the same message, except for one word.

The first sign said:

"Hand hygiene prevents *you* from catching diseases."

The second sign said:

"Hand hygiene prevents *patients* from catching diseases."

Changing a single word in the message resulted in substantial modifications in behavior. When professionals were reminded that use of hand sanitizer would help patients, they were more likely to pump the dispenser. An altruistic intrinsic motivator was more powerful than the suggestion of personal benefit.

This is not to say that extrinsic motivators don't work: They can, at least in the short term. A large U.S. academic medical center had hand sanitizer utilization rates of less than 50% at baseline. To reach levels above 90% in time for their scheduled regulatory accreditation visit, the organization decided to introduce a financial incentive for using hand sanitizer. If the organization reached its goal, all clinicians would receive a financial bonus. It worked. Within several months, the use of hand sanitizer before and after touching patients exceeded 90%.

It would have been cheaper to put up signs (and more prudent in the long run).

Paying professionals to do what they would do normally for altruistic reasons can also have profound, unintended negative consequences. It sends a message that money or another incentive is required to motivate individuals to provide high-quality care for patients. The use of extrinsic motivation to perform basic patient-safety practices, such as hand sanitation, is fundamentally flawed and turns a core professional value into a financial transaction in a way that is both demeaning and dangerous. Health care leaders should target the heart, not the bank account.

BURNOUT AND MODELS OF COMPENSATION

How health care professionals are paid also impacts their relationship to their work as well as their risk of burnout. Although most nurses are paid on an hourly wage basis (unless they are in management), there are many types of physician compensation models. Most systems fall into one of three general categories: salary, salary plus an incentive, and pure productivity (Figure 29.1).

In a national study, one of us (Shanafelt et al, 2014) reported the risk of burnout is lowest among physicians paid a fixed salary, increases among those given a base salary along with a bonus based on productivity, and is highest among those in a pure productivity-based compensation model. Similarly, in national studies of greater than 7,500 U.S. surgeons, a pure productivity-based compensation model was found to increase the risk of burnout by approximately 35%, after adjusting for all other personal and professional factors (Shanafelt et al, 2009).

These observations likely result, in part, from incentivizing overwork among a group of professionals who already work excessive hours. Incentivizing overwork also magnifies problems with work-life integration. Compensation models heavily weighted toward productivity-based pay change the relationship between professionals and their work. For example, many physicians working in such models refer to their compensation structure as "eat what you kill," which is a crass and unprofessional way to view caring for the health and well-being of other human beings.

In some productivity-based compensation models, health care professionals are rewarded with greater personal compensation depending on the medical care they recommend (they are rewarded for "generating downstream revenue"), which introduces a potential financial conflict of interest and can also increase burnout. Orthopedic surgeons deciding whether or not to recommend a spine operation should make that decision based solely on whether it is in the patient's best interest,

	Model		
	Salary	**Salary + Incentive**	**Productivity**
Intended conse-quences	Intrinsic motivation Focuses on value without financial conflict of interest with patient Favors cooperation over competition Emphasizes collaboration over independence Focuses on contribution to overall mission, including education, administration, research, and quality improvement Lowest burnout risk Prioritizes team over individuals	Favors value and moderates financial conflict of interest with patient Reduces financial risk of salary to the organization Favors cooperation over competition and collaboration over independence Greater burnout risk Dual focus on quality and production	Extrinsic motivation Focuses on volume Fairness in pay Minimizes financial risk of salary to the organization Prioritizes production over quality and patient satisfaction Highest burnout risk Potential threat to teamwork
Potential unintended conse-quences	RVU underperformance may be "rewarded" Risk of inequity in pay if the model is poorly managed Salary may be a financial risk to organization if demand or performance inadequate Salary may be a financial risk to organization if not structured properly or inadequate demand	Patient experience incentive may result in overuse of diagnostic tests, procedures, and drugs Risk of inequity in pay if the model is poorly managed Salary may be a financial risk to organization if not structured properly or inadequate demand	Risk incentivizing overwork and increasing burnout Transactional approach to care Financial conflict with patient and stated values of the organization Productivity at cost of patient experience and quality Cognitive dissonance Favors competition over cooperation Emphasizes independence over collaboration Prioritizes individuals over the team
Safeguards and mitigation strategies	Leadership conversations about performance to ensure fairness/equity Peer pressure Culture Transparency Minimum productivity thresholds	Leadership conversations based on intrinsic rewards Culture Transparency Counterbalancing quality measures Ceiling of maximum reward Counterbalancing measures to promote self-care and personal resilience	Counterbalancing quality measures Ceiling of maximum reward Counterbalancing measures to promote self-care and personal resilience

© MAYO 2019

Figure 29.1. Compensation Model Consequences. RVU indicates relative valve unit.

not on whether their personal compensation will increase if they recommend surgery. An oncologist recommending whether to pursue salvage chemotherapy should not have a financial interest in recommending more treatment or selecting one treatment over another. Although these principles have led to self-referral laws that prevent physicians profiting from some of the medical testing and imaging they own or recommend, the more pervasive conflict of interest, such as the examples above, are often widely promulgated through the productivity-based compensation models of many health care organizations.

Productivity-based compensation models, which focus on extrinsic motivation, may also cause individuals to view their job as transactional rather than as an altruistic calling. They also emphasize volume over quality and outcomes.

Salary plus an incentive approaches are hybrid models that blend a base salary with a productivity bonus. The intent of these approaches is often to mitigate the negative consequences of pure productivity-based models, while simultaneously ensuring equity and encouraging productivity/access. Whether such models strike a happy medium or devolve to "the worst of both worlds" depends on the implementation. Increasingly, safeguards are being introduced to serve as a counterbalance to the productivity-over-quality mindset. This is often accomplished by incorporating quality, patient satisfaction, and self-care measures (e.g., taking a minimum number of vacation days) along with the number of relative value units (RVUs) (the amount of work required for a physician to treat a patient) into the formula to determine the amount of the incentive people will receive.

Another innovative structure for such hybrid models is to base the incentive on team-based metrics for quality and productivity rather than individual metrics. This fosters teamwork and collaboration rather than competition (e.g., cherry picking certain types of patients to hit RVU-incentive targets) and fosters group efforts and accountability for improving quality.

Case Study: Production Models and Collegiality

A procedural-based specialty division at an elite academic medical center used a salary plus RVU-based incentive program. The compensation model had a profoundly negative impact on the morale in the division. The desire to maximize income was so strong that some physicians would cherry pick patients being referred for certain high-RVU procedures (i.e., quick procedures with high assigned RVUs). More complex cases that were more time intensive but had similar RVUs were so undesirable that nobody wanted them. The model also led to having individuals within this academic department build their own referral silos from the community (regardless of their area of subspecialty expertise) rather than function as a team of specialists applying and sharing the collective duties and expertise of the specialty, which was the premise behind community referrals to this academic center.

The system also led to faculty members overscheduling the number of procedures they could perform in their assigned procedure-room time block so that they could maximize personal RVUs (e.g., they would schedule 10 procedures into a morning block in which only seven or eight procedures could be performed). This led to morning blocks constantly running several hours into the afternoon, such that their colleagues who were assigned afternoon procedure-room times (typically the junior colleagues) nearly always started at least an hour late. This delay resulted in having physicians (and patients) regularly stay late for these elective procedures. This situation created tremendous friction and interpersonal conflict among team members. Over time, compensation inequity also developed.

Predictably, high turnover developed among the junior faculty. In addition, over several years, the staff collectively lost the surgical skills needed to perform one complex but relatively low-reimbursement procedure that was necessary for the center to function as a destination tertiary referral center. No one wanted those cases, and they filled up their calendars with the higher RVU cases. The division ultimately had to recruit a surgeon from another institution to bring that skill back to the institution. Further, to attract someone qualified and prevent the same thing from happening again, they had to give that person a separate, customized compensation plan distinct from everyone else's (potentially creating even more inequity).

Ultimately, in this case, the unintended consequences of the hybrid salary plus RVU incentive–compensation system led to an environment characterized by failing to meet patients' needs, discourteous behavior to colleagues, inequity, social isolation, poor team work, low morale, burnout, and turnover that were a disservice to patients, physicians, and the organization.

FINANCIAL PRESSURES

Productivity-based compensation models create financial pressures for health care professionals. The average debt of a graduating medical student is just shy of $200,000. Pressure to pay off that debt can increase stress and negatively influence the doctor-patient relationship. At a recent gathering of physicians, nurses, APPs, and administrators one of us attended, a physician stated, "I was so relieved when I was finally out of education loan debt. Until that point in my career, patients had a number on their forehead that was preceded by a dollar sign." Such financial pressures drive cognitive dissonance.

Many physicians and health care professionals with protracted training requirements also fall prey to a mindset of making up for lost time (delayed gratification). Physicians typically spend seven to 11 years in training after graduating from college and, during this time, often work extremely long hours with very modest pay. Most watch the friends they graduated with, even those who pursue other professional degrees, enjoy the financial benefits and security of beginning their career before they even complete their residency or fellowship. When these physicians finally enter practice in their early thirties, they often buy a home, a new car, and many of the things they and their families have done without for the previous decade. They often do so believing they can increase their income through productivity-based pay. These choices, however, further heighten financial pressures and encourage working excessive hours. Nurses and other health care professionals may also be impacted by such sentiments, leading them to pick up an excessive number of extra shifts. These financial pressures and an incentive to overwork can be even greater for young physicians living in areas with an extremely high cost of living (e.g., New York City, San Francisco, Seattle, Los Angeles, Boston, Chicago), which may compound the risk of productivity-based compensation models for organizations in these areas.

A Moving Target Income

In *target-income* theory, workers set a goal for the income that will support the lifestyles they aspire to and the debt load they have accumulated. Even if physicians initially set a realistic goal, that number will continually reset because of ever-changing payer reimbursements and payer mix. Approximately 10,000 Americans are now turning 65 years every day, which will continue for the next decade, causing the payer mix to shift to a larger proportion of Medicare payments. In most settings, this translates to lower reimbursement levels. For physicians and medical centers to keep even, they need to increase productivity. That usually means more work (increased volumes) for the same financial reward. This scenario can lead to a vicious cycle, resulting in burnout from higher workloads, problems with work-life integration, and cognitive dissonance.

The target-income theory and fee-for-service insurance do not match well with production models. Together, they are one of many root causes of overuse of medical services in this country. Financial rewards for greater RVU generation may lead to *up-coding* (i.e., payment coding for a more complex procedure or treatment than is indicated). A pure productivity-based compensation model also introduces the risk of cognitive dissonance and moral distress because the system is encouraging behavior (e.g., volume and up-coding over quality) that health care professionals would not choose for themselves or a loved one.

Patient Experience Metrics

Even patient experience metrics can create cognitive dissonance for health care professionals when misused. Financial incentives for better patient experiences may, on the surface, seem like a great idea. However, there are at least two unintended consequences:

1) Making sure "the patient leaves happy" may discourage nurses (and others) from speaking up when a patient is disrespectful, abusive, or uncivil (moral distress causes burnout).
2) Making sure "the patient leaves happy" may encourage physicians to prescribe antibiotics for viral infections and opioids for pain, instead of taking the time to explain what is best for the patient (moral distress causes burnout).

For example, the Pediatric Emergency Care Applied Research Network (PECARN) clinical prediction rule is best practice for determining whether a child with low-impact head trauma, brought to the emergency room by parents, would benefit from a computed tomography (CT) scan of the head. If used properly, the PECARN clinical prediction rule and clinical judgment will identify 100% of patients who need to be seen by a neurosurgeon, and those patients *will* be seen by a neurosurgeon. The PECARN clinical prediction rule saves money and time for the patient and the community. It also reduces ionizing radiation exposure and the associated future risks for patients.

However, the PECARN clinical prediction rule takes time for the emergency department physician to administer. If the family believes a head CT scan is needed and is expecting that recommendation, the emergency department physician will then need to spend time explaining why a CT scan is not in the patient's best interest. (The same is true for explaining why antibiotics are not needed for a viral infection or narcotics for certain types of pain.) The time it takes to have the conversation lowers productivity, may result in lower patient satisfaction scores, and may reduce the administrative code complexity (no CT scan) of the patient visit—all of which decrease compensation in a productivity-based compensation system.

The easiest thing to do and one that helps make sure "the patient leaves happy" is to order the head CT. The right thing to do is not the easy thing to do in many of our systems of care. Professionals often get paid less for doing what is in the best interest of the patient. In a productivity-based compensation system, they may actually have a financial incentive to order an unnecessary test or procedure. This not only can create cognitive dissonance for the ordering provider but also moral distress for the other members of the health care team observing routine use of inappropriate testing.

We believe that patient experience metrics are best used to give providers feedback that will enable them to provide better care. Use of metrics should be coupled with targeted training (e.g., communication skills, creating an efficient agenda for the patient visit that addresses primary concerns, emotional intelligence training). A variety of nonfinancial approaches can be used to make progress (e.g., the confidential sharing of information on how a professional's score compares to those of colleagues locally and nationally) and awards given to top performers. If these techniques are used in a compensation formula, they should be one of multiple variables related to professionalism and should be for group, not individual, results. It is best to use incentives that encourage collaboration instead of competition.

Which Model Is Best?

Ultimately, there is no right or wrong model of compensation. It is important to recognize, however, that every compensation model has both intended and unintended consequences and that the model used may impact the well-being of patients and professionals and change the way health care professionals view their work. Organizations must consider all ramifications of the model used and apply appropriate safeguards and mitigation strategies (Figure 29.1).

Productivity models may incentivize overwork, increase rates of professional burnout, favor competition over cooperation, emphasize independence over collaboration, and prioritize individuals over the teamwork.

Salary models run the risk that some individuals (e.g., those who are not intrinsically motivated) might take advantage of the system (e.g., through laziness, spending too many work hours on personal issues, being less productive than colleagues). For these models, safeguards and mitigation strategies include supervisors holding people accountable to maintain equity and fairness or transparently communicating the productivity of each individual in the group to all members.

Hybrid models can strike a happy medium or incorporate the worst of both worlds.

The key is recognizing both the intended and potentially unintended consequences of each model, putting in appropriate safeguards and mitigation strategies to prevent undesirable consequences, and continually evaluating how the model is working and whether adjustments are needed.

Two Housekeepers

We will close this chapter with the stories of two housekeepers at different health care organizations that emphasize the importance of intrinsic rewards. In most organizations, housekeepers have a very narrow job description. Their tasks include changing soiled sheets, cleaning toilets, and sanitizing door knobs. Yet, with the right organizational attention to culture, values alignment, leadership development, camaraderie, and esprit de corps, housekeepers can find real meaning and purpose in their work.

A housekeeper at Mayo Clinic in Rochester, Minnesota, was selected randomly to be interviewed for the filming of a documentary on patient safety. The director asked her what she did for the organization. She said, "My job is to save lives." When asked to expand on this, the housekeeper told the interviewer that keeping the hospital clean and safe was integral to patient care. She shared that she and her team developed a checklist of all the important surfaces in each room to be sanitized as they changed and refreshed rooms. She reported that their work had been studied and found to have had a measurable impact on hospital-acquired infections. No one asked them to make these improvements. This was not in their job description. However, because the housekeeper saw her job as saving lives rather than cleaning rooms, patients received better care.

Another housekeeper, an employee at Intermountain Healthcare in Ogden, Utah, saw a patient crying in her hospital room. Rather than continue her cleaning, she started a conversation with the patient. The patient, who was bedridden, said that her father had just been admitted to the same hospital for pneumonia, but she had been unable to get in touch with him. The housekeeper took it upon herself to locate the patient's father and walk to his room. She then helped him call his daughter. They visited for about 10 minutes. At the end of the conversation, the housekeeper overheard the patient tell her father, "I love you." The housekeeper said that his face lit up like a Christmas tree. About 30 minutes later, an overhead page announced "code blue," followed by the father's room number. The father had passed away, but he had love in his heart, and his daughter took solace in having spoken with him right before the end.

Neither story would have had its ending had the housekeepers felt their job was to adhere strictly to the duties listed in their job descriptions or had their compensation model been predicated simply on the number of rooms they cleaned each day. In both cases, the housekeepers worked for employers whose organizational values were designed to connect employees to the underlying meaning and purpose of their work, empower them, and encourage discretionary effort. This type of care team benefits patients.

CONCLUSION

Intrinsic motivation and rewards are important elements of the ideal work environment for health care professionals. Behaviors and actions that promote and grow intrinsic motivation should be embedded into leadership behavior and the structure of organizations that desire a culture of dedication to their altruistic mission and values. To achieve their strategic objectives, health care organizations must develop teams of professionals who are intrinsically motivated, dedicated to each other, and committed to the organization's mission. Leaders' primary responsibilities are to connect staff to the meaning and purpose of their work and to help them evolve from looking at their work extrinsically as a job with outward rewards to seeing their work as a career and, ultimately, as a calling with intrinsic motivation. When health care work becomes a calling, as it did with the two housekeepers, the work environment is optimized and patients are the main beneficiaries.

SUGGESTED READING

Donnelly GE, Zheng T, Haisley E, Norton MI. The amount and source of millionaires' wealth (moderately) predict their happiness. Pers Soc Psychol Bull. 2018 May;44(5):684–99.

Drzymalski J, Gladstone E, Troyani L, Niu D. The 7 key trends impacting today's workplace: results from the 2014 TINYpulse employee engagement and organizational culture report [Internet]. 2014 [cited 2018 Dec 4]. Available from: https://www.tinypulse. com/2014-employee-engagement-organizational-culture-report.

Grant AM. The significance of task significance: job performance effects, relational mechanisms, and boundary conditions. J Appl Psychol. 2008 Jan;93(1):108–24.

Grant AM, Hofmann DA. It's not all about me: motivating hand hygiene among health care professionals by focusing on patients. Psychol Sci. 2011 Dec;22(12):1494–9.

Kahneman D, Deaton A. High income improves evaluation of life but not emotional well-being. Proc Natl Acad Sci U S A. 2010 Sep 21;107(38):16489–93.

Pink DH. Drive: the surprising truth about what motivates us. New York (NY): Riverhead Books; 2009.

Shanafelt TD, Balch CM, Bechamps GJ, Russell T, Dyrbye L, Satele D, et al. Burnout and career satisfaction among American surgeons. Ann Surg. 2009 Sep;250(3):463–71.

Shanafelt TD, Gradishar WJ, Kosty M, Satele D, Chew H, Horn L, et al. Burnout and career satisfaction among U.S. oncologists. J Clin Oncol. 2014 Mar 1;32(7):678–86.

Shanafelt TD, Hasan O, Dyrbye LN, Sinsky C, Satele D, Sloan J, et al. Changes in burnout and satisfaction with work-life balance in physicians and the general U.S. working population between 2011 and 2014. Mayo Clin Proc. 2015 Dec;90(12):1600–13.

Shanafelt TD, Mungo M, Schmitgen J, Storz KA, Reeves D, Hayes SN, et al. Longitudinal study evaluating the association between physician burnout and changes in professional work effort. Mayo Clin Proc. 2016 Apr;91(4):422–31.

30

CAMARADERIE ACTION: CULTIVATING COMMUNITY AND COMMENSALITY

TODAY: DISTRESS

George is an isolated family physician disconnected from meaning in his work. Recently, he has had some challenging cases and no opportunity to discuss them or express his angst and concerns with colleagues. He feels alone despite working with a dedicated team of nurses and advanced practice providers (APPs) at the clinic each day. The daily schedule is burdensome, and he dreads going to work each morning.

◆ ◆ ◆

Cultivating Community and Commensality (the act of sharing a meal together) is the first of three Camaraderie Actions that are validated means to achieving two of the eight Ideal Work Elements: community at work and camaraderie and intrinsic motivation and rewards. In this chapter, we explain the value of building community and supporting regular commensality as well as describe how to successfully implement these evidenced-based actions that will combat professional burnout and foster esprit de corps.

HEALTH AND HAPPINESS

What is the most significant determinant of poor health? Hypertension? Smoking? Obesity? Nope. It's lack of social connection (Holt-Lunstad et al, 2017). Social connectedness reduces the risk of early death by half (Holt-Lunstad et al, 2010)! As a result, the World Health Organization now identifies social support as a health determinant. Camaraderie is a manifestation of social connection that reduces isolation and helps immunize health care professionals against burnout.

Various tactics can build community and team connectedness. Leaders should consider the following ideas:

- Begin staff meetings with positivity.
  - Consider around-the-table personal updates.
  - Consider around-the-table sharing of "one good thing."
- Schedule monthly team events off campus.
- Before typing someone an email, consider walking down the hall or up a floor for a short face-to-face communication instead.

Happiness

People are not as happy as they once were. Research shows that during the last several decades in the United States happiness has been declining. Why is this so? Social scientists have reported that much of the decrease in happiness has been caused by a decrease in social connections and a loss of confidence in institutions. Commensality can help address both of these issues (Smith et al, 2015; Blanchflower and Oswald, 2017).

COMMENSALITY

Collegiality and social connections with peers are critical components of engagement, satisfaction, and well-being of health care professionals. However, increased clinical and administrative demands in health care can make creating these connections more challenging. Sharing a meal together is one way to build community and promote team performance and, if fostered by the organization, confidence and positive feelings about the institution. Throughout human history, people of every culture have developed rituals based on sharing meals together. There is something special about breaking bread with other people whether they are friends, colleagues, or family.

Staff social gatherings are relatively easy to make happen. With strategic use of space, such as a staff lunch room or surgical lounge, community and social connection can occur daily. When food is provided (e.g., to celebrate a unit milestone), even more socializing will occur.

While these types of gatherings are helpful for building casual social connectedness of staff, more structured situations can dramatically increase the impact of these events. Commensality with an intentional design can be used to encourage health care professionals to explore the virtues and challenges of their lives in the healing professions and to support one another. This approach is evidenced based and will promote engagement and reduce burnout. Commensality groups are designed to cultivate vital human connections by encouraging caregivers to gather for a complimentary meal and engage in conversation about their professional experiences. They have proven effective in two randomized controlled trials at Mayo Clinic (West et al, 2014).

The Mayo Clinic Experience

An Hour of Protected Time

Mayo Clinic has conducted several randomized trials of commensality and small group discussions (West et al, 2014; Luthar et al, 2017). In the first study, the investigative team enrolled 75 physicians and bought an hour of their clinic time every two weeks for nine months (West et al, 2014). Half of the physicians were randomized to use the hour in any way they chose. A free lunch was provided for them one day a week that they could pick up and eat it in their offices. The other half of the physicians were randomized to meet with a consistent group of seven other participants along with a facilitator. They ate lunch together and then engaged in a discussion of a specified topic at each meeting related to the experience of being a physician. Surveys were administered to participants electronically at baseline and at regular intervals (approximately every three months) to assess change in burnout and meaning in work.

At the end of the nine months, burnout scores improved in both groups relative to 450 peers who did not receive the hour of protected time. However, burnout scores improved more for the group who met with colleagues. In addition, meaning and purpose in work improved only in the group who met with colleagues. Among the group who could use the hour as they chose (most caught up on administrative work), burnout immediately returned to baseline once the intervention ended and they stopped receiving the protected time. Strikingly, the benefits (i.e., less burnout and improved meaning in work) for those randomized to meet with colleagues persisted for a year after the intervention ended.

A Commensality Intervention

A second randomized controlled trial built on the results of the first trial. Physicians could sign up with a group of six or seven colleagues to participate in a commensality intervention. Half of the groups were randomized to begin meeting for a meal (i.e., breakfast, lunch, or dinner) once every two weeks for six months. The meal cost was covered for up to $20 per participant. The second group was randomized to begin meeting after six months.

The physician selected to be the coordinator for each group was sent a list of five questions to bring to the meal, and participants were invited to pick the question they were most interested in discussing. They were asked to spend the first 15 minutes of the gathering allowing each of the participants to share their perspective or experience related to that question and then to use the remaining time to continue the discussion, move on to other topics, or simply enjoy one another's company.

Half the groups were randomized to begin their dinner meetings immediately, while the other half were randomized to a delayed start. For the first six months, they completed assessments (for which both groups were compensated) but did not meet. After six months, the groups crossed over, and the delayed-start groups began meeting. The findings from this trial were similar to those from the first study: decreased rates of burnout and improved meaning and purpose in work at the six-month time point for physicians who met with colleagues compared with those who didn't start meeting until the six-month time point.

Commensality Groups at Mayo Clinic

Thousands of health care professionals at Mayo Clinic have now participated. Health care professionals are invited to form and register their groups. Once registered, these self-selected teams of clinical caregivers gather socially to share a meal and choose from a predetermined list of discussion topics (see below) relevant to their lives, work, profession, or relationships. Mayo Clinic pays for the meals with a limit of $20 per person.

By supporting the formation of commensality groups and providing the meal, the message from the organization and senior leaders is, "We care about you. We know you and your colleagues face unique challenges and that only you understand all the demands of your work. We want to create space for you to support one another, and we will provide funding to encourage it."

LOGISTICS OF COMMENSALITY GROUPS

At Mayo Clinic, groups of six to eight clinicians meet for a meal (i.e., breakfast, lunch, or dinner) at a restaurant of their choice. Some groups cater the meal and rotate hosting the gathering in their home. Guidelines for meal expenses are aligned with the culture of the organization as well as its meal and beverage policies. Groups are asked to commit to meeting at least once a month (one or two group meals each month works well) for six months, although it is understood that participants may not be able to attend every meeting. After six months, the group can register again and continue meeting if they desire, split into multiple groups and draw in new participants (since group size is capped to preserve intimacy), or take a break.

Each group designates a group coordinator/leader who registers the group. The leader coordinates the date and location for meetings and communicates this information to the group members. Ideally, scheduling is performed several months in advance and in a consistent manner (e.g., the second Thursday of each month) to facilitate ease of planning for group members.

Group leaders receive a list of discussion questions before each meeting to guide the conversation. The group chooses one question to discuss at each session. The questions are provided for structure to help the group explore dimensions of professional life/work not often discussed in casual daily interactions and to avoid having the sessions devolve into gripe sessions. The first 15 minutes or more of each gathering should be dedicated to discussion that gives each group member an opportunity to give a perspective on the question. Discussions within each group are confidential.

Groups can be composed of members from a single profession or more than one profession; however, the structure selected will alter the focus of the sessions and their outcomes. Single-profession groups (e.g., all nurses, physicians, APPs) typically foster deeper conversations with greater vulnerability. Members of single-profession groups are often more willing to let their guard down and share some of their unique challenges. We have had both physicians and nurses share with us that much of what they discuss in a group of like colleagues is different than what they feel comfortable sharing when in a multidisciplinary setting.

We have also found that physicians in multidisciplinary groups will typically assume a "team leader" role and are far less willing to share their personal struggles in this situation. Likewise, nurses have shared with us that there are challenges related to personal shortcomings at work that they would be willing to discuss with peers but not with physicians present. In-depth discussions are also difficult in multidisciplinary groups when challenges may be unique only to one group (e.g., long work hours and call schedules for physicians vs. schedules and shift work in many other disciplines; moral distress for nurses who are required to implement physician orders whether or not they agree; role ambiguity for APPs).

Because of these issues, the focus of multidisciplinary commensality groups is more often on team building and members getting to know one another (i.e., there is limited vulnerability and sharing about struggles). These distinctions are not absolute and are influenced by the specific composition of the group, how long the individuals have been working in the profession, how long the individuals have known each other, and the emotional intelligence, self-awareness, and comfort level of being vulnerable among the participants.

Guidelines for Commensality Group Leaders

The following guidelines are designed to help the commensality group leaders ensure an environment that allows the group members to connect intellectually and emotionally as well as to explore the virtues and challenges of their profession in a casual, informal setting:

- Ask the group to keep the conversation confidential among group members to encourage openness and honesty.
- Ensure that all group members have an opportunity to share their experiences. Do not let any one group member monopolize the time. Should one member try to dominate, you might say:
  - "Let's hear from those who have not had a chance to share yet."
  - "Do others have a perspective or personal experience to share?"
- If you detect a group member is experiencing considerable distress, express your concern in private and help connect the person with the peer-support or counseling services available for health care professionals at your center.
- If the meeting is in a public setting (e.g., restaurant), remind the group that they are in a public setting and will want to be mindful of those around them.

Ground Rules for Participants

Participants should understand the key ground rules for the group, including:

- The conversation among group members is confidential.
- They are there to listen and share their own personal experiences, not give advice to others in the group.
- Their goal is to listen and offer support.
  - "Thank you for sharing your experience."
  - "I admire your courage to make a change."

Themes for Discussion Questions

The suggested discussion topics are intended to promote sharing, discovery, connection, and self-awareness. The group may want to identify and discuss other topics that have meaning to them. Topics typically center on the themes listed below.

Your Profession

- Why did you go into medicine, nursing, etc.?
- What gives you the most meaning in work right now?
- Think about a meaningful patient encounter in the last two weeks. What made it meaningful for you?
- What are you most grateful and appreciative for this week?
- How do you best navigate stress when you feel overloaded?
- What helps you recharge after a demanding situation in your personal or professional life?

- What personal growth have you experienced from working through professional challenges in the last year?
- What brings you joy in your practice?
- How do you stay connected to why you are a doctor, nurse, etc.?
- What do you need to flourish in your typical work week?
- What makes it all worthwhile for you despite the challenges?
- Think about a colleague or co-worker who is a source of support to you at work. What do you most appreciate about that person?
- Who is your role model? What do you admire about that person?
- Who do you turn to for coaching or support?
- Think about an important mentor who had an impact on your career. How did they impact you?
- Think about a time you made a medical error. Describe how it affected you. How did you eventually move forward?

Professional Growth

- What do you need to keep things fresh and experience professional growth? How are you able to meet this need?
- Share a lesson your patients have taught you.
- What did you learn this week?
- Think of a mistake you made in the last year. What did you learn from it?
- What's something new that you tried in the last few weeks that was challenging or hard?
- How do you keep going when things get tough?
- What do you hope to accomplish before the end of your career that you have not yet achieved?
- If money was no object and you had the flexibility to spend your professional efforts doing what was most fulfilling to you, what would you do?
- What matters to you most in life? Can you think of a tangible example of something you do (or would like to start doing) that demonstrates you are living in a manner congruent with this value?
- Have you ever been burned out? How did you know?
- Think of a time in your career when you felt burned out. How did you recover?
- How do you prevent burnout from occurring or recurring in your professional life?
- What wisdom have you learned from your professional experience that you would pass on to a junior colleague?

Managing the Day to Day

- What do you do to make it a good day at work for those around you?
- What techniques, strategies, or approaches have you discovered that help make it a good day for you?
- What helps you stay present in the moment when you are with a patient?
- What self-care do you engage in during the work day to sustain your energy and concentration?

Work-Life Integration

- What are your current challenges related to work-life integration? What tactics have helped you effectively meet both your personal and professional priorities?
- How have you created firewalls that prevent work from excessively spilling over into home life? Which have been most helpful for you?
- What hobbies or recreation bring you joy? How do you create time to do these things?
- Can you share a lesson your children have taught you?
- What are the personal repercussions of your work as a health care professional on your family?

Relationships

- What is the best way for you to connect with your patients?
- What is the best way to connect with your colleagues?
- How do you stay compassionate with others despite the emotional demands of your work?
- How have you preserved connections with friends despite a demanding schedule?
- How do you protect time away from work to spend with your spouse or partner?
- How do you protect time to be with or connect with your children in your current routine?

Self-Care

- How do you balance your career with other important elements in your life?
- Think of a trade-off you made that you now regret. What did you sacrifice that you wish you had not?
- Think of a trade-off you made that you are grateful for. What did you sacrifice and what did you gain?
- What is most helpful to you in managing your stress?
- What role does forgiveness have in your life?
- Are you able to be as kind or compassionate to yourself as you are to your colleagues?
- How do you know when you need to take a step back from work to recharge?
- What is the greatest source of stress for you at work? How do you mitigate or manage this source of stress?
- What do you do to recover from exposure to grief and patient suffering at work?
- What helps you cope when bad things happen?
- How do you strategically use vacations and time away from work to restore yourself?

OUTCOMES

Numerous wonderful outcomes result from these sessions. By hearing about the challenges others have experienced, participants learn that they are not alone in their struggles. They gain insights into how colleagues have navigated challenges similar to those they face, which can provide new ideas and approaches for meeting their challenge. The sessions also remind participants of what they love about their work. They remind them that they have the privilege of working with a remarkable group of colleagues and allow them to cultivate a group of peers with whom they can be vulnerable and honest about the most difficult parts of their work as health care professionals. The group often becomes a community that shares struggles and sensitive issues as they arise and that supports its members.

THE MAYO CLINIC EXPERIENCE REVISITED

After the second randomized trial demonstrating the efficacy of commensality groups, the Mayo Clinic Board of Governors had enough evidence. Before them was an intervention proven in two randomized trials to reduce burnout and promote engagement and it cost, on average, about $200 per participant each year (most individuals attend approximately two-thirds of the sessions). The Board acted swiftly. They approved commensality groups as a standard offering at Mayo Clinic in November 2016. A website was created to facilitate registering groups.

The skeptics said no one would sign up because everyone was already too busy and would not want to spend even more time away from their family or personal activities. Within the first 18 months, 50% of the approximately 2,400 eligible individuals on Mayo Clinic's campus in Rochester, Minnesota, had joined a group, and there was 30% to 40% participation on the Arizona and Florida campuses. Efforts to expand the groups to other health care professionals are being explored.

We discovered that the format also catalyzes participation. Professionals who never would have participated individually were invited to join a group by colleagues they respected and with whom they wanted to spend time. Colleagues drew one another into community, which resulted in high participation.

Oxytocin

Oxytocin is the trust-building hormone. Its levels increase when people are together in person—in meetings, socializing, shaking hands, or sharing meals. Webinars, email, and conference calls may be efficient ways to accomplish work; however, face-to-face meetings are necessary to build camaraderie and bonding of teams and to increase oxytocin levels. Although the half-life of oxytocin is just minutes, the trust built from face-to-face interaction can last forever—if you don't break it.

CONCLUSION

Humans have a social need for community and camaraderie. In today's health care environment, high-functioning teams are critical to delivery of high-quality medical care. Collegial and mutually respectful interactions are particularly important in health care because of the demanding, stressful, and high-stakes nature of the work. Leaders should be intentional in the actions they use to help build teams and foster community. Cultivating Community and Commensality, the first of three Camaraderie Actions, builds space for colleagues to connect and support each other on a deeper level than afforded in day-to-day work. When your organization supports commensality, the return on investment is high: a greater sense of community that enhances professional fulfillment, reduces burnout, and promotes esprit de corps (Box 30.1).

TOMORROW: FULFILLMENT

George recently joined a group breakfast meeting with six supportive colleagues who meet every month. The gathering provides him a safe place to talk about the virtues and challenges of his life as a family physician. Hearing about what provides meaning at work for his colleagues has reminded him of some of the things he loves about medicine. He can't believe his institution picks up the check for breakfast. George is no longer socially isolated and cynical. There are still plenty of challenges, but he now sees daylight instead of darkness.

Box 30.1 The Playbook

- Establish a commensality program.
  - o Provide individuals the ability to sign up in teams.
  - o Help provide a basic structure, questions, and guidelines for groups that facilitate discussion of important aspects of experiences as a health care professional.
  - o Pay for the meals, if possible, to demonstrate organizational commitment.
- Schedule monthly work-unit team events off campus.
- Begin staff meetings with positivity.
  - o Consider around-the-table personal updates.
  - o Consider around-the-table sharing of "one good thing."
- Before typing an email, consider walking down the hall or up a floor for a short face-to-face communication instead.

SUGGESTED READING

Bartolini S, Bilancini E, Pugno M. Did the decline in social connections depress Americans' happiness? Soc Indic Res. 2013;110(3):1033–59.

Blanchflower DG, Oswald A. Unhappiness and pain in modern America: a review essay, and further evidence, on Carol Graham's happiness for all? NBER working paper No. 24087 [Internet]. 2017 [cited 2019 Apr 16]. Available from: https://www.nber.org/papers/w24087.

Holt-Lunstad J, Robles TF, Sbarra DA. Advancing social connection as a public health priority in the United States. Am Psychol. 2017 Sep;72(6):517–30.

Holt-Lunstad J, Smith TB, Layton JB. Social relationships and mortality risk: a meta-analytic review. PLoS Med. 2010 Jul 27;7(7):e1000316.

Kirsch P, Esslinger C, Chen Q, Mier D, Lis S, Siddhanti S, et al. Oxytocin modulates neural circuitry for social cognition and fear in humans. J Neurosci. 2005 Dec 7;25(49):11489–93.

Kniffin KM, Wansink B, Devine CM, Sobal J. Eating together at the firehouse: how workplace commensality relates to the performance of firefighters. Hum Perform. 2015 Aug 8;28(4):281–306.

Luthar SS, Curlee A, Tye SJ, Engelman JC, Stonnington CM. Fostering resilience among mothers under stress: "authentic connections groups" for medical professionals. Womens Health Issues. 2017 May-Jun;27(3):382–90.

Smith TW, Son J, Schapiro B, National Opinion Research Center (NORC) at the University of Chicago. General social survey final report: trends in psychological well-being, 1972-2014 [Internet]. 2015 [cited 2019 Apr 16]. Available from: http://www.norc.org/PDFs/GSS%20Reports/GSS_PsyWellBeing15_final_formatted.pdf.

West CP, Dyrbye LN, Rabatin JT, Call TG, Davidson JH, Multari A, et al. Intervention to promote physician well-being, job satisfaction, and professionalism: a randomized clinical trial. JAMA Intern Med. 2014 Apr;174(4):527–33.

West CP, Dyrbye LN, Satele D, Shanafelt TD. A randomized controlled trial evaluation the effect of COMPASS (Colleagues Meeting to Promote and Sustain Satisfaction) small group sessions on physician well-being, meaning, and job satisfaction [abstract]. J Gen Intern Med. 2015;30:S89.

31

CAMARADERIE ACTION: OPTIMIZING REWARDS, RECOGNITION, AND APPRECIATION

TODAY: DISTRESS

Victoria feels unappreciated. She is a physician practicing in an academic medical center and has always devoted extra hours to medical students, families, and patients. She views medicine as a calling, and this investment of time is meaningful to her even though it is uncompensated. Lately, she has been pressured by her administrators to squeeze in more patients and be more "productive." The hospital treats her as a revenue center, and she has begun to feel that she is working for an organization without a soul. Victoria still cares about her patients but no longer cares much about the success of the organization. Most days, showing up for work just feels like chasing a paycheck.

$$\bullet \, \bullet \, \bullet$$

The actions that compose the second of three actions in the Camaraderie Action Set are Optimizing Rewards, Recognition, and Appreciation. These actions focus principally on improving professional well-being by respecting and nurturing intrinsic motivation and acknowledgment; this is a foundational piece of the esprit de corps puzzle.

INTRINSIC AND EXTRINSIC MOTIVATORS

Leaders directly impact discretionary effort by inspiring commitment, providing recognition, and offering growth, responsibility, challenging work, and development opportunities for their people. Health care professionals want to be appreciated for their work, be a part of a high-performing team, and experience a sense of purpose in work. All of these intrinsic motivators (e.g., driven by internal rewards) can be delivered consistently with coordinated leadership, aligned values (see also Chapter 18, "Agency Action: Creating a Values Alignment Compact"), and an organizational approach that values partnership in decision making (see also Chapter 29, "Camaraderie Ideal Work Element: Intrinsic Motivation and Rewards").

Rewards, recognition, and appreciation systems that are primarily based on extrinsic motivators (e.g., driven by external rewards such as money and fame) can help an organization achieve some objectives but can also lead to unintended consequences, including cognitive dissonance, moral distress, a self-centered (rather than collaborative) focus, deleterious increases in workload, overuse of tests and procedures, and unhealthy work-life integration.

Mayo Clinic has made a concerted effort to design recognition systems that focus on intrinsic motivation. All Mayo Clinic leaders are assessed on their recognition and appreciation practices through the annual survey, which includes the Leader Behavior Index, that is sent to all staff.

Leaders demonstrate appreciation for staff in ways that go beyond a simple thank you. Programs such as a robust benefit to support travel for professional development and continuing education, the Spirit of Caring Fund, Values Council programs, Karis Awards, and the Professional Development Assistance Program are just a few ways that Mayo demonstrates genuine concern for and commitment to its staff. For example, the Karis Award (*karis* from the Greek word for caring) was established to formally recognize the many caring people across Mayo Clinic who live out the organization's values in an extraordinary way as they serve patients, visitors, and colleagues. The award is part of the Mayo Recognition Program. None of the approaches in the Recognition Program rewards with money. They are ways of investing in people, helping them grow professionally, and authentically thanking them.

Case Study: Intrinsic Motivation and a 75-Cent Pin

In the early 2000s when Mayo Clinic was establishing its Quality Academy, the question of how to train leaders and staff in the principles of continuous quality improvement was debated. Should staff and leaders be *required* to undergo basic training to receive certification or should such learning just be *encouraged* by connecting the work to the meaning and purpose of flawless patient care.

The decision was made to use the latter approach and have senior leaders model the behaviors they desired for colleagues. The logic was that the intrinsic motivation of "doing your work and improving your work" was sufficient to catalyze an internal social and cultural movement. In addition to the intrinsic motivation of professional development and improving the work environment, the program did have one tangible reward: a 75-cent pin that was to be worn on the health care professional's name tag.

The strategy worked!

The first name tag pins were earned and donned by the chief executive officer and the chief administrative officer. After six years of offering training, role modeling, and encouraging health care professionals to get certified in the basic principles of quality improvement, more than 42,000 health care professionals (of 64,000) certified as bronze, silver, gold, or diamond quality-improvement fellows. They used their discretionary time to study and complete improvement projects because they believed in the purpose of the work—to create a safer and higher-quality care delivery system for their patients and a more professionally fulfilling work environment for themselves.

They didn't do it for the pin.

Collateral Damage From Extrinsic Rewards

Research shows that gifts from pharmaceutical companies impact the prescribing patterns of physicians (Wood et al, 2017). Gifts are a form of extrinsic rewards, and the study results showed that, except for pediatricians, providing physicians gifts led to prescribing of more costly pharmaceuticals, more prescriptions per patient, and a higher proportion of name brand prescriptions. The larger the gift from Big Pharma to the physician, the more these outcomes occurred, thus negatively impacting patients and society—and the physicians themselves.

Blood Donation

Countless people donate blood every day. The motivation to donate is a sincere desire to help an anonymous person in need with the gift of blood. Studies show that when people who have donated blood are offered a financial incentive to donate, something unfortunate happens (Mellstrom and Johannesson, 2008). They stop giving blood. The financial remuneration changes an altruistic gift (and intrinsic motivation) to an anonymous patient in need into a financial transaction (and extrinsic motivation). The donation has lost its meaning and purpose.

Hygiene Factors and Motivators

Another way to look at the issue of intrinsic and extrinsic motivation is through the two-factor theory, which distinguishes between *motivators* and *hygiene factors* (Herzberg, 1964). Salary, benefits, title, seniority, job security, policies, management practices, work conditions, and vacation days are considered hygiene factors. Hygiene factors do not motivate people, but they can result in dissatisfaction if they are absent or administered unfairly (e.g., inequitable wages). Hygiene factors do not drive esprit de corps. By nature, they are extrinsic because they are not part of work itself. They tend to be of greater importance to individuals who relate to their work as a job or career rather than as a calling.

Unlike hygiene factors, intrinsic motivators are inherent to work, important to the individual, and can increase fulfillment. Such intrinsic motivators are important to individuals who relate to their work as a calling. They endow esprit de corps.

MOTIVATORS: A WAY FORWARD

Whenever possible, organizations and leaders should embrace the opportunity to employ intrinsic motivators. Leaders must deliberately consider and determine the best rewards, recognition, and appreciation for health care professionals in their organization. The following five-step approach may be helpful in the decision-making process:

1) Review your rewards, recognition, and appreciation programs.
2) Systematically assess alignment:
   • Are the programs aligned with the best interests of patients?
   • Are the programs aligned with the stated vision of the organization?
   • Are the programs aligned with the well-being of professionals?
3) Choose best rewards, recognition, and appreciation programs for your institution and circumstances.
4) Assess leader performance of staff recognition and appreciation using the "recognize" component of the Leadership Behavior Index (i.e., Does my leader express appreciation and gratitude in an authentic way?).
5) If the current approach is not the ideal long-term solution, identify opportunities, strategy, and a timeline to transition from an extrinsic to intrinsic motivation model.

COMPENSATION SYSTEMS: THE CHALLENGES

Health care professionals are remunerated using a variety of compensation systems. Many health care professionals, such as nurses, physical therapists, and technologists, typically receive an hourly wage based on the number of hours worked. Other professionals, such as pharmacists, nurse practitioners, and advanced practice providers, generally have a fixed salary.

Greater variation in compensation structure exists for physicians. Physicians are typically paid in one of three ways: 1) a salary independent of productivity or hours; 2) a salary plus incentive bonus; or 3) a productivity system wherein the compensation is based entirely on output (e.g., relative value unit [RVU] generation or taking extra shifts). As described in Chapter 29 ("Camaraderie Ideal Work Element: Intrinsic Motivation and Rewards"; Figure 29.1), each system has advantages and disadvantages.

Unintended Consequences From Productivity-Based Compensation Models

The unintended consequences of many compensation programs are often at the root of burnout. Multiple studies of health care professionals have found that burnout is lowest among salaried employees and highest among professionals who are compensated on productivity alone (see Chapter 29, "Camaraderie Ideal Work Element: Intrinsic Motivation and Rewards"). Such models transform physicians' altruistic motivations to a simple financial transaction and incentivize individuals already working excessive hours to "kill themselves chasing the carrot."

Human Costs of Compensation Systems

Organizations must consider the human costs of various compensation systems as part of the overall approach to addressing professional burnout. Consequences of production-model compensation systems include stressors that can increase the likelihood of burnout, partial quitting (i.e., part-time work), turnover, reduced patient satisfaction, and lower-quality health care. The stressors include:

- Increased competition
- Decreased collaboration
- An individual rather than team focus
- Decreased time with patients
- More tests and procedures
- Cognitive dissonance
- Decreased time with colleagues
- Decreased time with family/friends
- Problems with work-life integration
- Moral distress for other members of the care team

Thus, production models of compensation get three strikes:

1) They can harm patients (e.g., overuse of tests and treatments such as chemotherapy at the end of life or spine surgery that does not improve quality of life).

2) They are not aligned with the stated mission of most medical institutions (e.g., providing the best care to patients).
3) They negatively impact the well-being of health care professionals (e.g., moral distress, cognitive dissonance, financial incentives that may conflict with what is best for patients and incentivize overwork) and teams.

Organizations concerned about burnout of health care professionals and about quality of care should be cautious and prudent with the use of productivity-based compensation models.

COMPENSATION SYSTEMS: A WAY FORWARD

It is important for leaders to intentionally determine the best compensation model for health care professionals in their organization. Consider amending physician compensation systems to align with the values and mission of your organization and to a system that nurtures the well-being of your professional staff. Then, develop strategies to mitigate the unintended consequences of the compensation model you select.

The following seven-step approach may be helpful in the decision-making process:

1) Review your existing compensation programs.
2) Systematically assess alignment:
   - Is the model aligned with the best interests of patients?
   - Is the model aligned with the stated vision and mission of the organization?
   - Is the model aligned with the operational plan of the organization (e.g., are you incentivizing volume when you really need value)?
   - Is the model aligned with the best interests of professional well-being?
3) Choose the best compensation model for your institution and unique circumstances.
4) If the program chosen is not the ideal long-term solution, identify opportunities, strategy, and a timeline to transition from an extrinsic to intrinsic motivation model.
5) For your chosen compensation model:
   - Consider the unintended consequences for patients.
   - Consider the unintended consequences for the mission.
   - Consider the unintended well-being consequences for health care professionals.
6) Build in appropriate safeguards and counterbalances to reduce the negative impact on patient, mission, and professional well-being.
7) Create continuing professional education opportunities that promote well-being through their rewards, recognition, content, and format (see next section).

As mentioned in Chapter 29 ("Camaraderie Ideal Work Element: Intrinsic Motivation and Rewards"), there is no right or wrong way to compensate people, but safeguards and mitigation strategies need to be included to prevent detrimental, expected, and unintended consequences.

Case Study: Dr. Joseph Cacchione, M.D., Executive Vice President of Ascension Medical Group; Baligh Yehia, M.D., Chief Medical Officer, Ascension Medical Group

Ascension Medical Group, described in Chapter 17 (Agency Action: Introducing Control and Flexibility"), historically compensated its physicians in a productivity-based, RVU-driven model. As health care evolved toward focusing more on quality outcomes and caring for populations, Ascension made the decision to look at new ways to compensate physicians—not only to ensure that better quality care would be provided but also to aid in restoring satisfaction for physicians who all too often felt as though they were on a treadmill.

In 2017, leaders began work to change the Ascension model to compensate physicians for more than their productivity. Physicians would also be compensated for delivering great outcomes and being good citizens within the medical group and the greater community. The enhanced model allowed physicians to be compensated for the totality of their contributions and performance.

As would be expected with such a transition, the migration required multiple changes in management tactics, including socialization and input from key stakeholders, most of whom were physicians. It was important for the physicians to understand why the changes were made and how they helped the organization meet the goals of the Quadruple Aim: to deliver exceptional health outcomes, an exceptional experience for the people served, and an exceptional experience for providers, at an affordable cost.

Fundamentally, Ascension believes that moving away from a purely RVU-driven compensation model is the best way to align the values of the organization and its care providers with the needs of its patients. The leadership team has demonstrated courage in tackling a potentially contentious issue and doing so in a transparent way that began with honest and frank conversations with clinicians on the "why." In addition, a deliberate implementation program was undertaken to allow for transition rather than abrupt change. Finally, a comprehensive performance-review tool was embedded in the new compensation plan, and leaders were required to be trained on its implementation. This new tool required a change in management philosophy to assist leaders in understanding the impact of performance review and to help working physicians in understanding the new paradigm for compensation.

CONTINUING PROFESSIONAL EDUCATION

Offering opportunities for continued professional development (i.e., time and financial support for continuing medical education) is an example of an effective intrinsic motivation strategy. Professional education has an important role in an organization's portfolio of burnout-reduction strategies. For health care professionals working in a rapidly changing environment, continuing education programs are about talent development and nurturing of the organization's most valuable resource. Providing time and support for continuing professional education demonstrates an organization's commitment to clinicians' professional development as well as a tangible example of their commitment to quality. Such programs also increase retention and an institution's appeal to new talent (i.e., "We want you to stay current and develop greater expertise so you can provide better care for patients.").

For all of these reasons, providing time and support to attend continuing education programs should be a component of professional compensation.

Well-designed continuing education programs are relevant (i.e., improve the day-to-day quality of work), efficient (i.e., part of the workday or time to participate provided), and important for professionals to maintain state-of-the-art knowledge and competence. Many programs can be designed to engage clinicians where they work. Continuing education programs can also incorporate topics that help advance the organizational journey toward esprit de corps (Box 31.1). Constructing the experiences so that clinicians can spend time interacting and eating together incorporates commensality into these efforts, which can magnify the benefits.

For example, a one-day course on how to develop and use coaching skills would help team members:

- Develop skill in a thoughtful discipline that involves asking questions and listening to understand. This caring technique helps patients, health care professionals in training, and colleagues discover for themselves the best way forward.
- Connect with their colleagues through highly interactive training.
- Create networks with co-workers that help sustain the culture of the organization.

Continuing education and programs to maintain certification also have the potential to provide intensive training in other domains that foster the organizational journey to esprit de corps, such as leadership development, teamwork, emotional intelligence, communication skills, and process improvement methodology. These types of programs have the potential to integrate organizational efforts to improve quality, patient satisfaction, and collegiality. By fostering multidisciplinary learning, they can break apart silos and promote boundarylessness.

Thus, investing in well-designed and coordinated continuing professional education can be a powerful force in optimizing rewards, recognition, and appreciation to nurture esprit de corps.

Box 31.1 Topics for Continuing Medical Education That Promote Clinician Well-being and Esprit de Corps

- Leadership development
- Change management
- Process improvement
- Teamwork and team function
- Emotional intelligence
- Communication skills
- Professionalism
- Coaching
- Mentorship
- Self-care
- Self-awareness
- Work-life integration
- Self-compassion
- Cultural competence

DESIGNED BY PATIENTS

If patients designed professional compensation systems, they would eliminate production-based compensation models that focus on volume. They would choose a compensation model that does not introduce a potential financial conflict with their interests. They would want a system that focused on value and quality. Patients would invoke a salary system in which physicians were not paid more or less on the basis of the care they recommended and would not reward them for spending less time with patients or seeing so many patients that they become burned out, jaded, and cynical. If there was any variable pay, it would be based on group performance for providing quality care.

CONCLUSION

The second Camaraderie Action is Optimizing Rewards, Recognition, and Appreciation. It connects with and fuels intrinsic motivation and also influences community and collegiality. Embracing compensation and acknowledgment systems based on intrinsic motivators is part of the foundation for cultivating esprit de corps. Consider what patients want the system to reward (Box 31.2).

TOMORROW: FULFILLMENT

Victoria has regained the passion that attracted her to medicine. Her leaders regularly express genuine appreciation for her willingness to go the extra mile for her patients and students. The new salary system only has compensation at risk for three patient-centered quality outcomes that her group co-created with senior leadership. The incentive thresholds in these areas are group goals that all team members work toward together. Once again, Victoria feels like a professional with a calling. Her heart is warm, and her pocketbook has all it really needs.

Box 31.2 The Playbook

- Review your compensation and recognition programs.
  - o Identify opportunities to transition from extrinsic to intrinsic motivators.
  - o Three questions:
    - ■ Is the system aligned with the best interests of patients?
    - ■ Is the system aligned with the stated vision of the organization?
    - ■ Is the system aligned with the best interests of professional well-being?
- Consider the unintended well-being consequences of your compensation and recognition systems.
  - o Change the system or discuss ways to manage negative impact on well-being or build in appropriate safeguards and counterbalances to reduce undesirable consequences.

(continued)

Box 31.2. (*Continued*)

- Create continuing professional education opportunities that promote professional development as well as serve as a tangible example of commitment to quality. Such programs should:
  - Be relevant (i.e., improve the day-to-day quality of work).
  - Be efficient (i.e., include as part of the work day time to participate provided).
  - Make it easier for professionals to maintain state-of-the-art knowledge and competence.
  - Include topics that foster the organizational journey to esprit de corps (e.g., leadership development, teamwork, emotional intelligence, communication skills, and process improvement methodology).
- Develop a habit of gratitude.
  - Handwrite one appreciation note to someone every day.
  - Start every meeting with a sincere public recognition of someone.

SUGGESTED READING

Hackman JR, Oldham GR. Motivation through the design of work: test of a theory. Organ Behav Hum Perform. 1976;16(2):250–79.

Herzberg F. The motivation-hygiene concept and problems of manpower. Pers Adm. 1964;27(1):3–7.

McMahon GT. The leadership case for investing in continuing professional development. Acad Med. 2017 Aug;92(8):1075–7.

Mellstrom C, Johannesson M. Crowding out in blood donation: was Titmuss right? J Eur Econ Assoc. 2008;6(4):845–63.

Shanafelt TD, Balch CM, Bechamps GJ, Russell T, Dyrbye L, Satele D, et al. Burnout and career satisfaction among American surgeons. Ann Surg. 2009 Sep;250(3):463–71.

Swensen SJ. Esprit de corps and quality: making the case for eradicating burnout. J Healthc Manag. 2018 Jan/Feb;63(1):7–11.

Swensen SJ, Duncan JR, Gibson R, Muething SE, LeBuhn R, Rexford J, et al. An appeal for safe and appropriate imaging of children. J Patient Saf. 2014 Sep;10(3):121–4.

Wood SF, Podrasky J, McMonagle MA, Raveendran J, Bysshe T, Hogenmiller A, et al. Influence of pharmaceutical marketing on Medicare prescriptions in the District of Columbia. PLoS One. 2017;12(10):e0186060.

32

CAMARADERIE ACTION:
FOSTERING BOUNDARYLESSNESS

TODAY: DISTRESS

Amanda is a talented nurse who is worn out and frustrated. She works in an organization where distinct walls exist between doctors and nurses. She feels as though her high-demand work life is controlled by someone else. Decisions are made without the benefit of her expertise, perspective, and input. She does not feel part of a team, and she is actively looking for another job.

◆ ◆ ◆

Boundarylessness is the final Camaraderie Action. This action is principally focused on improving professional well-being by cultivating leader behaviors and organizational processes that foster collaboration without boundaries. Boundarylessness means negligible communication and interaction barriers between roles, ranks, departments, professions, titles, hospitals, and clinics. Boundarylessness fosters greater social capital (trust and interconnectedness) and promotes esprit de corps.

PANDO

What is the oldest (and largest) living organism on planet Earth?

A tree named Pando!

Pando is an 80,000-year-old quaking aspen in Fishlake National Forest in Utah. However, Pando (Latin for "I spread") is actually an integrated community of tens of thousands of trees with a single, unified root system—and no boundaries for continued growth.

As a species, the quaking aspen is both resilient and adaptable. It has the widest natural range of any tree in North America. It lives at elevations from sea level to the tree line and is among the first species of tree to emerge after forest fires, a result of its unified root system. Its bark has a thin layer of chlorophyll for year-round photosynthesis (even in winter when other deciduous trees are dormant).

For organizations to thrive, they need to be like Pando. Patient-centered institutions need a single root system that connects its people and has no counterproductive boundaries between its units and departments or between its clinics and hospitals. Members of the health care team must work together co-creating the best processes of care and superlative patient experiences. No one on the team knows everything necessary for the ideal care strategy for a given patient, but together they do.

This chapter is about the interrelationship of co-creation and boundarylessness and how they form the infrastructure to grow esprit de corps.

CO-CREATING VALUE AND ELIMINATING BOUNDARIES

In health care, boundaries are everywhere—boundaries between different professions, specialty disciplines, roles, teams, ethnicities, genders, ranks, and titles. There are boundaries between different types of organizations (e.g., hospitals, clinics, nursing homes). And there are boundaries associated with old and new ways of thinking. To achieve the most effective organization and the best patient care, boundaries need to be eliminated to allow co-creation of value by diverse teams of health care professionals and administrators. Co-creation is about working together, planning together, and dreaming together on behalf of patients. To achieve boundarylessness, the best question to ask health care professionals is one we learned from Donald M. Berwick, M.D., M.P.P. (president emeritus and senior fellow of the Institute for Healthcare Improvement): "How will it help the patient?"

A Boundarylessness Well-being Coalition

Working across organizational boundaries is one of the critical success elements for the work of a chief wellness officer (CWO) charged with mitigating burnout of health care professionals. Analyzing the scope of work for organizational groups, departments, divisions, and offices will allow the CWO to assemble a coalition of collaborators with staggering potential for change. Once boundaries are eliminated, coalition members will find areas of common ground that they can work on together to achieve the best quality patient care and outcomes, decrease burnout, and create esprit de corps. Below is a short list of potential coalition members and an example of the types of interests they share with the group.

Chief Quality Officer

Common ground: Quality is the systematic removal of needless waste, variation, and defects in processes of care. Needless waste, variation, and defects of care processes and workflow are also major staff frustrations that result in patient adverse events and cause burnout.

Director, Leadership and Organization Development

Common ground: Much of what the Intervention Triad offers are opportunities to partner with leadership development professionals and use proven leadership development experiences to effect change (e.g., Leader Behavior Index, identifying and removing pebbles, Ask-Listen-Empower [and Repeat]).

Chief Human Resource Officer

Common ground: Efforts to promote staff satisfaction and enhance morale provide chief human resource officers opportunities to enrich professional development and reduce staff turnover.

Department and Division Chairs and Chiefs

Common ground: Recruiting and retaining the best staff, developing professionals, and maximizing the potential of team members are universal goals of department and division chairs and chiefs and dividends of reducing burnout.

Patient Experience Officer

Common ground: Improved patient outcomes, quality, and experience are the result of growing esprit de corps and a central interest of every patient experience officer.

Chief Executive Officer and Chief Nursing Officer

Common ground: Chief executive officers (CEOs) and chief nursing officers have a shared interest in efforts to enhance professionalism and mutual respect, cultivate community, promote satisfaction, enhance morale, provide opportunities for professional development, reduce turnover rates, and maximize the potential of team members.

Chief Financial Officer

Common ground: For the chief financial officer, there are financial dividends (the business case) for addressing professional burnout among health care professionals.

So at the end of the day what may have seemed to a CWO like a small staff and meager budget for addressing the formidable challenge of mitigating professional burnout is now a social movement within the organization aligned around fostering boundarylessness, a common vision, and collaboration. The benefits will accrue to health care professionals and, importantly, also to the patients they serve.

Daily Care-Team Huddles

Daily, unit-level, care-team huddles around a whiteboard are a simple and effective participative management tactic to promote boundarylessness at the work-unit level. Huddles are short, 10- to 15-minute meetings that provide a platform for multidisciplinary teams to convene and review the goals, action items, safety risks, problems, and solutions—all of which are recorded on the huddle board.

The following steps describe the process we recommend for initiating daily care-team huddles:

1) Schedule daily care-team huddles for the entire team at a consistent time before the day's work begins. Having the huddle at the start of the shift allows everyone on the team to be on the same page. This saves time throughout the day because everyone has the information needed to function effectively and efficiently as a team.

2) Gather the team around a huddle whiteboard. The layout of the huddle board should be designed in a manner that is aligned with the goals of the organization and the requirements and tasks of the unit. Include an agenda. Show work-unit

metrics, charts, lists of new ideas, and action plans. The information on the board should guide the conversation in the huddle.

3) Start by discussing patient safety. Each member of the team should be encouraged in this psychologically safe setting (i.e., open and nonconfrontational) to take a turn in communicating risks, patient care near misses, safety events, equipment failures, patient concerns, and rapid responses. This is an opportunity for shared learning for the entire team. Huddles also allow the team to discuss care for patients in the unit or for patients who will be contacted that day. Discussion can include key decision points, what will be needed for each patient (e.g., nurse education time), who will perform each task, and when tasks will be completed. From the huddle, each team member will be able to plan for the day's events. This process is much more efficient for the entire team because it reduces interruptions during the day by addressing anticipated questions of staff, patients, and families.

4) Review staffing and supplies to ensure correct coverage and equipment to provide safe and high-quality care.

5) Review progress on operations, action plans, tactics, and improvement projects. Health care professionals should be invited to share improvement ideas. Huddles prompt colleagues to be transparent about current status, thus reinforcing goals and putting in place the best plans, resources, and timeframes to accomplish goals.

6) Close with an invitation to share additional ideas and recognize and thank team members for their contributions.

7) Incorporate positive events in the huddles. Consider beginning or ending each huddle with an invitation for team members to share something positive that happened on the unit during the previous 24 hours.

Functions of Daily Care-Team Huddles

Giving voice and visualization to issues and ideas among teams validates the importance of every team member (regardless of role, rank, or title) and engenders camaraderie, progress, timely project execution, and continuous improvement. Daily care-team huddles help prevent difficulties that can occur when one health care professional assumes that all other team members are aware of everything everyone is doing. Huddles bring members together with the potential to build on ideas, solve problems, and develop efficient workflow processes and plans (i.e., to co-create). When executed properly, daily care-team huddles enhance social connectedness, bolster positivity, and promote community at work and camaraderie, build trust and respect, foster control and flexibility, and cultivate meaning and purpose in work. They break down the boundaries that prevent multidisciplinary groups from flourishing.

Daily care-team huddles can help eliminate repercussions from *working in silos* (i.e., not sharing information), such as duplicated, competing, or wasted efforts; making decisions on the basis of incomplete information; and operating without knowledge of staffing, equipment, or other roadblocks.

Tiered-Escalation Huddles

Tiered-escalation huddles use a process of structured escalation to improve daily care-team huddles and promote boundarylessness. They mitigate or remove both the horizontal (e.g., between roles and disciplines on teams) and vertical boundaries (e.g., between roles and disciplines in the organizational hierarchy [all the way to the executive suite]) seen in most organizations.

The tiered-escalation huddle works like this:

1) Start with daily care-team huddles with point-of-care teams gathered around the huddle boards.
2) Escalate (i.e., communicate) the important messages or problems the care team members are unable to address themselves to the next-level tier. Relevant events and issues that cannot be solved or require awareness at higher levels are reported up through additional tiers on the basis of set escalation protocols involving different levels of management.
3) Escalate the most critical information and matters that require system-level action immediately to the most senior executives.

In the traditional hierarchical organization, leaders often receive information about an event from follow-up aggregated reports weeks or months after the event occurred. The tiered-escalation huddle provides all leaders awareness of critical events in real time and allows leaders to align the organization on what is most important.

Huddles are designed to have clinicians work across, blur, or eliminate:

- Interpersonal point-of-care team boundaries (e.g., physician, nurse, social worker).
- Role, rank, and title boundaries in all tiers.
- Boundaries between the point-of-care team and leaders to whom they report (including the CEO, chief medical officer, chief nursing officer).
- Horizontal boundaries across departments, hospitals, and clinics as like units learn from each other and diffuse best practices and safety solutions to each other.

Functions of Tiered-Escalation Huddles

Tiered-escalation huddles leverage co-creation to break down boundaries. The huddle process connects the point-of-care teams to top executives every day of the year. Tiered-escalation huddles meaningfully impact the timeliness of critical action plans that resolve urgent (and intractable) safety, practice, and access issues. The voices of clinicians break down the boundaries from bedside to headquarters, and the huddle process engenders a culture of trust, respect, and partnership. It builds immunity to burnout. Health care professionals know that leadership is listening to them, empowering them to address issues proactively and to escalate those outside of their sphere of influence.

Done well, the process of tiered-escalation huddles answers the age-old company question, "Does management care?" Yes!

A tiered-escalation huddle also has an important secondary function. It allows leaders from across the system to build a sharing culture and collaborate on issues that affect one another. When leaders share practices that do and do not work well, system-wide consistency, transparency, and performance improve. Best practices developed in one area can be rapidly replicated in other areas, improving outcomes and reducing inappropriate variation in quality and cost.

Case Study: Daily Tiered-Escalation Huddles

Intermountain Healthcare leadership established tiered-escalation huddles as a new way of working, with the intention to nurture a learning organization with high social capital.

Leaders learned early on that issues and ideas needed to be escalated beyond the local frontline managers, and if necessary, to the executive level. So the health system implemented daily tiered-escalation huddles that begin with frontline clinicians (tier one) and end with the executive leadership team (tier six). The huddles occur every day before 10:30 AM and last for approximately 15 minutes. Through this process, the clinical teams are able to get critical data and issues to the appropriate level, ensuring that leaders in a position to resolve the problems are able to do so in a timely way.

The executive leadership team stands before its system-level huddle board to receive reports on issues from group leaders, hospital CEOs, and members of shared services, such as information systems, legal, and communications. Matters requiring immediate and collective attention of top executives are reported, with a particular focus on removing barriers that interfere with the highest-quality patient care. Communication back to frontline leaders is immediate. And, as actions determined at the huddle are completed, accountable leaders report the follow-up in subsequent tier six huddles to close the loop on escalated action items.

One of the most important benefits of this process is the early identification of trends that allow for timely interventions (initial corrective actions occur within 24-48 hours). Hospital-acquired infections, downtime of information systems or equipment, power outages, injury of health care professionals, patient falls, capacity and access issues, and other performance indicators are tracked daily. For example, senior leaders can address capacity issues at one facility by coordinating diversions to other facilities. Safety events can be investigated immediately, with system-wide alerts sent to prevent similar events.

After less than one year of daily tier six huddles at Intermountain Healthcare, the gains were measurable. Leaders addressed safety and capacity issues more effectively. Patient and customer-service issues were identified and resolved faster. The process of tiered escalation huddles yielded better care and service for patients. It also made the work of health care professionals more meaningful and appreciated. From an investment of just 10 to 15 minutes each day, the entire team works together more effectively, and senior leaders understand what point-of-care professionals know and how to support them.

Case Study: Boundaryless Relationships With Community Organizations (Personal Communication, Barry E. Egener, M.D., Medical Director of the Northwest Center for Physician-Patient Communication)

Health care relationships with community, government, and other organizations are examples of boundarylessness. Such collaborations can improve population health. The creation of Unity Center for Behavioral Health in Portland, Oregon, is an example of boundaryless collaboration among local health care systems to address a community need as well as a common interest. Unity Center is a behavioral health services center with the first emergency department (ED) in Oregon and Southwest Washington explicitly designed to deliver immediate psychiatric care for people experiencing a mental health crisis. Unity Center was created with the goal of reducing the *boarding time* of patients with behavioral health issues in hospital EDs. The wait for patients in crisis previously averaged between 40 and 60 hours for some of the busiest area EDs.

In 2014, four health care systems in Portland, Oregon (Adventist Health, Kaiser Permanente, Legacy Health, and Oregon Health & Science University), came together to solve the issue of long boarding times, one of the most challenging impacting health care today nationally. By combining resources and co-creating value, the four health systems reduced the average wait time for a bed from upwards of 60 hours to a mere eight!

The four health systems have a total of 10 hospitals that now have access to a higher level of specialized mental health care for patients experiencing a behavioral health crisis. With a combination of emergency, inpatient, and community-based outpatient services, Unity Center provides comprehensive psychiatric emergency care with 85 adult inpatient beds and 22 inpatient beds for adolescents aged nine through 17.

Unity Center is a revolutionary model for providing crisis mental health services because it spreads the cost and leverages the investment as well as the expertise and the range of human, technological, and systemic resources of the major stakeholders to meet a pressing need in the community. The collaboration between the four health system partners ultimately benefits human health and well-being and lowers costs in health care as well as law enforcement and the legal system (the social structures of last resort for persons with mental illness).

While this community-focused effort of health care organizations has clear benefits to the systems that created it and the patients it serves, there are internal benefits as well. In fact, the well-being of clinicians is improved. The substantial reduction in boarding time has an important impact on local area EDs and the people who staff them. Professionals are less stressed because they are not confronted by patients with psychiatric crises whose conditions cannot be adequately treated in the ED, and the patients do not return repeatedly. Psychiatric crises in the ED also affect the experience of other patients who wait longer for their emergency care because staff are preoccupied with patients with mental health issues. Cross-organizational collaboration has reduced this burden for all participating organizations and professionals.

Because Unity Center partners across boundaries with dozens of community-based organizations to connect patients with social services and follow-up care, patients continue to receive the support they need after leaving Unity Center. This is the epitome of boundarylessness. Collateral benefits for society include less homelessness and better morale for correctional facility employees, who are not equipped to help these patients. Everyone benefits.

LEADER CHARACTERISTICS

How do leaders foster boundarylessness? They do this by:

- Seeking a shared purpose and advocating for win-win scenarios.
- Visiting and harvesting ideas from diverse improvement teams, work units, and other organizations.
- Being generous with attention and making connections with those they lead.
- Sharing resources and co-creating solutions.
- Utilizing systems thinking to frame challenges for those they lead.
- Respecting people in different roles and units and seeing the possibilities of working together.
- Prioritizing the mission and highest good rather than the parochial self-interest of their group.

When boundaries are removed, common ground and resolve grow like the roots of the great tree, Pando, strengthening an organization around a shared vision.

CONCLUSION

Leaders play a central role in modeling and facilitating engagement and connectedness across boundaries. They should establish the expectation for both adoption and active diffusion of practices and bidirectional learning. Deploying the huddle process is one way of doing so. Boundarylessness practices demonstrate humility, respect for all, and the power of teamwork. Organizations that foster boundarylessness can help to create esprit de corps by enabling the possibility of *E pluribus unum*: out of many, one (Box 32.1).

TOMORROW: FULFILLMENT

Amanda is "all in" at work. Everyone working on her unit functions as a valued part of a true team. Together, they huddle every morning, co-create the day's work, and discuss the best way to take care of patients and the prospects they have to improve their work life. The power-distance index between the doctors and nurses still exists, but it is so modest that it has totally disappeared as an issue for her. Amanda feels respected, appreciated, and valued; she is no longer looking for a new job.

Box 32.1 The Playbook

- Establish one huddle system in an area with eager and willing colleagues.
  - Think big, start small, act fast.
    - Gain experience
- Connect with one leader to explore common ground and collaboration.
  - Chief quality officer
  - Director, leadership and organization development
  - Chief human resource officer
  - Department and division chairs and chiefs
  - Patient experience officer
  - Chief nursing officer
- Determine how boundarylessness could improve your work life.
  - Are there boundaries that limit your joy, engagement, or results?
    - These boundaries could be between rank, professions, hospitals, clinics, nursing homes, ethnicities, specialty disciplines, gender, roles, titles, teams—or boundaries between old and new ways of thinking.
    - Discuss the boundaries with appropriate colleagues and create a shared action plan to achieve a future state.

SUGGESTED READING

Egener BE, Mason DJ, McDonald WJ, Okun S, Gaines ME, Fleming DA, et al. The charter on professionalism for health care organizations. Acad Med. 2017 Aug;92(8):1091–9.

Swensen S, Pugh M, McMullan C, Kabcenell A. High-impact leadership: improve care, improve the health populations, and reduce costs. IHI White Paper. Cambridge (MA): Institute for Healthcare Improvement; 2013.

33

APPLYING THE ACTION SETS TO ADDRESS THE UNIQUE NEEDS OF MEDICAL STUDENTS, RESIDENTS, AND FELLOWS

We need to protect the workforce that protects our patients.
—Timothy Brigham, M.Div., Ph.D.

An entire book could be written on the unique needs and opportunities of future health care professionals in training. The focus of this chapter is to explore how the Action Sets of Agency, Coherence, and Camaraderie can apply to trainees. Although some of the tactics differ among the groups, all aspects of the Action Sets are relevant to the well-being of trainees. The actions that are most applicable to the needs of a particular education program should be carefully selected and implemented.

BURNOUT BEGINS IN MEDICAL TRAINING

Evidence indicates that future physicians (i.e., premedicine undergraduate students) usually begin their training with better mental health profiles than those pursuing other professions. They typically have chosen a career in health care out of an altruistic desire to heal and serve humanity. They view the profession as a calling. They have less burnout and depression as well as more favorable scores for emotional health, physical health, and overall quality of life than those pursuing other professions (Brazeau et al, 2014).

Sadly, this favorable profile rapidly erodes during their training. Studies of medical students show that depression increases during the first two years of school. Burnout begins to increase in years three and four and crescendos during residency. At the time of transition to graduate medical education, approximately 50% of students experience burnout (Dyrbye et al, 2014). National studies involving over 15,000 resident physicians suggest that 75% experience professional burnout before they even complete their education (West et al, 2011). The very training that should augment their altruism, compassion, and commitment is instead extinguishing it. Clearly, unique systemic issues need to be addressed for medical students, residents, and fellows (hereafter called trainees when discussed as a group).

The following factors predispose trainees to emotional and psychological distress during the training process:

- Dramatic lifestyle shifts from college to medical school as well as from medical school to residency and fellowship
- Limited control over their work environment

- Transitioning to a new city/community, often geographically distant from personal support systems
- Sleep deprivation from frequent night call and fluctuating work schedules
- Frequent transitions to new work settings (e.g., different hospitals and clinics) with each rotation
- Short-term assignments without "ownership" of issues or opportunities to improve the environment
- Frequent rotations among specialties, which result in a student feeling like a perpetual novice
- Negligible control over attending physician behavior and unit/rotation culture
- Heavy academic workload/clinical caseload
- Perceived need of the trainee to excel among an exceptional peer group or risk being unable to pursue desired specialty or practice opportunities
- Uncertainty about future career opportunities (e.g., specialty, location, practice setting)
- First-time feelings of responsibility for the survival and outcome of patients (sometimes without adequate experience or expertise)
- First experiences with terrible diseases as well as patient suffering and death
- Inadequate preparation and training to deal with the emotional burden of caring for patients and families
- Cognitive dissonance between their altruistic ideals and the reality of medical practice
- Repetitive and menial tasks
- Frenetic, intense pace of training
- Time pressure and demands
- Challenges with work-life integration
- Stress related to educational debt
- A fundamentally unhealthy 80-hour work week that affords inadequate time for friends and family, fitness, and sleep

Organizations that have the privilege of training health care professionals must pay attention to the occupational distress of the training process for trainees and the educational environment for faculty. By implementing relevant aspects of the Action Sets in the Intervention Triad, organizations can prevent burnout and foster esprit de corps for trainees.

APPLICATION OF THE ACTION SETS

Agency Actions

As described in earlier chapters, Agency is the capacity of individuals or teams to act independently. When possible, trainees should be given voice, input, flexibility, and control.

Awareness

Leaders in medical education must be responsible for raising awareness about occupational distress among trainees. Faculty and trainees must learn to identify the signs of professional distress (including burnout, depression, sleep deprivation, moral injury, suicidal ideation, and substance abuse) among their peers and within themselves. They should understand where and how to refer or seek appropriate care. They should also be encouraged to alert appropriate staff when there are concerns that a peer or colleague may be displaying signs of any distress.

Promote Universal Wellness

Training programs should make a commitment to promoting well-being among all trainees and should work with learners to create a compact for the shared responsibility for well-being. A training program has the responsibility to help trainees develop self-care habits, strengthen personal resilience skills, and set appropriate boundaries of work-life integration (see Chapter 34, "Nurturing Well-being"). This culture can be achieved in various ways, including:

- Offer courses about wellness, resilience, and meaning and contentment. The courses should be subsidized or free to all trainees and faculty and offered at times that accommodate trainee schedules to facilitate participation.
- Hold quarterly meetings for small groups of like trainees, during which education leaders check in on stress, work-life integration, and the training experience of the various groups. The groups should be small enough to facilitate an open and psychologically safe conversation about shared experiences. At these sessions, individual plans for self-care and well-being should be discussed.
- Have all learners meet one-on-one with a psychologist at the beginning of their training to discuss wellness promotion. By doing so, the trainees will also establish a relationship with someone whom they can call if distress develops later in the course of their training. Ideally, these psychologists should also participate in the quarterly small group meetings so that they remain visible and continue to cultivate relationships with learners.
- Create a well-being policy and plan that supports optimal emotional health for trainees. Mayo Clinic Alix School of Medicine has a comprehensive program in place that includes measurement, education, pass-fail grading, mentor/advisor relationships, social network builders, self-care training, and a safe haven refuge (Dyrbye and Shanafelt, 2016; Goldman et al, 2018).
- Reduce the stigma associated with seeking professional assistance for psychological and emotional concerns. This is often best achieved by having faculty share about their experiences with distress, seeking help, and navigating stressful times in their own professional journeys. Such vulnerability by faculty normalizes trainee experiences and makes seeking help acceptable. They further establish for the trainees that their role models are not "super human," that it is OK to be imperfect, and that they should seek help when needed.

Access to Help

Organizational culture plays a central role in setting expectations for well-being. If the leadership and culture promote self-care and support of one another, trainees will be happier and less likely to burn out or have other serious problems during their training. Training institutions should systematically measure trainee well-being in a confidential and anonymous manner at regular intervals and provide access to self-screening tools for burnout, depression, and other forms of distress. Tactics that may be of value include:

- Support for and easy access to affordable, safe, confidential, proactive mental health resources, assessments, counseling, and treatment, including urgent and emergent care.
- Safe haven for compassion fatigue or adverse events counseling.
- Flexibility and adequate time off.
- Self-care training.

Case Study: Improving the Training Environment

The Graduate Medical Education Office at Dartmouth-Hitchcock has developed a robust set of interventions to improve the training environment for residents and fellows. Their effort resulted in measurably improved well-being. The interventions included:

- Providing education for faculty, residents, and fellows on how to identify the symptoms of burnout, depression, and substance abuse.
- Providing information on where and how trainees experiencing issues could seek appropriate care.
- Encouraging residents, fellows, and faculty to alert designated personnel when they had concerns that a colleague may be displaying signs of burnout, depression, substance abuse, or suicidal ideation.
- Providing access to tools for anonymous online self-screening for burnout, depression, and substance abuse.
- Providing access to confidential and affordable mental health assessment, counseling, and treatment, including access to urgent and emergent care 24 hours per day, seven days per week.
- Requiring each residency and fellowship program to create a wellness policy and plan to support optimal resident (and faculty member) well-being.

Removing Pebbles

Trainees deal with many unique frustrations related to different rotations, schedules, transitions, curricular factors, group dynamics, financial stress, and logistics (e.g., parking at different locations, access to the electronic health record). Seeking to understand and address unique situational needs and challenges of trainees is an effective means to nurture Agency and reduce negativity of the workplace environment. Leaders should organize and support "what frustrates you" conversations with trainees, followed by open discussion about what could be done to address these issues. These conversations might look like the following:

- Meet with the group and start the conversation (see Chapter 16, "Agency Action: Removing Pebbles").
- Ask: "What are the pebbles in your shoes?"

- Listen: Hear and really understand frustrations.
- Empower: "Let's remove them together."
- Repeat.

Make trainee concerns visible and transparent by using an electronic or manual whiteboard feedback system, with a running list of the status of each improvement effort (e.g., escalated within the organization, improvement in progress) and a place to contribute input on changes to test going forward. Leaders may need to take more responsibility for driving this process for trainees than they do with health care professionals who are in practice because 1) trainees have extensive other responsibilities and time demands and 2) improvement efforts may need to extend longer than the duration of the trainees' time on the rotation or in the training program. Ownership and responsibility for the whiteboard improvement work should therefore reside with the appropriate deans, program directors, clerkship directors, and other faculty members with clear accountability for results. The whiteboards should be placed where all trainees and leaders can view them so that progress of the improvement work is transparent.

Senior Resident Leadership Development

Senior residents are the leaders of teams, and their attention to the welfare of the junior residents, interns, and medical students on their team is critical to well-being. It makes sense that education leadership should model the desired behaviors and attend to the leadership development of senior residents. The program could feature the five leader behaviors (include, inform, inquire, develop, recognize) and consider how these behaviors are appropriately demonstrated within the resident team (see Chapter 15, "Agency Action: Measuring Leader Behaviors" and Chapter 23, "Coherence Action: Selecting and Developing Leaders").

Senior residents as team leaders could promote esprit de corps by assisting other members of the team when the workload is heavy (e.g., helping with admissions, carrying the intern's pager so that person can take a break, investing in the learning and professional development of the team by teaching or bringing articles). Programs should consider investing in such leadership training for residents as they progress through their training and help them become effective leaders of the team and better physicians for their career.

Coherence Actions

Coherence is an organizational state in which the parts fit together in a united and thoughtfully constructed whole. To be coherent, educational programs must holistically approach the interrelated goals of learning and well-being.

Education Program Structure, Curriculum, and Culture

The education program's structure, curriculum, and culture have central roles in the well-being of trainees. Results from a systematic review showed that trainees were more satisfied with programs that included block scheduling; continuity programs for patient care (i.e., diagnosis to treatment to resolution); trainee, staff team, and community building activities; and dedicated faculty with a special interest and training in education and mentorship (Stepczynski et al, 2018).

A thoughtfully designed curriculum with these elements contributes to the Coherence of an education program. In contrast, curriculum without Coherence drives student distress. Strategic reforms to address gaps based on student and faculty-generated input have been shown to significantly improve student well-being (Slavin, 2018). Validated restructuring targets include course content, contact hours, scheduling, grading, electives, learning communities, and required resilience and mindfulness exercises. Such alterations can also improve community and cohesion (i.e., the social connectedness) among students.

Case Study: Organizational Culture at Saint Louis University School of Medicine

At Saint Louis University School of Medicine, education leaders pursued a decade-long effort to improve their organizational culture in order to advance medical student well-being. Their efforts resulted in a remarkable reduction in depression and anxiety among first-year students and confirmed that interventions and sustained attention make a difference (Slavin, 2018).

The focus of their intervention centered on three tactics:

1) Improve the learning environment by reducing preventable sources of stress in training systems, evaluation, and curriculum
2) Establish opportunities for students to connect to the meaning and purpose of their work through interactions with patients, families, and colleagues
3) Offer training in stress management and personal resilience and provide resources and promote emotional and psychological support

Work-Hour Limitations

Although long work hours contribute to professional distress, efforts to reduce duty hours for resident physicians have not universally improved patient care or resident wellness. Fewer duty hours may also negatively affect education value (Bolster and Rourke, 2015). If not done appropriately, reducing hours can create new challenges, such as excessive work when on duty because the team is smaller, fragmentation of learning, loss of continuity with patients that can erode meaning in practice, and missed learning opportunities when residents or fellows are forced to leave at the end of their maximum time on duty, even when they are in the midst of a high-value learning experience.

Measurement

To ensure Coherence, improvements in well-being need to be measured with validated instruments in a confidential or anonymous fashion and benchmarked with results at peer institutions (see Chapter 9, "Assessment").

Trainee surveys should measure:

- Well-being of the individual (e.g., burnout, professional fulfillment, sleep-related impairment).
- Impact of the structure of the learning environment (e.g., schedule, hours, supervision, support) on well-being.
- Effectiveness of the program leaders and clinician educators.

Heat maps can be developed to show where trainees are experiencing greater amounts of distress (e.g., rotations, hospitals, specialty disciplines), after which prioritized opportunities for improvement should be addressed.

Leadership Accountability

Of course, measurement without remediation is meaningless. An accountable senior leader must review the survey data and heat maps, and co-assemble a plan to address work environment and leadership issues.

1) Determine the educational, clinical work unit, and specialty leaders who are responsible and accountable for individual trainees.
2) Perform an annual review of each program and clerkship director on the basis of:
   - Feedback from students, residents, and fellows for all physician leaders regarding the work environment, culture, and psychological safety. Feedback should be 360 degrees and shared with leaders in the spirit of helping them become better leaders with a style that enhances trainee well-being.
   - Esprit de corps and professional distress of units for which they are accountable.

The results will determine the remediation indicated and may include executive coaching, leadership development, or leader rotation, as indicated.

Camaraderie Actions

Leaders in medical education share a responsibility to nurture community at work and camaraderie among trainees. Within education programs, use of pass-fail grading has been shown to reduce competition and promote collaboration and should be considered wherever feasible (Rohe et al, 2006). In addition, programs should support and fund meals and discussion groups for medical students, residents, and fellows. Commensality groups are a validated means to improve social isolation, meaning and purpose, emotional exhaustion, and cynicism. Approaches to foster community, including commensality groups, are discussed in Chapter 28, "Camaraderie Ideal Work Element: Community at Work and Camaraderie," and Chapter 30, "Camaraderie Action: Cultivating Community and Commensality." It should be noted that requiring trainees to participate in community-building opportunities (rather than providing it as option) and failing to provide coverage for clinical duties may undermine effectiveness (Ripp et al, 2016).

Case Study: The Dream Team Project (Personal Communication, Christopher R. Peabody, M.D., M.P.H.)

Every physician remembers the jarring transition from medical school to residency training. Idealistic new physicians start their residency with enthusiasm and with definite goals for their future. During their training, however, the enthusiasm often fades. Even with much more responsibility, residents have little autonomy, experience intense work demands, and may become emotionally exhausted, cynical, and uncertain they are making a difference. They often experience a defining *crucible moment*.

The Dream Team project, which is embedded at five medical centers in the San Francisco Bay area, aims to change this downward trajectory. The Dream Team is a values-based peer group established by resident physicians to improve self-care, work control, and support for career development. During the first week, as part of orientation, participants are asked to write a one-page reflection about their goals for residency and to describe their dreams for the future. They are then grouped with four or five colleagues with the explicit purpose to develop a longitudinal strategy to hold each member accountable for their goals and dreams. The project is designed to help residents find peers who will challenge and help hold them accountable if they appear to lose their bearing or deviate from their previous beliefs and values. Dream Teams are designed to augment traditional mentorship programs, support professional aspirations, and prevent burnout.

Dream Teams help residents navigate challenges, hold on to their values, and preserve altruism and aspirations. The teams are supported so that they have protected time to meet and discuss shared strategies for work-life integration, career development, and emotional support. Dream Team members have found more joy in their work and are regularly and thoughtfully reminded why they chose health care in the first place.

CONCLUSION

Although medical students, residents, and fellows have some drivers of professional distress that differ from those of practicing clinicians, the themes of Agency, Coherence, and Camaraderie are equally relevant. As described, actions in the Intervention Triad can be adapted and used as a framework to decrease burnout and promote esprit de corps among trainees as part of a comprehensive educational program initiative to address unique needs of the target group (Box 33.1).

Box 33.1 The Playbook

- Build senior leadership, faculty, and trainee awareness of the impact of burnout on medical student, resident, and fellow well-being.
- Pursue universal wellness promotion.
  - Offer courses at times that accommodate trainee schedules about wellness, resilience, and meaning and contentment.
  - Hold quarterly meetings for small groups of like trainees during which education leaders check in on stress, work-life integration, and the training experience of the various groups.
- Reduce stigma.
  - Pursue sustained and concerted strategies for trainees to seek help for psychological and emotional concerns.
  - Have faculty share their experiences with distress, seeking help, and navigating stressful times in their own professional journeys as one effective approach to normalize help seeking and reduce stigma.
- Provide access to help.
  - Support and ensure easy access to affordable, safe, confidential, proactive mental health resources, assessments, counseling, and treatment, including urgent and emergent care.
- Improve the learning environment.
  - Reduce preventable sources of stress in training systems, evaluation, and curriculum. To the extent possible, consider how to create predictability and reduce chaos.
  - Determine the faculty and leaders who are responsible and accountable for individual trainees and their well-being. Assess their performance and address opportunities for improvement.
- Provide leadership development training for senior residents in the five leader behaviors (include, inform, inquire, develop, recognize) and consider how these are appropriately demonstrated within the resident team.
- Launch programs that build social community.
- Regularly measure the well-being of trainees using validated instruments in a confidential or anonymous fashion.
  - Provide trainees access to self-assessment tools that provide links to resources for those with distress.

SUGGESTED READING

Bolster L, Rourke L. The effect of restricting residents' duty hours on patient safety, resident well-being, and resident education: an updated systematic review. J Grad Med Educ. 2015 Sep;7(3):349–63.

Brazeau CM, Shanafelt T, Durning SJ, Massie FS, Eacker A, Moutier C, et al. Distress among matriculating medical students relative to the general population. Acad Med. 2014 Nov;89(11):1520–5.

Dyrbye L, Shanafelt T. A narrative review on burnout experienced by medical students and residents. Med Educ. 2016 Jan;50(1):132–49.

Dyrbye LN, West CP, Satele D, Boone S, Tan L, Sloan J, et al. Burnout among U.S. medical students, residents, and early career physicians relative to the general U.S. population. Acad Med. 2014 Mar;89(3):443–51.

Goldman ML, Bernstein CA, Konopasek L, Arbuckle M, Mayer LES. An intervention framework for institutions to meet new ACGME common program requirements for physician well-being. Acad Psychiatry. 2018 Aug;42(4):542–7.

Mata DA, Ramos MA, Bansal N, Khan R, Guille C, Di Angelantonio E, et al. Prevalence of depression and depressive symptoms among resident physicians: a systematic review and meta-analysis. JAMA. 2015 Dec 8;314(22):2373–83.

Ripp JA, Fallar R, Korenstein D. A randomized controlled trial to decrease job burnout in first-year internal medicine residents using a facilitated discussion group intervention. J Grad Med Educ. 2016 May;8(2):256–9.

Rohe DE, Barrier PA, Clark MM, Cook DA, Vickers KS, Decker PA. The benefits of pass-fail grading on stress, mood, and group cohesion in medical students. Mayo Clin Proc. 2006 Nov;81(11):1443–8.

Slavin S. Reflections on a decade leading a medical student well-being initiative. Acad Med. 2019 Jun;94(6):771–4.

Stepczynski J, Holt SR, Ellman MS, Tobin D, Doolittle BR. Factors affecting resident satisfaction in continuity clinic: a systematic review. J Gen Intern Med. 2018 Aug;33(8):1386–93.

West CP, Shanafelt TD, Kolars JC. Quality of life, burnout, educational debt, and medical knowledge among internal medicine residents. JAMA. 2011 Sep 7;306(9):952–60.

34

NURTURING WELL-BEING

TODAY: DISTRESS

Heather is one of the most meticulous and respected pathologists in her department. Over the years, Heather's workload has gradually increased. She sits all day in a windowless reading room. She keeps a box of granola bars in her desk and usually eats one for lunch in her office alone so she can continue to work. Heather has lost the joy she experienced in her early years of practice. She is socially isolated at work and no longer has time to go to department meetings or lectures. She has started to wonder if her effort really matters. The long hours have also caused friction with her husband. She wakes up in the morning dreading having to go to work.

◆ ◆ ◆

This chapter focuses on our twelfth action—the importance of organizational efforts to nurture individual health care professionals as they enhance their holistic well-being (hereafter "well-being") (i.e., optimized wellness, resilience, and contentment). Enhancing personal well-being is a shared responsibility between individuals and organizations. Individuals must cultivate personal well-being. Organizations can help by providing training and resources, and by making it easy for health care professionals to participate despite their demanding professional life and work schedules. When individual well-being is bolstered, health care professionals are more fulfilled, have greater meaning and purpose in work, and are better able to tolerate negativity.

Three Sisters

For centuries, the Iroquois and Paiute tribes have grown corn, pole beans, and squash by planting the seeds together in the same mound of dirt. They call this method "the three sisters" because the three plants grow better as a family. In other words, the yield of crops growing together is much greater than the yield of the three grown separately (Figure 34.1).

The first sister, corn, provides a natural pole for the beans to climb. The second sister, beans, adds nitrogen to the soil through its roots—improving the fertility of the plot for years to come. The bean vines also climb the cornstalk, stabilizing the plant and making it less vulnerable to wind damage. The third sister, squash, provides living mulch with its shallow roots, and its broad leaves provide shade to retain soil moisture and stunt the growth of emerging weeds.

Growing together, the three sisters provide structure, fertilization, and mulch, which improve crop performance. Their interdependence leads to more efficient use of resources, provides safety, and results in better yields (i.e., outcomes). To thrive,

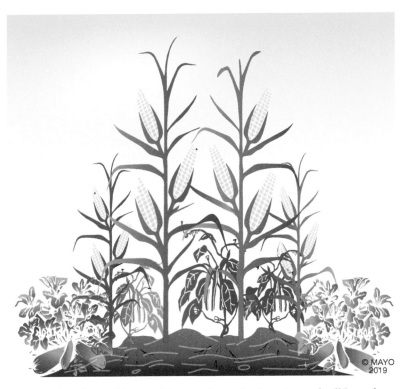

Figure 34.1. The Three Sisters. We extend the metaphor to the three sisters of well-being for health care: wellness, resilience, and contentment.

health care professionals need a similar interdependency, which we call the *three sisters of well-being* (i.e., wellness, resilience, and contentment).

Together these three sisters produce something greater than the individual components: well-being. To further the analogy, this growth can only be achieved if all three sisters of well-being share the same *mound of dirt* (i.e., these three dimensions must work synergistically to optimize well-being).

WELLNESS, RESILIENCE, AND CONTENTMENT

Wellness, resilience, and contentment are key to the sustainability of professionals, quality of care, and well-being. Our framework for the interrelationships of the three dimensions is summarized below.

Wellness refers to being in good physical and mental health. Wellness involves sleep, exercise, fitness, nutrition, rest, and preventive as well as indicated medical care.

Resilience is the flexibility and capacity to recover rapidly from stressful encounters. Resilience gives humans the ability to adapt to and recover from the challenges and disruptions that are a part of life. For some components of resilience, individuals have limited or no control (i.e., genetics and personality traits). However, many aspects of resilience can be strengthened and developed: self-compassion, cognitive flexibility, moral code, growth mindset, forgiveness, religion, spirituality, mindfulness, and gratitude.

Contentment requires an understanding of one's values and having a sense of peace of mind and fulfillment. Contentment involves good spiritual, emotional, and intellectual health as well as work-life integration (i.e., nurturing relationships, hobbies, and avocational activities that cultivate growth as well as contentment).

THE INTERRELATIONSHIP OF
WELL-BEING AND BURNOUT

So how does well-being relate to burnout? Well-being is a holistic construct characterized by healthy levels of social, physical, and mental resources that can be replenished. In contrast, burnout is characterized by a depletion of social, physical, and mental resources caused by unrealistic professional demands. A person's energy, engagement, and enthusiasm are determined by the difference between their *burn rate* (i.e., how rapidly their resources are depleted) and their *replenishment rate* (i.e., how rapidly their resources are restored) of social, physical, and mental resources (Figure 34.2). For example, adequate sleep, breaks, rest, exercise, and nutrition are about replenishing reserves. Optimal well-being occurs with a low burn rate and a high replenishment rate. Resilience helps mitigate the depleting factors that contribute to burnout (Figure 34.3).

On the flip side, persons who diligently replenish may avoid burnout even though they may not be particularly resilient. Similarly, resilient persons who do not replenish may be able to withstand challenges and persevere longer than most. Diligently attending to both resilience and replenishment is necessary for health care professionals to nurture their well-being in a sustainable way over the course of their career.

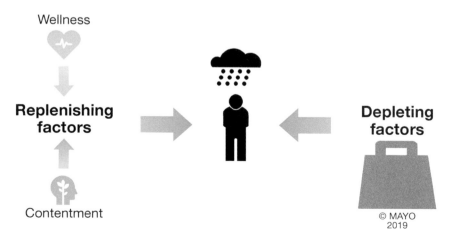

Figure 34.2. Effects of Replenishing and Depleting Factors. In this scenario, the depleting factors are excessive and well-being is low.

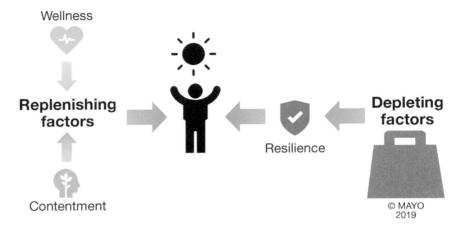

Figure 34.3. Impact of Resilience on Replenishing and Depleting Factors. Resilience helps mitigate the depleting factors and well-being improves.

Five Organizational Scenarios for Well-being

Consider the following five organizational scenarios:

1) The first organization has high levels of professional burnout and low esprit de corps. It has neglected to attend to the factors that promote well-being or to mitigate depleting factors. It has not implemented the Intervention Triad (Agency, Coherence, Camaraderie) (Figure 34.4).
2) The second organization has moderate levels of professional burnout and modest esprit de corps. This organization focuses on factors that promote well-being

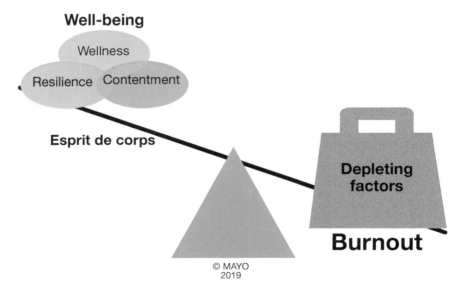

Figure 34.4. Organization Not Attending to the Well-being of Health Care Professionals or Mitigating Depleting Factors. Depleting factors outweigh replenishing factors.

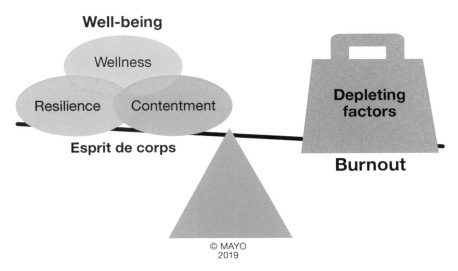

Figure 34.5. Organization Focused on Promoting Well-being Without Mitigating Depleting Factors.

but has not mitigated depleting factors. It has not implemented the Intervention Triad. Its focus on cultivating wellness and resilience (replenishing factors) has allowed it to realize measurable improvements in professional distress, but the risk of burnout remains needlessly high (Figure 34.5).

3) The third organization has mild levels of professional burnout and modest esprit de corps. It has prioritized efforts to reduce depleting factors but has not attended to promoting well-being. The organization invests in reducing inefficiencies, improving workflows, and enhancing the operational aspects of the work environment without specifically attending to the well-being of its professionals (Figure 34.6). It has not implemented the Intervention Triad. This type of organization has a needlessly high risk for burnout of health care professionals.

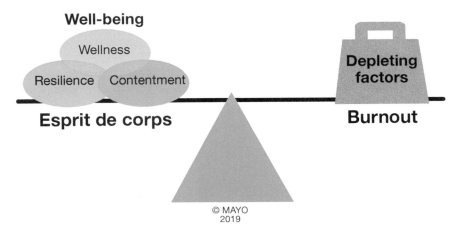

Figure 34.6. Organization Focused on Reducing Depleting Factors Without Attending to Well-being.

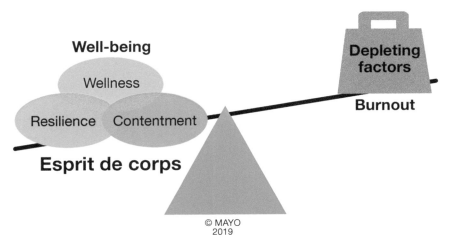

Figure 34.7. Organization Focused on Reducing Depleting Factors and Promoting Well-being Without Implementing the Intervention Triad.

4) The fourth organization has moderate levels of professional burnout and much improved esprit de corps. Leaders and professionals have prioritized efforts to reduce depleting factors and have attended to personal well-being of health care professionals but have not implemented the Intervention Triad. This type of organization may have made substantial progress with both burnout and esprit de corps, but it still has not come close to its full potential because it has not created an environment, culture, and community of health care professionals with aligned purpose who support each other (Figure 34.7).

5) The fifth organization has very low levels of professional burnout and high esprit de corps. The fulcrum has shifted to a more favorable position because the organization successfully implemented actions from the Intervention Triad (which reduce workplace negativity and grow workplace positivity). The leaders and professionals have substantially reduced depleting factors and attended to personal well-being of health care professionals (Figure 34.8).

This last scenario is ideal. Leaders support professionals and their environment to create the ideal workplace. They work collaboratively on the Intervention Triad to 1) decrease depleting factors; 2) increase clinician wellness, resilience, and contentment; and 3) create an environment of esprit de corps with interventions that optimize the balance of Agency, Coherence, and Camaraderie.

PRACTICES FOR CREATING WELL-BEING

Various evidence-based practices can be used to help promote the well-being of health care professionals. All are primarily dependent on developing personal resilience and attending to self-care. Achieving success in each practice area can be helped with identification of a role model or mentor. Below we present several select, validated practices that can strengthen one of the well-being subdimensions (i.e., wellness, resilience, and contentment) (Figure 34.9).

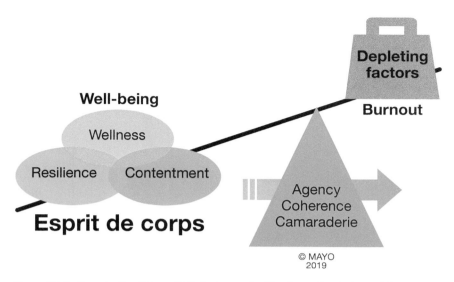

Figure 34.8. Organization Using a Holistic Approach of Implementing Actions of the Intervention Triad. This approach shifts the fulcrum to the right, further mitigating burnout while reducing depleting factors and promoting well-being. This is the ideal state for organizations and health care professionals and can be reached by following the Blueprint for cultivating esprit de corps.

Wellness

Individual wellness can be improved in several ways. Wellness depends on many factors (Box 34.1). Organizations should sponsor accessible wellness programs and encourage health care professionals to take advantage of them. Four important wellness factors that are straightforward to achieve are adequate sleep, sunlight, movement, laughter, and midday breaks.

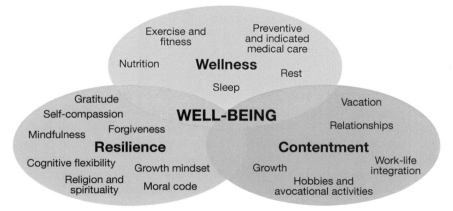

Figure 34.9. Practices That Create Wellness, Resilience, and Contentment: The Three Sisters of Well-being for Health Care.

> **Box 34.1.** Wellness Practices
>
> - Sleep
> - Exercise
> - Fitness
> - Nutrition
> - Sunlight
> - Laughter
> - Preventive care
> - Indicated medical care
> - Wellness role models

Sleep

Adequate sleep is fundamental to wellness. To the extent possible, persons should rest as much as the body needs. Health care professionals who work for 17 hours straight have been shown to develop temporary cognitive and technical impairments comparable to the level of impairment induced by elevated blood alcohol levels (Williamson and Feyer, 2000). We do not allow health care professionals to come to work drunk, and we should not tolerate environments or work schedules that cause them to be impaired due to sleep deprivation. For physicians and other health care professionals, unhealthy habits and patterns of sleep deprivation are promulgated early in the training years and are often extended into the practice years.

Sleep deprivation is a depleting factor that has a major impact on health and contributes to burnout. The amount of sleep received impacts metabolic function, which has ramifications for weight gain and the risk of developing diabetes. Inadequate sleep may also negatively impact the immune system as well as increase the risk for serious illnesses such as heart disease, cancer, and depression.

Organizations need to bring schedules for health care professionals (including health care professionals in training) in line with those of other high-performance professionals, such as commercial airline pilots. The recommended amount of sleep (seven to eight hours) must become a professional priority.

Sunlight

Sunlight is good for humans. Sunlight positively influences physical and mental health (including moods and emotions) as well as performance and may increase longevity. Studies indicate that patients who have natural light in their hospital rooms have shorter lengths of stay and require fewer narcotics for pain (Rogers, 2008; Park et al, 2018). Nurses who are exposed to sunlight on their shifts make fewer medication errors. Sunlight works through endogenous generation of a combination of nitric oxide, melatonin, glutamate, serotonin, and vitamin D. When you take a break or walk during the workday, consider stepping outside.

Movement

Movement is also important and can be combined with getting some sun. Exercise has been shown to positively affect physical and mental health (Sharma et al, 2006; Chaudhury et al, 2009). Those who exercise have fewer work absences, more and better social relationships, better immunity, less heart disease, and, like those who get sunshine, longer lives and better performance (Penedo and Dahn, 2005; Laskowski, 2016). In an interesting study, radiologists who interpreted computed tomography scans while walking at one mph on a treadmill had higher detection rates of clinically important findings than those who read images while seated (Fidler et al, 2008).

The key is to infuse movement throughout your day. Thirty minutes of intense exercise in the gym at the end of the day does not make up for the fallout of an eight-hour sedentary work day.

Laughter

Laughter is another healthy habit, and humor appears to increase life span (Romundstad et al, 2016). Laughter improves breathing and circulation, stimulates the immune system, boosts aerobic capacity, and increases positive emotions, such as excitement, self-assurance, and joyfulness. At work, laughter enhances health care professionals' morale, confidence, and resilience as well as reduces stress. As journalist Norman Cousins said, "Laughter is inner jogging."

Midday Breaks

Stress, interruptions, pressure to stay on schedule, and decision fatigue among health care providers should be acknowledged and managed. There is evidence that the time of day patients are seen makes a difference in their experience and outcomes. Physicians, for example, order fewer indicated, preventive cancer screening examinations for patients seen later in the day compared with number of screenings ordered in the morning. At the end of the afternoon, ordering rates were 10% to 15% lower than for appointments around 8:00 AM (Hsiang et al, 2019). Breaks can enhance performance!

Midday breaks can make a difference in these patterns. Opportunities should be created for health care professionals to have midday breaks and rest (e.g., a short meditation session or nap, stretching exercises, five minutes outside on a bench with some deep breaths).

Resilience

Everyone faces stress each day. To mitigate stress, individual resilience should be increased. Resilience depends on many factors (Box 34.2), and organizations should sponsor and encourage programs that allow individuals to enhance their resilience. Five fundamental contributors to resilience that can be strengthened include 1) self-compassion with cognitive flexibility and growth mindset, 2) mindfulness, 3) religion and spirituality, 4) forgiveness, and 5) gratitude.

Box 34.2 Resilience Practices

- Self-compassion
- Growth mindset
- Gratitude
- Mindfulness
- Moral code
- Cognitive flexibility
- Forgiveness
- Religion and spirituality role models

---

1) Self-compassion With Cognitive Flexibility and Growth Mindset

Health care professionals need to treat themselves with the same compassion and standards that they have for a patient or loved one. Too often, health care professionals hold themselves to a perfectionistic, unrealistic ideal. If you ever feel you are falling short or are having a difficult time, first pause and ask yourself how you would treat a colleague in the circumstance. Then, treat yourself with the same kindness and compassion that you would treat them. Self-compassion and related cognitive reframing techniques, cognitive flexibility, and management of the impact of excessive cognitive workload and cognitive dissonance are important resilience skills (Hsiang et al, 2019). These skills can also help health care professionals reframe their perfectionistic tendencies to instead focus on a commitment to excellence, growth, and improvement. The practice of self-compassion is a key ingredient of resilience.

2) Mindfulness

Mindfulness is a type of self-awareness and meditation that involves focusing intently on the present. Meditation can help train the mind to be relaxed, focused, and less judgmental and can effectively reduce stress and bring a sense of calm to the day. Mindfulness meditation has been shown to have a profound and synergistic effect on clinician well-being, resilience, burnout, empathy, and psychosocial orientation.

The nature of professional-patient relationships is central to healing. Studies have suggested that the ability of health care professionals to practice empathy and be aware of patient-relationship dynamics (Beach and Inui, 2006) improves with greater mindfulness. Mindfulness meditation has also proved effective in reducing negative feelings, rumination, and anxiety.

During the day, the mind naturally wanders. On average, people are distracted for approximately half of each day (Sood, 2015), and most of that distraction is actually focused on negative or neutral thoughts. This scenario can result in stress, anxiety, and loss of energy. Mindfulness training is a win-win for a health care organization and should be encouraged. If your organization doesn't offer this training, at least take regular breaks from work. Take a walk with natural light. Breathe deeply in and out 10 times. Clear your mind. Find something that works for you. Smile.

3) Religion and Spirituality

For many, religion and spirituality include forgiveness, gratitude, purpose, personal growth, community, service to others, and a moral code. A moral code is an internalized set of values that guide a person's ability to judge what is right and wrong and to act accordingly with regard to ethical behavior. A strong moral compass can help one connect to the meaning and purpose in work and result in greater resilience to burnout.

4) Forgiveness

Anger predisposes people to depression, anxiety, inadequate sleep, high blood pressure, and heart attacks. Forgiveness is one way to reduce the overall effects of anger. Research has shown that forgiveness can have a positive impact on health (Davis et al, 2015; Sood, 2015) (e.g., reduced blood pressure, lower stress levels, improved relationships). Forgiveness is a skill that can be learned and developed.

5) Gratitude

Gratitude and appreciation have been shown to drive a host of desirable outcomes (Sansone and Sansone, 2010; Epstein and Krasner, 2013). Gratitude and appreciation can:

- Cultivate social connectedness
- Boost energy
- Lift mood
- Increase optimism
- Enhance well-being
- Bring happiness and good feelings
- Add positive memories
- Improve self-esteem
- Aid relaxation
- Promote optimism
- Elevate psychological and social well-being
- Improve physical health
- Refine quality of patient care

Studies have suggested that simply recording five things you are grateful for in the previous seven days once each week can have profound positive effects on health. In a controlled trial, this simple habit improved optimism, positivity, and physical symptoms, and changed exercise patterns (increased 30 to 90 minutes/week) (Emmons and McCullough, 2003). Studies in which people recorded what they were grateful for on a daily basis had similar effects and improved sleep patterns (Sansone and Sansone, 2010; Epstein and Krasner, 2013). Gratitude is good for you!

Incorrect assumptions often prevent expressions of gratitude. People tend to believe that others already know what is appreciated about them. They believe that expressing gratitude doesn't make much of a difference and will make others feel awkward. However, studies show that people are often surprised by what others appreciate about them and rarely feel awkward when gratitude is expressed (Kumar and Epley, 2018). Notably, studies indicate that expressing gratitude increases the positivity and happiness of *both* the person receiving gratitude and the person expressing the gratitude (Emmons and McCullough, 2003).

Contentment

Many of the approaches to develop contentment help replenish the social, physical, and mental resources we use each day (Box 34.3). As with the other two subdimensions of well-being, organizations should sponsor programs to help cultivate contentment and encourage health care professionals to take advantage of them. Two approaches are described below.

Work-Life Integration

Achieving work-life integration requires attention to firewalls, boundaries, and choices about workload as well as to social support, self-care, and avocational interests. Excessive workload and job demands are consistent drivers of burnout among health care professionals. Reduced burnout and enhanced satisfaction are strongly associated with reductions in professional work effort. Clearly, institutions should offer greater flexibility to clinicians for when, how, where, and how much they work. But workload is a shared responsibility.

Most health care professionals have some control over how much they work:

- Some have the choice to reduce their hours in a volume-determined compensation system in return for a smaller paycheck.
- Some have the opportunity to work part time.

Box 34.3 Contentment Practices

- Work-life integration
- Relationships
- Vacation
- Hobbies
- Avocational interests
- Growth
- Contentment role models

Either of these options can allow health care professionals to meet their personal, family, and professional responsibilities. If you have these options, it may be worth it to cut back. Evidence suggests that reducing work hours can help individuals prevent or recover from burnout (Shanafelt et al, 2016).

How about leaders? A leader who works harder and clocks more hours will be more effective, right? Nope. It turns out that the opposite is true. Research shows that healthy work-life integration also improves the effectiveness of leaders (Smith et al, 2016). Leaders rated as "more effective" had work-life integration scores substantially higher than those judged by team members as "less effective." Thus, work-life integration applies to leaders, too, and should be considered a performance improvement strategy (as well as good role modeling for those they lead).

Taking vacation time is an important aspect of work-life integration. Time away helps workers refresh and renew their energy and commitment. Yet many organizations incentivize workers not to take vacations (e.g., they give people financial compensation to "sell" unused paid time off back to the organization rather than use the time). This practice is shortsighted and ultimately contributes to burnout, depletion, and turnover. Organizations should actually consider doing the opposite and incentivize people to take vacation and use paid time off. In the United States, about half of workers do not take all of their allotted vacation days each year (U.S. Travel Association, 2018)! Just because you can work more does not mean that you should.

Friends and Family

Decades of research show at-home and work communities are powerful predictors of human resilience and mortality (Holt-Lunstad et al, 2010). Good relationships with friends and family have extensive benefits for wellness and well-being and are important for making life worth living.

Health care professionals who experience community at work and camaraderie are more satisfied, more committed to the organization, more productive, more engaged, and more accountable for their performance. These health care professionals have lower levels of exhaustion and burnout. Social connectedness also strongly influences longevity. Everyone should intentionally invest time in those people who matter most to them. Time spent with friends and family is precious and costs nothing. As William W. Mayo said many years ago, "No one is big enough to be independent of others."

A MISTAKE TO AVOID

It should be emphasized that burnout is mainly caused by systems, leaders, and characteristics of the work environment, not by a deficiency in personal well-being or resilience. When leaders begin the quest to address burnout in their organizations, they often make the mistake of starting individual-focused programs that imply the cause of burnout is due to a lack of resilience on the part of the health care professional. Staff are encouraged to "take better care of themselves" and are given the option of participating in programs that include some of the validated means to bolster resilience (such as those discussed in this chapter). With this, many leaders believe their work is done. However, this approach leaves staff with an unintended message: They are at fault for their burnout because they have not taken care of themselves.

Organizational and occupational scientists refer to this as the "strong worker" mindset, and it was debunked as an inaccurate and flawed framework decades ago. Unfortunately, many health care organizations still do not understand the deficits of this approach. Health care professionals, however, immediately recognize efforts that focus primarily on personal resilience as a hollow and insincere effort or, worse yet, they feel as though they are being blamed for the failings of the organization and systems. They know that the system problems and the work environment are driving their burnout. Thus organizations must begin by addressing the system issues under their control before engaging individual professionals in the shared responsibility of caring for themselves.

Elite Athletes

Elite athletes religiously attend to all well-being subdimensions discussed in this chapter. Why? To improve their performance! Their physical, emotional, and psychological health is top tier. They sleep, rest, eat healthy foods, have an off season, visualize their goals, develop routines to reduce stress, and take care of themselves because they want to fuel optimal performance. The best athletes intentionally surround themselves with positive and supportive friends and family—because it helps their performance.

Even with a superior organizational design, excellent leaders, and the best facilities, a medical center cannot flourish without fit clinicians. To deliver the best possible care, health care professionals must be healthy: physically, emotionally, and psychologically. Leaders in health care organizations must attend to helping their people replenish.

CONCLUSION

Well-being programs designed to increase wellness, resilience, and contentment (the three sisters of well-being) are important for health care organizations to implement. Like corn, beans, and squash, they accomplish more when executed together and nurtured in a work ecosystem. Sponsoring programs to bolster individual well-being and encouraging health care professionals to take advantage of the programs are important pieces to place in the esprit de corps puzzle (Box 34.4).

TOMORROW: FULFILLMENT

Heather has a smile on her face. A few months ago, she made some changes in her lifestyle. She walks to work every day (except on the days she rides her bike). She reconnected with an old friend and asked her to lunch. Now every Thursday a group of five women meet for lunch if they are in town. Heather gave up processed foods and eats a Mediterranean diet (most of the time).

She tried yoga . . . not for her.

She tried the laughter club . . . not for her.

But self-compassion training hit the mark. She now uses a number of self-awareness and cognitive reframing practices. She also regularly takes a short break in the afternoon to slow down her mind. This approach really works for her. There are still issues that the hospital leaders need to address, but Heather has rediscovered joy in practicing medicine. She has control of her life again, has reconnected with her husband, and wakes up in the morning eager to walk (or ride her bike) to work.

Box 34.4 The Playbook

- Create a portfolio of subsidized or free offerings to help individuals care for themselves. Include distinct programs targeting wellness, resilience, and cultivation of contentment.
- Make the courses flexible and accessible to the unique schedules and time demands of health care professionals.
- Invite participation with colleagues.
- Evaluate and update policies and practices that may discourage people from taking their vacations.
- Encourage health care professionals to take the initiative to form one new well-being habit right away.
- Model the behaviors you want to see in colleagues.

SUGGESTED READING

Barsade SG, O'Neill OA. What's love got to do with it? A longitudinal study of the culture of companionate love and employee and client outcomes in a long-term care setting. Adm Sci Q. 2014;59(4):551–98.

Beach MC, Inui T; Relationship-Centered Care Research Network. Relationship-centered care: a constructive reframing. J Gen Intern Med. 2006;21 (Suppl 1):S3–S8.

Beecher ME, Eggett D, Erekson D, Rees LB, Bingham J, Klundt J, et al. Sunshine on my shoulders: weather, pollution, and emotional distress. J Affect Disord. 2016 Nov 15;205:234–8.

Chaudhury H, Mahmood A, Valente M. The effect of environmental design on reducing nursing errors and increasing efficiency in acute care settings: a review and analysis of the literature. Environ Behav. 2009;41(6):755–86.

Davis DE, Ho MY, Griffin BJ, Bell C, Hook JN, Van Tongeren DR, et al. Forgiving the self and physical and mental health correlates: a meta-analytic review. J Couns Psychol. 2015 Apr;62(2):329–35.

Emmons RA, McCullough ME. Counting blessings versus burdens: an experimental investigation of gratitude and subjective well-being in daily life. J Pers Soc Psychol. 2003 Feb;84(2):377–89.

Epstein RM, Krasner MS. Physician resilience: what it means, why it matters, and how to promote it. Acad Med. 2013 Mar;88(3):301–3.

Feder A, Nestler EJ, Charney DS. Psychobiology and molecular genetics of resilience. Nat Rev Neurosci. 2009 Jun;10(6):446–57.

Fidler JL, MacCarty RL, Swensen SJ, Huprich JE, Thompson WG, Hoskin TL, et al. Feasibility of using a walking workstation during CT image interpretation. J Am Coll Radiol. 2008 Nov;5(11):1130–6.

Gardiner M, Lovell G, Williamson P. Physician you can heal yourself! Cognitive behavioural training reduces stress in GPs. Fam Pract. 2004 Oct;21(5):545–51.

Holt-Lunstad J, Smith TB, Layton JB. Social relationships and mortality risk: a meta-analytic review. PLoS Med. 2010 Jul 27;7(7):e1000316.

Hsiang EY, Mehta SJ, Small DS, Rareshide CAL, Snider CK, Day SC, et al. Association of primary care clinic appointment time with clinician ordering and patient completion of breast and colorectal cancer screening. JAMA Newtw Open. 2019 May 3;2(5):e193403.

Kelley JM, Kraft-Todd G, Schapira L, Kossowsky J, Riess H. The influence of the patient-clinician relationship on healthcare outcomes: a systematic review and meta-analysis of randomized controlled trials. PLoS One. 2014;9(4):e94207.

Krasner MS, Epstein RM, Beckman H, Suchman AL, Chapman B, Mooney CJ, et al. Association of an educational program in mindful communication with burnout, empathy, and attitudes among primary care physicians. JAMA. 2009 Sep 23;302(12):1284–93.

Kumar A, Epley N. Undervaluing gratitude: expressers misunderstand the consequences of showing appreciation. Psychol Sci. 2018 Sep;29(9):1423–35.

Laskowski ER. Walking throughout your day keeps depression (and a host of other health problems) away. Mayo Clin Proc. 2016 Aug;91(8):981–3.

Lindqvist PG, Epstein E, Nielsen K, Landin-Olsson M, Ingvar C, Olsson H. Avoidance of sun exposure as a risk factor for major causes of death: a competing risk analysis of the melanoma in Southern Sweden cohort. J Intern Med. 2016 Oct;280(4):375–87.

Lyubomirsky S, King L, Diener E. The benefits of frequent positive affect: does happiness lead to success? Psychol Bull. 2005 Nov;131(6):803–55.

Park MY, Chai CG, Lee HK, Moon H, Noh JS. The effects of natural daylight on length of hospital stay. Environ Health Insights. 2018;12:1178630218812817.

Penedo FJ, Dahn JR. Exercise and well-being: a review of mental and physical health benefits associated with physical activity. Curr Opin Psychiatry. 2005 Mar;18(2):189–93.

Rogers AE. The effects of fatigue and sleepiness on nurse performance and patient safety. Patient safety and quality: an evidence-based handbook for nurses. Rockville (MD): Agency for Healthcare Research and Quality; 2008. Available from: https://www.ncbi.nlm.nih.gov/books/NBK2645/.

Romundstad S, Svebak S, Holen A, Holmen J. A 15-year follow-up study of sense of humor and causes of mortality: the Nord-Trondelag Health Study. Psychosom Med. 2016 Apr;78(3):345–53.

Sansone RA, Sansone LA. Gratitude and well being: the benefits of appreciation. Psychiatry (Edgmont). 2010 Nov;7(11):18–22.

Seligman MEP. Flourish: a visionary new understanding of happiness and well-being. New York (NY): Free Press; 2012.

Shanafelt TD, Dyrbye LN, West CP, Sinsky CA. Potential impact of burnout on the U.S. physician workforce. Mayo Clin Proc. 2016 Nov;91(11):1667–8.

Sharma A, Madaan V, Petty FD. Exercise for mental health. Prim Care Companion J Clin Psychiatry. 2006;8(2):106.

Smith DN, Roebuck D, Elhaddaoui T. Organizational leadership and work-life integration: insights from three generations of men. Creighton J Interdiscipl Leadersh. 2016;2(1):54–70.

Sood A. The Mayo Clinic handbook for happiness: a four-step plan for resilient living. Boston (MA): Da Capo Press; 2015.

U.S. Travel Association. State of American vacation [Internet]. 2018 [cited 2019 May 3]. Available from: https://www.ustravel.org/research/state-american-vacation-2018.

Williamson AM, Feyer AM. Moderate sleep deprivation produces impairments in cognitive and motor performance equivalent to legally prescribed levels of alcohol intoxication. Occup Environ Med. 2000 Oct;57(10):649–55.

SECTION IV

The Journey

35

SUMMARY

You treat a disease, you win, you lose. You treat a person, I guarantee you, you'll win, no matter what the outcome.
—Patch Adams, M.D.

A BETTER STORY

Mike, Sally, and Jennifer

Work environments and interpersonal relationships either promote or degrade well-being of health care professionals. Remember Mike, Sally, and Jennifer from Chapter 2 ("Consequences of Professional Burnout")? They were all burned out: Mike, the general internist who could no longer provide the best care for his patients or spend enough time with his family; Sally, the medical-surgical nurse who was mentally and physically exhausted from juggling too many tasks and from the cognitive dissonance of administering chemotherapy to a patient whom she knew wouldn't benefit; and Jennifer, the hospital administrator in a volume (rather than value)–oriented medical center whose dream had been to collaborate with health care professionals to benefit patients—something her current job did not allow.

Today, Mike, Sally, and Jennifer are thriving. They work in systems and cultures intentionally designed to sustain their passion and altruism for the care of people in need: their patients. Their leaders realized they were losing talented professionals to other medical centers and were dismayed by shortfalls in quality of care and patient experience. They used the simple, practical, validated, and evidence-based actions described in the Intervention Triad to help their organization, teams, and individual health care professionals find fulfillment in delivering the best possible care to patients. In fact, nurses, doctors, and administrators are now competing to join their organizations.

The senior leaders in their organizations grew to realize that esprit de corps for their people was inseparable from superlative quality of care and a financially durable organization. Today, they embrace cultivating esprit de corps and quality of care as essential to their patient-centered business strategy. As a result, the rate of burnout has decreased, and professional fulfillment has blossomed in its place.

MILKWEED SEED

In 1944, one of our mothers (S.J.S.) was 13 years old. She, along with thousands of other U.S. teenagers, walked the ditches and fence lines of Midwest farmland to collect milkweed seeds, one milkweed pod at a time. Milkweed is a crucial component of the monarch butterfly's habitat, but in 1944, the milkweed plant also served an important role in the World War II struggle against Nazi Germany and Imperial Japan.

At a pivotal time during the war, the Japanese gained control of the Dutch East Indies, where the United States procured its supply of floss—the material used to make life preservers for airmen and sailors. Flotation devices were critical to Allied success because so much of the war was fought on or over the seas. Fortunately, there was an acceptable, buoyant, alternative to floss: milkweed seed. But unfortunately, there was no industrial supply.

Almost everyone in the United States was engaged one way or another in supporting the war effort. Citizens participated with victory gardens, scrap metal drives, rationing cards, blackouts, war bonds, and higher taxes. And schoolchildren across the country collected tons and tons of milkweed seed, enough for the needed life preservers for U.S. sailors.

This model of collective and absolute engagement holds important lessons for health care. In decades of experience with health care organizations worldwide, we have learned that the most successful ones have fully engaged people who *do their work, improve their work,* and *care for each other.* When all three of these workplace principles coexist, esprit de corps is more likely to result. We have also learned that esprit de corps can exist only when authentic, caring partnerships develop between the health care professionals doing the work and their leaders, whose support enables and empowers professionals to improve their work.

As in the collective effort of World War II, everyone must be engaged.

OPTIMISM

Optimism means hope with evidence. We are optimistic about the prospects of organizations engaging their health care professionals, mitigating burnout, and cultivating esprit de corps because the evidence, tactics, and experience necessary to transform our hope into reality already exist.

Health care professionals and their organizations have been granted the privilege of caring for people and their communities. That honor is best served when they can work in an environment of esprit de corps—one where the common spirit of the group members inspires enthusiasm, devotion, and a strong regard for the honor of the team as well as the common good, mutual respect, camaraderie, trust, and shared responsibilities among all clinicians.

Esprit de corps is more than the absence of burnout, just as health is more than the absence of disease. Esprit de corps is about nurturing social connections along with meaning and purpose in work. It is predicated on trust between team members and leaders. It is about physical, emotional, spiritual, and psychological resilience. It is about optimized care delivery at the work-unit level, achieved and maintained through the voice, input, and ownership of the health care professionals working on that unit.

Esprit de corps is necessary to cultivate because:

- Everyone aspires to work in an organization with palpable esprit de corps.
- Every patient desires to be cared for in an organization with tangible esprit de corps.
- The pathway to achieving the organizational mission starts with esprit de corps.

We choose to frame this important opportunity for health care organizations in a positive way. We believe it is more fruitful to look for solutions in the spirit of abundance rather than scarcity. Thus, we don't look at burnout as a problem to diagnose and fix; rather, we make the case that cultivating esprit de corps along with quality should be the fundamental strategy of all patient-centered medical organizations. Burnout will disappear as we improve quality and achieve esprit de corps.

THE APPROACH

The Blueprint we presented for creating esprit de corps (Figure 35.1) is an evidence-based formula that has been validated in both health care and business sectors. The process is threefold and addresses the fundamental needs of people by:

1) Creating the Ideal Work Elements.
2) Decreasing negativity (by mitigating the drivers of burnout [Figure 35.2]) and increasing positivity (by cultivating leader behaviors and organization processes that promote well-being).
3) Bolstering individual wellness, resiliency, and contentment (by increasing tolerance of negativity and decreasing depleting factors).

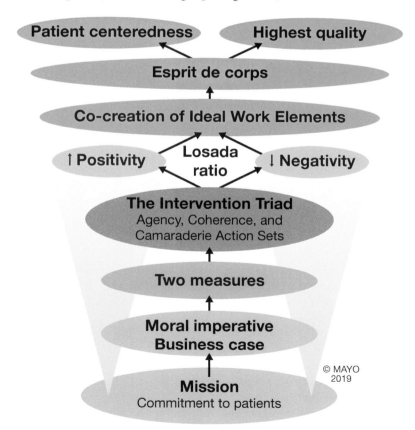

Figure 35.1. The Blueprint for Achieving Esprit de Corps.

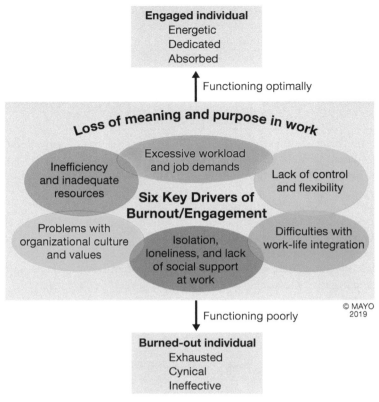

Figure 35.2. Drivers of Burnout.
(Modified from Shanafelt T, Noseworthy JH. Executive leadership and physician well-being: nine organizational strategies to promote engagement and reduce burnout. Mayo Clin Proc. Jan 2017;92[1]:129-46; used with permission of Mayo Foundation for Medical Education and Research.)

The Ideal Work Elements

We have presented an organizational framework and tactics that leaders and health care professionals can deploy to reduce professional burnout and cultivate esprit de corps. To do so, organizations must satisfy the social and psychological needs of professionals by creating a work ecosystem with the following eight Ideal Work Elements (Figure 35.3):

1) Community at work and camaraderie
   - Health care professionals will thrive with a supportive community, camaraderie, and the fellowship of commensality.
2) Control and flexibility
   - Health care professionals need some degree of flexibility over how they work, where they work, when they work, and how much they work (to the extent that this helps advance the organization's patient-centered mission).

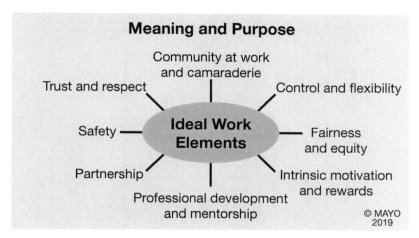

Figure 35.3. The Ideal Work Elements.

3) Fairness and equity
   - Health care professionals need a fair and just culture that acknowledges human limitations and employs a framework of compassionate improvement, not shame and blame. They should be supported when they experience a patient adverse event (whether the root cause was a systems failure or anticipated human factors error).
4) Intrinsic motivation and rewards
   - Health care professionals are by nature intrinsically motivated and should receive rewards, recognition, and appreciation that acknowledge their character—not superficial, ephemeral, and extrinsic rewards.
5) Partnership
   - Health care professionals should be led with the principles of participative management and embraced as partners involved in co-creation and continuous improvement of their work environment.
6) Professional development and mentorship
   - Health care professionals need someone to take an interest in their careers and feel that someone has their back when challenges arise.
7) Safety
   - Health care professionals need to feel psychologically and physically safe at work.
8) Trust and respect
   - Health care professionals need to feel trusted by the leaders of the organization and to feel included and valued by all other team members, regardless of gender, race, discipline, orientation, creed, or tradition.

The Intervention Triad

The Intervention Triad uses an evidence-based systems approach, which is grounded in established research from the fields of organizational psychology and social science. The three Action Sets of the Intervention Triad (Figure 35.4) that we

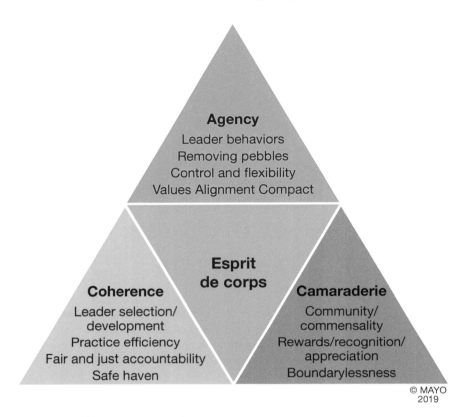

Figure 35.4. The Intervention Triad.

have presented include tactics that when successfully implemented help co-create fulfilling jobs for health care professionals. Some of the actions mitigate the drivers of burnout and reduce negativity. Others cultivate the leader behaviors and processes that enable professional well-being by increasing positivity. Some actions help strengthen individual resilience by augmenting professionals' tolerance of negativity.

Collectively, the Actions promote Agency, Coherence, and Camaraderie and are integral to the comprehensive Blueprint—to cultivate the Ideal Work Elements, address the drivers of professional burnout, and nurture esprit de corps.

Although more research is needed to further define the optimal organizational environment, we know enough today to make substantive improvements now. Time and attention from leaders and clinicians are the predominate resources required to implement the tactics. The model incorporates a strategy for creating symbiotic health care professional–organization relationships to mitigate burnout and achieve esprit de corps. The esprit de corps checklist can be used as a guide for ensuring that you have accounted for all parts of the Blueprint (Box 35.1).

We also hope that family members or concerned friends, after reading this book, better understand occupational burnout.

Box 35.1 Summing Up

How does an organization achieve esprit de corps? We have outlined the strategy in this book. The checklist below can be used to ensure that you are accounting for all parts of the Blueprint. Refer back to the first two sections, "Foundation" and "Strategy," to review the principles you will need to apply to make progress and to the third section, "Execution," to find information on the three validated Action Sets of the Intervention Triad (Agency, Coherence, and Camaraderie) that organizations, leaders, and individuals can use to create an ideal work environment.

The Esprit de Corps Checklist

✓ ☒ Imagine the ideal future state.
- Meet with staff to focus on the positive: What would the ideal state look like (i.e., the eight Ideal Work Elements)?
- Assess the current state through dialogue.
- Recognize the gap between the current and future states.

✓ ☒ Get executive leadership buy-in.
- Use the ideal future state observations to start the conversation.
- Include the moral/ethical imperative.
- Consider the business case.

✓ ☒ Appoint a chief wellness officer (or equivalent) to be part of the executive leadership team.
- Form a center or program that includes a small team of individuals (led by the chief wellness officer) dedicated to developing, catalyzing, and guiding the organization-level strategy and work, participating with local leaders to implement it.
- Form a coalition of leaders assigned to such areas as quality, safety, and patient experience; quality improvement; leadership and organization development; and human resources. Ensure that practicing physicians, nurses, and advanced practice providers are involved.

✓ ☒ Assess the current state of esprit de corps and leader behaviors through survey measurement.

✓ ☒ Prioritize each of the opportunities in the Intervention Triad (Agency, Coherence, Camaraderie) on the basis of group dialogue and survey results.

✓ ☒ Assess organizational readiness to execute the Action Sets of the Intervention Triad on the basis of the prioritized opportunities.

✓ ☒ Assess whether critical success factors are in place (organizational readiness) using the worksheet in Chapter 8 ("Getting Senior Leadership on Board") (Box 8.1).

✓ ☒ Develop a Project Management (Action) Plan for implementation of the prioritized actions of the Intervention Triad.

✓ ☒ Implement the Project Management (Action) Plan.

✓ ☒ Measure progress toward the ideal state with an annual survey.

✓ ☒ Repeat the necessary steps in the Plan until esprit de corps is achieved.

Will, Ideas, and Execution

The Institute for Healthcare Improvement has a simple mantra to describe the essential elements for strategic improvement: will, ideas, and execution. You must have the desire to improve (i.e., will), solutions for how to change to the status quo (i.e., ideas), and the ability to make it real (i.e., execution):

> *Will* is wanting to change the anguish and needless suffering of friends, colleagues, and patients and recognizing both the business case and moral imperative to act.
>
> *Ideas* include the Ideal Work Elements and tactics of the Agency, Coherence, and Camaraderie Action Sets.
>
> *Execution* is up to you. It can be done. We have led the execution of each of the interventions described in the Action Sets in diverse health care institutions.

Are you ready to lead the implementation at your organization?

36

CONCLUSION

Never doubt that a small group of thoughtful, committed citizens can change the world; indeed, it's the only thing that ever has.
—Margaret Mead

PANDO

Earlier we shared with you the story of Pando, the oldest and largest organism on planet Earth (Chapter 32, "Camaraderie Action: Fostering Boundarylessness"). For us, Pando is the metaphor of esprit de corps. By itself, a quaking aspen can live for a century. But as a community, it can thrive for millennia! We believe the prospect of achieving esprit de corps is fulfilled by growing a single, unifying root system that feeds our people, teams, and organizations—with each health care professional contributing to the system. A robust root system is not only good for patients, but it is also what organizations require to thrive and last.

As our roots become more connected . . .
We experience more camaraderie.
We develop more trust.
We become more resilient.
Our care for each other improves.
Teamwork is fostered.
We improve workflow, team dynamics, communication, and broken processes.
Compassion fatigue starts to evaporate.
Cognitive dissonance wanes.
Joy returns to our practice.

MAKE A DIFFERENCE

The two of us have spent most of our careers working clinically in the fields of leukemia and lung cancer. Our aspiration has been to make a difference in the lives of afflicted patients and their families.

Our work with esprit de corps and burnout is different. This work is about healing our colleagues and our profession. The creation of esprit de corps has the potential to make a difference on a broader scale, with lasting impact for patients, health care professionals, leaders, organizations, and the communities we serve. As leaders and health care professionals, we must partner and embrace mitigating burnout and cultivating esprit de corps for everyone who cares *for* patients, for the benefit *of* patients.

By cultivating esprit de corps, we as leaders and clinicians have the opportunity to help colleagues experience meaningful work each and every day.

It may not be particularly inspiring for you to make a difference in an organization.

It may not be particularly inspiring for you to make a difference for people you don't know.

But one thing we know for sure is that it will be inspiring for you to make a difference for the people you know, the professionals you work with, and the patients you serve together.

Join us in this journey.

INDEX

Figures, boxes, and appendixes are indicated by *f, b,* and *a* following the page number